7-13 Music 17.50

MusicMedicine Volume 2

Rosalie Rebollo Pratt, Ed.D.
Ralph Spintge, M.D.
Editors

AF709947

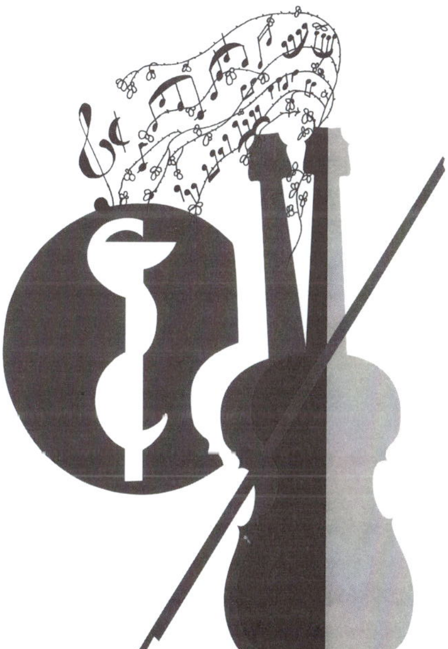

International Society for Music in Medicine
V. International MUSICMEDICINE Symposium

San Antonio, Texas
17–19 March, 1994

Barcelona Publishers
www.barcelonapublishers.com

MusicMedicine, Volume 2

Rosalie Rebollo Pratt, Ed.D., Ralph Spintge, M.D., Editors

© Copyright 1996 International Society for Music in Medicine. All rights reserved. International protection secured under Berne, UCC, Buenos Aires and bilateral copyright treaties. No part of this publication may be reproduced, stored in a retrieval system, or transmitted—in any form or by any means now known or later developed—without prior written permission except in the case of brief quotations embodied in critical articles and reviews.

Cover concept: International Society for Music in Medicine
Cover design: Linda Brown
Typesetter: Gary K. Lee
Printer: McNaughton & Gunn, Saline, Michigan
1st printing: September, 1996
Printed in USA
ISBN: 0-918812-89-5

For further information and catalogs, contact:

Barcelona Publishers
www.barcelonapublishers.com
4 White Brook Road
Gilsum, NH 03448
1-800-345-6665

TABLE OF CONTENTS

Section 3. Performing Arts Medicine

Section 4. Professional Issues and Theoretical Perspectives in MusicMedicine

INTRODUCTION

MusicMedicine, Volume 2 includes 33 papers that were presented at the Fifth Inter national Symposium on MusicMedicine. The areas of interest covered by the writers are four: Music, Physiology, and Physics; Music, Specific Populations, and Therapy; Performing Arts Medicine; and Professional Issues and Theoretical Perspectives in MusicMedicine. Thus, the theoretical, practical, and philosophical matters that underlie the field are addressed by the acknowledged leaders in MusicMedicine. As symposia continue to gather more information about the theory, practice, and philosophy of the field, the body of knowledge will grow to form a cohesive foundation that defines more and more clearly the principles of this specialty in healthcare.

We are now at a point where enough scientific research has put us at the threshold of designing doctoral-level programs that will generate generalizable research information. It is clear that such a degree program is a priority. It is also very clear that more research must include teams of professionals from several disciplines. Research conducted by a music psychologist, educator, or therapist, in conjunction with a physician or biologist is informed by the richness of the various disciplines. There are many examples of such interdisciplinary research efforts in the papers contained in this volume. They represent the work of scientists who have reached out to break down barriers among disciplines and to forge new bonds that are strengthened by the enlightenment each of the investigators brings from a particular field.

What is striking about this volume is its scope. MusicMedicine has penetrated all the broad areas of traditional medical practice, ranging from the well-being of the unborn infant to the needs of the elderly suffering from various forms of dementia and physical frailty. Effects of music on brain function; internal rhythm; connecting mind and body; rehabilitation; pre-, peri-, and post-surgery; pain relief; problems associated with repetitive stroke injury; and sound and vibration therapy are examples of the breadth of this new specialty within Medicine.

Healthcare is changing throughout the world as all societies and cultures are desperately seeking to find treatments and interventions that are within the grasp of the average human being. Costly, elaborate machines and technology aimed at remediation are simply not available to most people. On the other hand, music is shared by everyone in any part of the world. By harnessing the salubrious effects of music and presenting them in ways that are accessible to most people, a great contribution is made to preventive medicine, which is now the emphasis in medical practice worldwide. As we find ways to minimize the need for invasive and costly procedures by showing people how to use music to access their own natural painkillers and stress-reducing mechanisms, we also demonstrate ways in which patients can empower themselves and take more control over their well-being and health.

The thrust in MusicMedicine today also shows the willingness of the professionals involved to make of this new field an alchemy of the riches found in both the arts and sciences. If we use Sir Francis Bacon's metaphor about health being a matter of re-tuning the harp of the body and bringing it into consonance, we are once again reminded of the wisdom of those who began eastern and western medical traditions. These traditions were built on holistic diagnoses and treatments and an integration of the healing and fine arts. The field of psychoneuroimmunology has validated this perspective and enabled us to see clearly and scientifically the ways in which music can be used to affect selected physiological measures. Principles from the field of Biofeedback have been integrated with MusicMedicine to show how music listening and training to control autonomic nervous system responses can actually help people to cope with rehabilitation, pain, stress, and invasive treatments.

We are indebted to all the people who contributed to this book. Their research and commitment to the field of MusicMedicine is exemplary of dedication and scientific effort. We gratefully acknowledge their efforts in revising manuscripts to make the entire volume more uniform and cohesive.

The Editors wish to acknowledge the special efforts of members of the Editorial Board—Roland Droh, Charles T. Eagle, Donald A. Hodges, and Terry M. Mikiten—for their many hours of reading manuscripts. Special thanks are due to Norman Goldberg, President of MMB Music, our publisher, who has stood by all of us in this field and invested much time and many resources into the effort. We also want to thank Gary Lee, also of MMB Music, for his unfailing patience and good will in helping us solve problems attendant to text conversion.

Finally, our deepest gratitude is extended to Dr. Roland Droh, whose philosophy, pioneer spirit, and unwavering vision has guided us all toward contributing our finest efforts to the field of MusicMedicine.

Rosalie Rebollo Pratt, Provo, Utah, March 1995
Ralph Spintge, Lüdenscheid, Germany, March 1995

PREFACE

This volume is aimed at establishing a broader consensus about the therapeutic value of music in medical treatment. MusicMedicine is a multidisciplinary field that includes, but is not limited to, scientific findings derived from the disciplines of biology, ethnology, ethology, mathematics, medicine, music education, music theory, music therapy, musicology, music psychology, physics, physiology, psychology, and socioanthropology, all of which contribute to the growing body of knowledge about how and why music affects humans.

MusicMedicine is gaining increasing interest from the scientific and medical communities. It should be noted, however, that it is still a relatively "young" field. Accordingly, central concepts, as well as advanced standards for research, education, and therapy, are still in the process of being refined. Also, there is a continuing search for a central theory to bring together the parts gleaned from research and practice, and from the many disciplines involved. Finally, terminology (e.g., MusicMedicine, music in medicine, music and medicine, etc.) has yet to be standardized.

The Editorial Board selected, edited, and organized papers submitted specifically for this volume. Those included are revised versions of presentations given at the Fifth International Symposium on MusicMedicine, held in San Antonio, 17–19 March 1994. A process of peer review was used to insure cohesiveness of thought and high quality of research, without excluding ideas that were perhaps less conventional. Thus, in addition to the more strictly scientific papers, manuscripts also were accepted that had a thorough theoretical framework relevant to MusicMedicine. All papers were reviewed and edited for contents, validity, style, and language, following the style format suggested by the American Psychological Association. Members of the Editorial Board and Executive Board of The International Society for Music in Medicine gratefully acknowledge the enormous contributions of Dr. Rosalie Rebollo Pratt, who made this multidisciplinary, multinational publication possible.

Music has played an important role in human healing for thousands of years, and this volume is another step forward in unraveling the mysteries of the power of music. In spite of differences in professional and cultural backgrounds, all authors included in this book are united by their interest in understanding the profound effects of music upon humans and in having music play a more integrated role in health care.

The Editorial Board (as appointed by The International Society for Music in Medicine)
Roland Droh
Charles T. Eagle
Donald A. Hodges
Terry M. Mikiten
Rosalie Rebollo Pratt
Ralph Spintge

AUTHORS

Dr. med. Hans-Henning Abel is a physician, physiologist, and specialist in sports medicine at the Sportkrankenhaus Hellersen, where he is also the Director of the Clinical and Sports Physiology Lab. Dr. Abel is the co-founder of the Music Medicine Associates Research Group.

Dr. med. Leo Anthenien has been, since 1989, the Medical Director of the Psychiatric Center Oberwallis, District Hospital, Oberwallis, Brig, Switzerland.

Jorge I. Auñón, Ph.D., is the former Chair of the Department of Electrical Engineering, and Interim Dean of the College of Engineering at Colorado State University, Fort Collins, Colorado.

Jennifer Benjamin is a Graduate Research Assistant in the Department of Movement Science, Division of Kinesiology, the University of Michigan, Ann Arbor.

Susan H. Brown, Ph.D., is Assistant Professor in the Department of Movement Science, Division of Kinesiology, the University of Michigan, Ann Arbor.

Carlo Capone, M.D., is a fellow in Child Neurology, Neuropediatric Unit, Univ. of Parma; trained in Neurophysiology, Goteborg Univ. (I. Petersen's lab, 1980); Groningen University (H.F.R. Prechtl's lab (1982). His main interests include Developmental Neurophysiology and Chronobiology.

Kris S. Chesky, Ph.D. is a professional musician; Adjunct Faculty at the College of Music, University of North Texas; Associate Faculty, University of Texas at Arlington; and President of Sirkorp, Inc.

J. David Cooke, Ph.D., is Dean of the Faculty of Applied Health Sciences at the University of Western Ontario, London, Canada.

Giuseppe Cossu, M.D, is Associate Professor of Pediatric Neurology, Univ. of Parma; Moscow Univ. (A. R. Luria's lab, 1975–1977) Neuropsychology; and currently with the Neuropsychology Unit, Radcliffe Infirmary, Univ. of Oxford. His main research field is Developmental Neurolinguistics.

William J. Dawson, M.D, is Assoc. Professor (Clinical) of Orthopaedics at Northwestern Univ. Medical School; Chief of the Performing Arts Section, Evanbrook Orthopaedic and Sports Medicine Associates in Wilmette, IL; and Section Chief of Hand Surgery (orthopaedics) at the Evanston Hospital.

Dr. med. Eric Dayer is the Medical Director of the Immunological Department of the Central Institute of Hospitals in Wallis, Sitten, Switzerland.

Dr. med. Roland Droh is the Head of the Department of Anaesthesiology at the Sportclinicum Hellersen in Germany, Dr. Droh is the President of The International Society for Music in Medicine (ISMM) and a leader, lecturer, and writer in the field.

Charles T. Eagle, Ph.D., is Professor Emeritus of Southern Methodist University in Dallas, Texas. Dr. Eagle is also a Vice-President of ISMM, the creator of the *Music psychology index* and *CAIRSS*, a researcher, lecturer, and author.

Dr. med. Joseph Escher has been the Medical Director of the Medical Clinic of the District Hospital, Oberwallis, Switzerland since 1971. He has been University Lecturer at the University for Music and Theater in Hamburg since 1992.

Carmen Faienza, M.D., is a Full Professor of Pediatric Neurology and Psychiatry, University of Parma, Italy, whose special interests include Developmental Neurology and Neurophysiology, Epilepsy, Chronobiology, and Biomusicology.

Oliver Filz, D.I. in Computer Sciences, is a neuroscience researcher specializing in signal analysis, affiliated with the Austrian Academy of Sciences in Vienna.

Reinhard Flatischer is a composer, percussionist, and rhythm therapist who, after formal music study in Vienna, traveled throughout India, Korea, Cuba, and Brazil to learn the rhythmic traditions of these countries. He presents his music project, *Megadrums,* on concert stages throughout the world.

Jens-Stefan Geier is a doctoral student in musicology and psychology at the University of Osnabrück.

Arthur W. Harvey, D.M.A., is a well known educator, lecturer, and writer, who has held the posts of Director, Center for the Advancement of Arts in Medicine, Sarasota, Florida; Associate Professor, University of Hawaii at Manoa; and Executive Director of Music for Health Services Foundation.

Donald A. Hodges, Ph.D., is Professor of Music, Director of the Institute for Music Research, and Coordinator of Music Education at the University of Texas, San Antonio. He is the editor of the *Handbook of music psychology* and specializes in neuromusical research.

Leigh Anne Hunsaker, Ph.D., University of North Texas, teaches trumpet at Hardin-Simmons University in the Dallas/Fort Worth metropolitan area.

Julene K. Johnson is a doctoral candidate in Applied Cognition and Neuroscience at the University of Texas at Dallas. She also has degrees in flute performance and music therapy from Southern Methodist University.

George V. Kondraske, Ph.D., is Professor of Biomedical and Electrical Engineering, Founding Dir. of the Human Performance Inst., Univ. of Texas at Arlington; Adjunct Faculty in neurology and otorhinolaryngology, Univ. of Texas Southwestern Medical Center, Dallas, and Texas Women's Univ.

Jill Petersen Lex, M.A., is a recent graduate of Brigham Young University, Department of Music. Her thesis topic concerned the effects of music and biofeedback training on the cardiac chronotropic control of women in childbirth.

Raymond MacDonald, B.Sc., is currently an academic tutor and Ph.D. candidate, Psychology Dept., Glasgow University. He is also a Visiting Lecturer in communications and music at Glasgow Caledonian University and St. Andrew's College of Education, respectively.

Cheryl Dileo Maranto, Ph.D., RMT-BC, is Professor of Music Therapy at Temple University, Philadelphia. She is the President of the World Federation of Music Therapy and Past President of the National Association for Music Therapy.

Revis Ann Massey, M.M.T., RMT-BC, received her master's degree in music therapy from Southern Methodist University in Dallas, where she is currently Adjunct Faculty. She is also employed at Dallas Music and the Juliette Fowler Homes, a residential treatment facility.

Gerald C. McIntosh, M.D., is a neurologist and specialist in neurologic rehabilitation who is Medical Director for Rehabilitation Services and Life Skills Rehabilitation Center as well as the Center for Biomedical Research and Neurologic Rehabilitation in Fort Collins, Colorado.

Donald E. Michel, Ph.D., RMT, is Professor Emeritus and former Coordinator of Music Therapy at Texas Women's University, Denton, and a National Life Honorary member of NAMT.

Terry M. Mikiten, Ph.D. is Professor of Physiology, Assoc. Dean at the Grad. Sch. of Biomedical Sciences, The Univ. of Texas Health Science Center, San Antonio. His interests include adaptive changes in the nervous system, cognitive neuroscience, creativity, and mind-brain interactions.

Robert A. Miller, Ph.D. received his doctorate in electrical engineering from Colorado State University in 1993. He is currently a Postdoctoral Research Fellow in the Center for Biomedical Research in Music, Colorado State University, Fort Collins, Colorado

Dr. prof. Renate Müller is Professor of Sociology of Culture and Education, Pädagogische Hochschule Ludwigsburg. She holds a master's degree in sociology and a doctoral degree in music education. Her research interests include sociology of music, youth culture, and sociocultural music education.

Patrick O'Donnell, M.A., has been the head of the Psychology Dept. at Glasgow University for 9 years and has a long history of research and publications in the areas of social and applied psychology with evaluation techniques being a special interest.

Hellmuth Petsche, M.D., is a neuroscience researcher and author who is former head of the Institute of Neurophysiology, University of Vienna, and is affiliated with the Department of Brain Research, Austrian Academy of Sciences in Vienna.

Rosalie Rebollo Pratt, Ed.D., is Professor of Music and Director of the Biofeedback Research Lab, Brigham Young University; a Certified Neurofeedback Specialist; writer and lecturer; Vice-President of ISMM; the Editor of *IJAM*; and a research specialist in AD/HD (Attention Deficit Disorder).

Darhyl Ramsey, Ph.D., is an Associate Professor of Music Education at the University of North Texas, where he teaches graduate and undergraduate courses. His advanced degrees are from the University of Iowa.

Maureen P. Reilly, Certified Nurse Anesthesiologist, is a doctoral student at the University of Texas Health Science Center, San Antonio. She holds degrees from Incarnate Word College and Texas Wesleyan University.

Ruth R. Rice, M.S., P.T., is a physical therapist at Poudre Valley Hospital and a Research Associate at the Center for Biomedical Research and Neurologic Rehabilitation in Fort Collins, Colorado.

Peter Richter, M.D., is a neurologist who is affiliated with the Austrian Academy of Sciences in Vienna.

Prof. Dr. Albrecht Schneider studied biology and musicology at Bonn and Cologne, Germany. Since 1983, he has been teaching Systematic Musicology at the University of Hamburg and was a Visiting Professor at UCLA in 1991.

Justine Sergent, Ph.D., died on April 11, 1994. Dr. Sergent was a world leader in the field of human brain mapping and was affiliated with the University of Montréal, Canada. She will always be remembered as an equally outstanding scientist and human being.

David Shannahoff-Khalsa is a scientist and yogic therapist. He is the Director of the Research Group for Mind-Body Dynamics at the Institute for Nonlinear Science, University of California at San Diego.

Cynthia Snodgrass, an ordained Episcopal priest, has served the Diocese of Southern Ohio in both pastoral and chaplaincy capacities. With her background in musicology, she has conducted research for the Fetzer Institute in the areas of music and healing and the spiritual traditions of sound.

Crispin Spaulding is a pianist and physician who heads the prevention program at Trøndelag Music Conservatory in Trondheim, Norway, and is a teacher of music teachers and students throughout the world.

Dr. med. Ralph Spintge, Director of the Interdisciplinary Pain Clinic at the Sportkrankenhaus Hellersen, is Executive Director of The International Society for Music in Medicine (ISMM); Associate Editor of the *International Journal of Arts Medicine (IJAM),* and international lecturer and author.

Astrid von Stein, M.D. in Germany, Semiotics in Bologna, is a neuroscience researcher affiliated with the Austrian Academy of Sciences in Vienna. She is a writer on cerebral representation of concepts by means of the EEG.

Joe Stuessy, Ph.D., is Professor of Music and Director of the Division of Music at the University of Texas, San Antonio. A graduate of the Eastman School of Music, Dr. Stuessy is the author of *Rock and roll: Its history and stylistic development.*

Michael H. Thaut, Ph.D., RMT, is Associate Professor in the Departments of Music and Electrical Engineering at Colorado State University in Fort Collins, Colorado.

Hanna K. Ulatowska is Professor of Communication Disorders at the University of Texas at Dallas. She specializes in the evaluation of language in neurogenic and elderly populations.

PROLOGUE
Outlook

Roland Droh

This book is the result of an effective worldwide cooperative effort among colleagues under the banner of the International Society for Music in Medicine. For the last 12 years, since the founding of the International Society for Music in Medicine, this mutual cooperation has supported and accelerated research and scientific study in the field of music in medicine. From our start in 1972, more than 22 years ago, the intent of our clinical studies was to find new answers for unsolved problems that include reduction of anxiety, pain, mental disorder, cardiovascular and respiratory arrhythmias, and the like. We sought to take these problems beyond the scope of chemistry, pharmacology, surgery, and so-called orthodox medicine, and search for an entirely new natural scientific and holistic approach. We anticipate completely new answers to fundamental questions in all medical fields, from diagnosis to therapy, by combining the knowledge of modern physiology and physics and the quite new mathematics of nonlinear functions for dynamic processes with the new tools of fast and highly sophisticated computers.

Music is a dynamic process in spacetime that itself is a dynamic process bent by energy and matter that is unlimited in the direction of imaginary time and limited in the direction of real time. Diseases are disturbed dynamic processes in time. By investigating the application of music and its effects on the human body, we expect to discover a window to the understanding of disease processes and to gain access to the neurovegetative system and its adaptive changes in spacetime. Our medical thinking today is still strongly determined by the linear thinking of Descartes, Newton and Leibnitz, although we are already living in the time of Hawking, Mandelbrot, Feigenbaum, Haken, Prigogine, and in the time *after* Einstein, Planck, Gödel, Escher, and Bach.

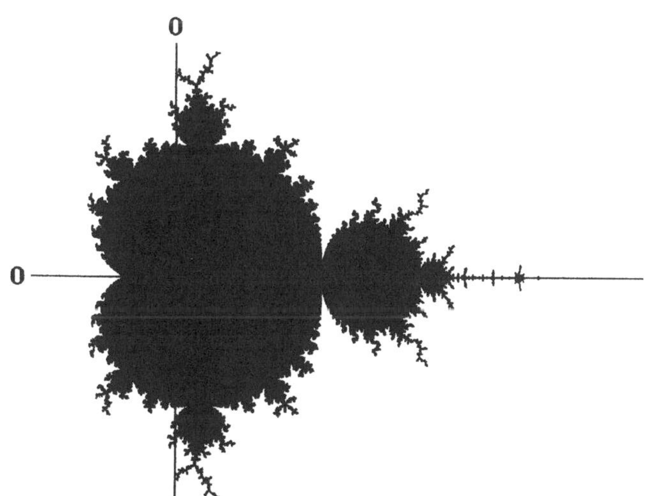

Figure 1. Mandelbrot graph

Western medicine (indeed, the whole western way of life) was basically founded on the principles of linear functions. However, the thinking of the future in dynamic, thermodynamic processes instead of steady states, tonus, and so on, has already started with the discovery of the nonlinear mathematical functions of the "chaos theories" and the nonlinear mathematical functions of the newest branch of mathematics founded by Hermann Haken and called "Synergetik", all of which bears importance for all living and nonliving natural processes.

Music is physics and mathematics; it is also feeling and hearing. It is art, intuition, rhythm, harmony, melody, and polyphony. All kinds of art, whether classical or prehistorical, such as Bach's three -and six-voice fugues and canons, or Peitgen's and Richter's beauty of fractals, or the paintings of Alta Mira depend on the structures, the rhythm, and the dynamic of our brain functions combined with the rhythms of the heartbeat, the vascular system, respiratory system, the hormonal release, etc. The brain function and its product are fractals of the structures of thinking, feeling, hearing, smelling, seeing, sleeping, and the like.

Music is based on linear and nonlinear mathematics. It is accompanied by order and disorder. It is rational, irrational, and imaginary. It is endless and limited in spacetime. It is an oscillating dynamic process and can affect resonances in living and nonliving nature. It is not only able to influence heartbeat, blood pressure, respiration, and the whole gamut of emotions, but it can also break glass and domes of cathedrals. It is a fundamental thermodynamic power in space and time. In the chaos of the Gestaltlosigkeit, and in the turbulence of disorder, music becomes an attractor of order, rhythm, dynamic processes, and control of social life and even the economy.

All that we do, such as speaking, reading, eating, drinking, going, thinking, sleeping, breathing, pulsating, playing music, dancing, climbing, rowing, trekking, even bone growth itself, all kinds of chemical and mechanical processes, all of living and nonliving nature follow certain cycles of rhythmicity in a wide range of different rhythms.

Certain energy states control certain patterns of dynamic processes and self organize systems on their own energy levels. Entropy is the death of everything, all processes in living and nonliving nature.

Music has the power of a strange attractor in the four-dimensional, perhaps the five-dimensional spacetime of dynamic processes. As far as we now know, music opens up a window to the neurovegetative system, which is the control center of the soul and body.

With the help of music, it seems possible to track an entrance to the secrets of the neurovegetative system and to locate with this particular pathfinder quite new dynamic parameters for the diagnosis and therapy of diseases of the neurovegetative system, the cardiorespiratory, humoral, immunological systems, and the like.

In summary, it can be said that music is a dynamic process in spacetime; it is a strange attractor in the chaos of the Gestaltlosigkeit; a self-organizing system; a power in the dimensions of the mathematical and physical laws of the nonlinear functions of "Synergetik" and of chaos theory; and a diagnostic and therapeutic pathfinder to the neurovegetative system. In the future, we expect that MusicMedicine, with a foot in the neurophysiological and mathematical sciences, will become a totally new branch of theoretical and practical medicine.

References

Basar, E. (1990). *Chaos in brain function.* Berlin: Springer Verlag.

Briggs, J., & Peat, F. D. (1989). *Turbulent mirror: An illustrated guide to chaos theory and the science of wholeness.* New York: Harper & Row.

Haken, H. (1981). *Erfolgsgeheimnisse der Natur, Synergetik die Lehre vom Zusammen-wirken. 1981.* Stuttgart: Deutsche Verlagsanstalt.

Haken, H., & Koepchen, H. P. (1991). *Rhythms in physiological systems.* Heidelberg: Springer Verlag.

Haken, H., & Haken-Krell, M. (1992). *Erfolgsgeheimnisse der Wahrnehmung, Synergetik als Schlüssel zum Gehirn.* Stuttgart: Deutsche Verlagsanstalt.

Hawking, S. W. (1988). *A brief history of time: From the big bang to black holes.* New York: Bantam Books.

Hawking, S. W. (1993). *Black holes and baby universes and other essays.* New York: Bantam Books.

Hofstadter, D. R. (1979). *Gödel, Escher, Bach: An eternal golden braid.* New York: Basic Books.

Peitgen, H.-O., & Richter, P. H. (1986). *The beauty of fractals, images of complex dynamical systems.* Berlin: Springer Verlag.

Droh, R., & Spintge R. (Eds.). (1983). *Angst, Schmerz, Musik in der Anaesthesie.* Basel: Editiones Roche.

Spintge, R., & Droh, R. (Eds.). (1985). *Musik in der Medizin: 2 Internationales Symposion 6–7 Oktober 1985.* Basel: Roche.

Spintge, R., & Droh, R. (Eds.). (1987). *Music in Medicine: Neurological basis, clinical applications, aspects in the humanities.* Berlin: Springer.

Spintge, R., & Droh, R. (1992). *Musik Medizin. Physiologische Grundlagen und praktische Anwendungen.* Stuttgart: Gustav Fischer.

Spintge, R., & Droh, R. (1992). *MusicMedicine,* vol. 1. St. Louis: MMB Music.

I.

MUSIC, PHYSIOLOGY, AND PHYSICS

PHYSIOLOGY, MATHEMATICS, MUSIC, AND MEDICINE: DEFINITIONS AND CONCEPTS FOR RESEARCH

Ralph Spintge

Introduction and Definitions

The last 15 years have brought substantial and steady progress in both research and clinical application of music in medicine. Today there is solid evidence that music has reproducible effects and valuable therapeutic properties. It is for this reason that we propose MusicMedicine (one word, two Ms) as the term to define the therapeutic use of music in medicine.

> *MusicMedicine comprehensively and essentially means scientific evaluation of musical stimuli in medical settings, especially through mathematical, physical, physiological, and medical research, as well as therapeutic application, in order to complement traditional medical treatment, with regard to the particular illness, medication, and procedures involved in each individual case* (see also Spintge & Droh, 1992a; Maranto, 1992; Pratt, 1995).

This approach is different from that of Music Therapy as part of psychiatric care or psychotherapy (Aldridge, 1993). We understand Music Therapy as the psychotherapeutic application of music, standing as a specialty of its own. There is, of course, a basic interrelationship between MusicMedicine and Music Therapy. In addition, our understanding of MusicMedicine is that it deals with occupational health problems of musicians and dancer.

However, the main question remains unanswered: Why is music effective and what are the effective parameters? There seems to be general consent that music may be the most effective emotional and aesthetic means of communication. There is no human civilization that has not produced and experienced music. The question is: How can we decipher the musical code for emotional communication?

Our clinical work leads us to believe that rhythm may be the most effective of musical elements. *Musical Rhythm is understood as structured sequence of metric, melodic, harmonic units over time within a piece of music, or, taken from a more biological point of view, as structured sequence of functional units over time within a dynamic system.* The vital role of rhythm is validated, for example, by our knowledge of the roots of music and healing. The history of human culture is always the history of religion, the history of healing, and the history of music as well. Music was part of the picture as far back as the Stone Age, 12,000 years ago (Soffer, 1985). Even the very oldest written documents about the existence of the healing arts displayed the use of music as part of a mystical, religious healing ceremony (4000BV, *Codex Hammurabi,* see overview, Spintge, 1992a). Later, music itself became a healing tool (Kuemmel, 1977). As we investigate the specific value music obviously offered early man, we should consider that the perception of time as a basic element of our existence is organized in rhythmic cycles such as day and night, the sequence of the four seasons, menstruation, and the like. From the beginning of human existence, the organization of time had, of course, a special survival value. Today, biorhythms are a new but well established branch of science. They govern the behavior of biological systems from the molecular level up to the macroscopic behavior of groups of individuals.

Is Rhythmicity the missing link between music and physiology and medicine? This is the topic of our present research (Abel, this volume; Koepchen, Droh, Spintge, Abel, Klüssendorf, Koralewski, 1993). *Rhythmicity is understood as structured coordination between different rhythms over time within a dynamic system, including interactive phenomena such as synchronization, extinction, amplification, and coupling.* The first results of research about Rhythmicity are presented in two papers in this book (Abel, Geier, Spintge, & Droh; Lex, Pratt, Abel, & Spintge). The basic concept upon which we are conducting our physiological studies is the following definition of MusicPhysiology:

> *MusicPhysiology as a natural science investigates the biological properties of Ars Musica, which itself expresses human emotions and feelings through a harmonically and rhythmically structured sequence of acoustic stimuli. All musical parameters show a certain degree of a time order or time structure in the course of the musical process. Thus MusicPhysiology seeks biological time structures in man that might be an equivalent resonating address to musical time structures.*

Figure 1 illustrates the concept of interrelationships among Physiology, Medicine, Mathematics/Physics, and Music, with Rhythmicity as the basic connecting principle. In more precise terms, this is *Anxioalgolytic* (anxiety and pain decreasing) *Music AAM* only.

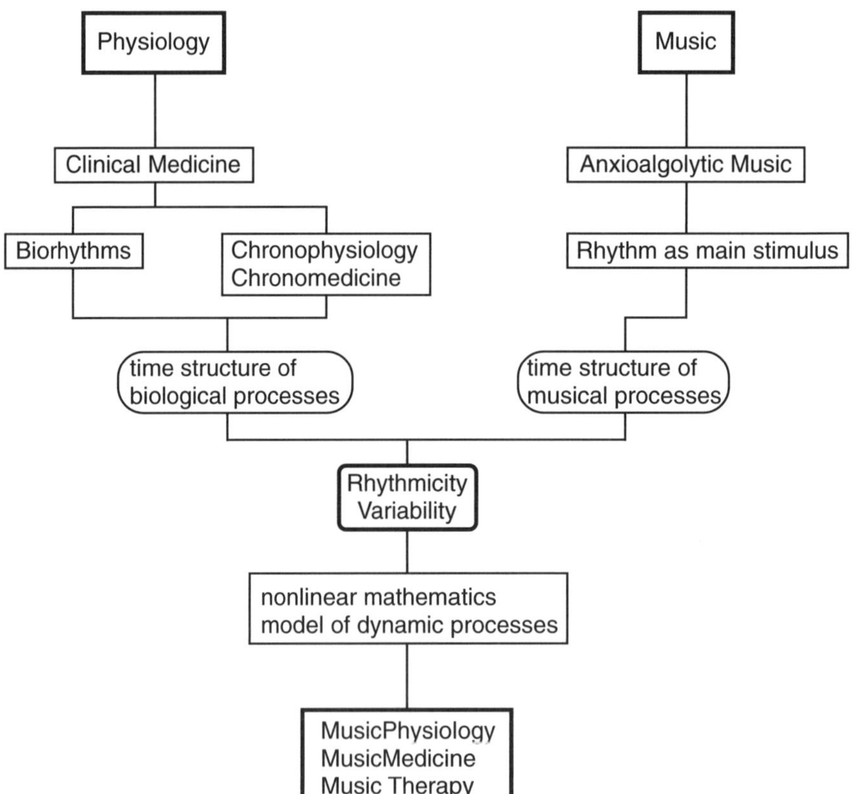

Figure 1. The basis of MusicPhysiology, MusicMedicine and Music Therapy – the interrelationship of Physiology, Medicine, Mathematics and Music with Rhythmicity as possible "missing link".

Music, Physiology, and Mathematics

Rhythms are one of the basic governing phenomena, perhaps even the basic ruling phenomenon, in all biologic systems (Haken & Koepchen, 1991). Only recently, research in rhythmicity has gained high interest in physiology, medicine, and mathematics. While musical rhythms are sui generis of interest to musicologists, musicians, music psychologists, and music therapists, music itself has long been recognized as a functional tool. Today, rhythm research has rapidly penetrated basic investigations in physics, physiology, and mathematics as well as in clinical medicine. This trend is supported by new methods of data acquisition and data analysis. Noninvasive methods to continuously observe dynamic physiological processes together with their computer-assisted evaluation, and new mathematical concepts for analysis of nonlinear biological systems, enable us to observe, describe, visualize, and predict as well the complex interactions of such different oscillating systems (Haken, 1978; Haken, 1986; Haken & Koepchen, 1991). For example, one such system could be music, and the other could be heart rate rhythmicity or electrical brain activity (EEG). It is remarkable that common principles of behavior and methods to describe their interaction mathematically have been substantiated in such different fields as physiology, laser physics, ecology, economics, traffic control, plant growth patterns, cardiology, and the like (Haken & Koepchen, 1990; Haken, 1992). In medicine, rhythm research has already covered an enormous range of phenomena such as heart rate variability (outcome prediction after cardiac stroke), autorhythmicity of blood vessels (control of blood pressure and perfusion), rhythmic sympathetic nervous activity (performance enhancement in high-competition athletes, control of chronic pain), rhythmogenesis of breathing patterns (sleep apnea syndrome, sudden infant death syndrome), synchronization and coordination in motor function (enhancement of performance in sports), circadian sleep rhythms, electrical brain activity, oscillation of perception, chemical communication in and within cells, and many more (Abel, Berger, Conze, Droh, Klüssendorf, Koepchen, Koralewski, Krause, Spintge, 1994; Haken, Kelso, & Bunz, 1985; Haken & Koepchen, 1991).

Although some research groups have tried to establish an overall mathematical model for music, we think it might be more rewarding to start with just one musical parameter, rhythm. A short outline of our musicophysiological concept is given below (for more details, see Koepchen, Droh, Spintge, Abel, Klüssendorf, & Koralewski, 1993). Biological life is a rhythmically organized process with frequencies extending over a wide range. Even molecules, the smallest components of life function, exert oscillatory chemical and functional variations. Human life, as part of the living world, is embedded in rhythmic orders, although we are consciously aware of a very limited part of all these rhythms. Most of the macroscopically observable rhythms are based on the mutual coordination of many single elements in a characteristic manner of self-organization. A nonlinear mathematical analysis of self-organization can be applied to these very different living systems. Since the interacting physiological rhythms result from synchronization and self-organization among oscillating subunits, this new kind of mathematics can quantify and analyze the complex biological rhythmicity.

Figure 2 shows the ranges of different internal physiological rhythms on the right. The rhythms of the outer environment and a physical time scale are depicted on the left. On the top, we find internal rhythms determined by the physico-chemical properties at the molecular level. At the bottom, we find the biorhythms that have evolved in adaptation to

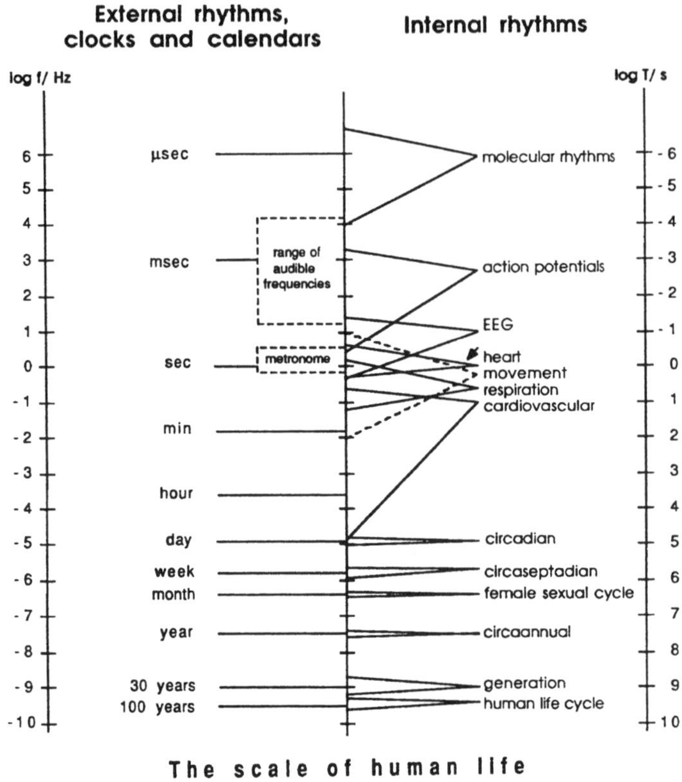

Figure 2. Range of frequencies of human physiological rhythms drawn upon a logarithmic scale with frequencies on the left and periods on the right scale. External rhythms acting from the outer world on the organism are depicted on the left side, internal rhythms on the right side. The triangles on the right side symbolize the most characteristic frequency and the range of occurrence of the respective rhythm. Note the broad frequency with extensive overlapping of neurovegetative and motor rhythms as compared with the small variability of the slower rhythms evolved in adaptation to external cycles.

cosmic rhythms in the course of evolution. The rhythms that are of particular importance to music are found in a medium range. At one end, we find the EEG rhythm; at the other end, the cardiovascular rhythm. The range between 1 Hz and 10^{-2} Hz is the domain of musical rhythms and it is here that we find the inner rhythms of heart beat with all its variations, of respiration, and of most of our normal motor behavior.

It is also remarkable that the range of frequencies installed in a metronome, used in musical studies, corresponds exactly to the frequency range of heart beats occurring between rest and physical work. Regarding physiological rhythmicity, this range has some characteristic features: The rhythms occur in systems with homeostatic feedback autoregulation of vital functions such as control of arterial blood pressure and blood gas concentrations. The result is that there is permanent competition between the homeostatic function of constancy and the rhythmic alteration (variability) of vital parameters, whereby both of these parameters limit each other. This holds true especially for the interactions between the vegetative (autonomic) and somatomotor systems. It is important to note that the rhythmic control of vegetative processes happens in a common network of neurons in the brain that are simultaneously responsible both for the state of general alertness in the brain and for the control of muscle tonus. Therefore, this neuronal network is involved in the central control of emotional behavior, including stress response. One of the interactions previously mentioned, called Entrainment, means that one rhythm synchronizes with another. The qualitative evaluation of entrainment is easily accomplished; for example, in the synchronization between motor action and respiration in rowers or runners. Quantitative analyses of these interactions is much more difficult.

Erich von Holst (1939) was the first to demonstrate the two principles that control the following complex physiological rhythmic phenomena: (a) the "Magneteffekt" (magnetic effect) and (b) the "Überlagerung" (superposition). The magnetic effect is the basis of entrainment and can be demonstrated in the form of statistically preferred phase relations even when synchrony has not been achieved. Usually, one rhythm is the leading rhythm, and the other is the dependent one. Superposition simply means that the amplitude of one rhythm is added to or subtracted from the other, without influencing the phase. Mostly, there is a mixture of magnetic effect and superposition. Von Holst has created the term "relative coordination" to describe these rules in their entirety. They are applicable not only to the interaction of different internal rhythms but also to the effect of the environment on internal rhythms. This has been demonstrated in the coordination of leg movements in running horses, infant suckling and respiration, and human hand movements (Haken, Kelso, & Bunz, 1985). The rhythms and oscillatory patterns that characterize life in general are properties that provide the flexibility and creative variability to sustain life in the face of challenging and life-threatening environmental conditions. From the medical viewpoint, it is imperative not only to know how these individual rhythms of physiological functions arise but also how outside rhythmic stimuli such as music affect rhythmic modulation. From this knowledge comes a certain degree of predictability of normal and abnormal physiological behavior (a) under various conditions of stress, (b) in chronic pain and disease, and (c) under physical workloads, with and without music, etc.

General Relationships between Physiological Functions and Music

We propose the idea that man has projected the essential rhythmic components of CNS-function (and of the rest of the organism) into a creation called music (and dance). The more we look into the specific self-organization of physiological functions, even down to the molecular level, the more we find steadily growing evidence for our assumption. We believe that abstract mental activity corresponds to musical structure; that rhythmic motor activity and neurovegetative rhythms of the CNS correspond to musical rhythm; and that man's emotional state corresponds to the emotional content of music. Starting with the last segment of this concept, we applied the methodology of psychophysiological research in emotion to the emotional impact of music in a specific situation, that is, anxiety. Our respective clinical results have already been published and have substantiated our hypothesis about the emotional part of the concept (Spintge & Droh, 1987; Spintge & Droh, 1992a; Spintge, 1994).

In physiology, research has uncovered the phenomenon of rhythmicity, which appears to be the missing link, or main mechanism behind the impact of music on human biology. The chief point here is that an enormous variety and variability of rhythmic phenomena in the organism can be reduced to a few principles, which, in turn, make the field accessible to scientific analysis and quantitative description. Our current research is focused on the control of neurovegetative mechanisms on internal physiological rhythmicity. *Neurovegetative rhythmicity is a means governed by the CNS that acts on inner organs and organ systems. Literature in the English language more frequently uses the term "autonomic", that is, independent of voluntary influence.* As previously mentioned, we can identify in the usual musical rhythms the rhythm of the heart beat as well as the rhythm of respiration in neurovegetative physiology, respectively. The rhythm of the heart beat originates in the pacemaker of the heart and is modified by central nervous influences (neurovegetative efferences), whereas respiratory rhythm is generated within the central nervous system. Thus, external rhythms, including musical rhythms, do not act on a passive or static organism but on a dynamic, complex, and primarily rhythmic system. All recordings of blood pressure, heart rate, peripheral blood flow, and recent direct recordings of sympathetic nerve activity taken from human subjects confirm that the same pattern of rhythmic variability, that is, rhythmicity, is present in healthy subjects.

It is a general principle that a pathological state is characterized by a loss of rhythmicity. Looking at the frequencies of rhythmic variability, there are two preferential frequencies in cardiovascular rhythmicity. One is in the range of 0.1 Hz (MFB = mid-frequency band), corresponding to a period of 10 sec. The other one is in the range of 0.25 Hz (HFB = high-frequency band). The HFB-range is also that of the usual respiratory frequency at rest. Relative coordination, previously mentioned, is illustrated by the well known respiratory cardiac arrhythmia, or respiratory sinus arrhythmia. It is easily detected by simply feeling the pulse during quiet breathing. During inspiration the HR increases; during expiration, the HR slows down. A preliminary quantitative, mathematical description of rhythmicity can be achieved through Fourier transformation. In this way, rhythmic changes can be displayed in the form of so-called power spectra. The peaks indicate the frequency content of the rhythmic process.

Figure 3 (taken from Koepchen et al., 1993, p. 52) shows the heart rate power spectrum with its preferential peaks in a sitting subject at rest. When we record a series of power spectra during the same session, that is, in 2-minute successive sections, no spectrum exactly equals the other. However, they have the same frequency contents, which means, in reality, the same power spectrum. The power spectra change in a manner related to changes in environmental conditions. This is, therefore, a mathematical tool to describe dynamic changes in biological processes, which provides us with a moving picture rather than one still shot. Since biological processes show nonlinear dynamic behavior, we are presently evaluating even more appropriate mathematical tools for analysis and description, such as phase-diagrams, fractals, and torus-attractors for multidimensional visualization of the respective processes. In cooperation with the Max Planck Institute Dortmund, the National Research Center Jülich, and the Institute of Theoretical Physics and Synergetics Stuttgart, we are attempting to apply algorhythms developed from Chaos Theory and Synergetics (Schiek, 1994).

The theoretical starting point from the mathematical (synergetic) perspective is the assumption that music as the so-called order parameter (Haken, 1986) enslaves the rhythmic control of the physiological systems in the organism. Synergetic mathematics tell us that

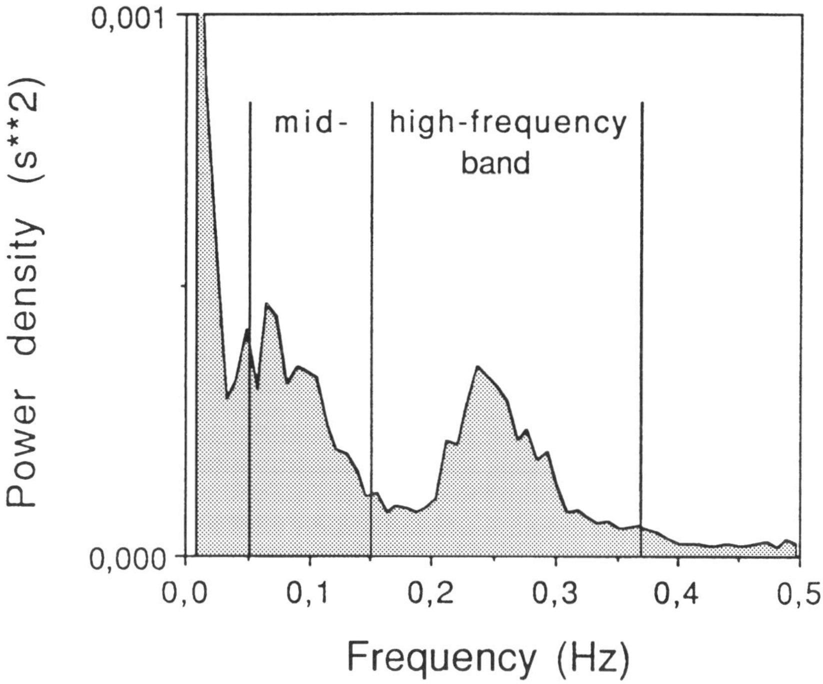

Figure 3. Typical power spectrum of spontaneous heart rate fluctuations in a normal young subject. Note the two peaks in the ranges around 0.1 Hz and 0.25 Hz. The latter corresponds to the frequency of respiration (so-called "respiratory sinus arrhythmia").

dynamic life processes follow the same principles as physical phenomena, that is, all these processes can be mathematically described and their evolutionary alternatives can be precalculated and, in specific situations, even predicted (Haken, 1978, 1983; Hofstadter, 1979). Small initial changes can alter a whole system. Thus, the design of specific initial changes can alter the direction in which the dynamic process evolves. This concept has already been successfully transferred to medical treatment of patients suffering from cardiac stroke. Their specific initial changes in the rhythmic pattern of the EKG seem to have a predictive value for treatment outcome. Why then could we not use music as an external stimulus to induce initial alterations that let the system (organism) behave in a desired manner? Although this concept is fascinating, it is still in the formative stage.

Mandelbrot (1977, 1991) introduced the concept of Fractal Geometry in order to describe shapes and forms in nature. These forms can be described as amorph, that is, stochastically fragmented, irregular, and self-similar. Especially when going from the macroscopic level of observation to the microscopic level (as in the example given by Droh in this volume). This principle can also be shown in an attempt to draw a map of the coastline of the United States, or when trying to draw a snow crystal, or the roots of a plant. The structure in all of these cases is (self-)organized by parameters that can be mathematically described and called, for example, strange attractors and order parameters (for details, see Haken & Wunderlin, 1991; Mandelbrot, 1977; Prigogine & Stengers, 1986). These modern mathematical concepts teach us that structure, self-organization, and behavior in non-living and living nature are governed by the same principles (Gerok, 1989). What may look like chaos is not chaos. Exactly 500 years ago, Johannes Kepler (1594) had already realized this when he perceived that the harmony of the universe exists with its harmonic interactions. Astrophysics teaches us that this universal harmony is in fact generated through chaos by some process of feedback (Cramer, 1989, p. 182). Even dynamic biological systems, though called open and, at first glance, appear governed by unpredictability and instability, can be mathematically described and, moreover, their behavior can be predicted insofar as we know "that the flap of a butterfly's wing in Hong Kong can create a thunderstorm in New York" (Briggs & Peat, 1989, p. 178).The possible consequences for a world picture, human philosophy, and religion are beyond the scope of this paper; There are megabrains in science, art, and the humanities who may be much better able to explain this. In any case, the question arises as to whether these concepts also hold true for the whole of human nature, and whether they hold true for brain function in general. And then, what about music?

There is Fractal Music and a developing modern school of fractal composition (Dodge & Bahn, 1986; Bohm & Peat, 1987). In classical music literature, the principle of self-similarity is used deliberately, without any precise knowledge about fractal geometry, of course, although a genius such as Bach must have had some intuitive feeling for the organization of dynamic processes and how they can be transformed into music and vice versa.

Can these concepts and theories from different disciplines be put together? Yes, I think so. And I am sure that MusicMedicine can be a vehicle for this new synthesis. Our ancestors declared that the task of an artist is to let nature look into a mirror. A mirror from Alice's Wonderland, full of playful uncertainty as in nature itself; a mirror that gives new life to the ancient tension between order and chaos, certainty and uncertainty, matter and spirit, nature science and the arts. (A marvelous essay on this topic can be found in Briggs & Peat, 1989.)

Back to Music in Medicine

The application of the already described physiological, physical, and mathematical models and concepts in man shows that, in a relaxed and painfree emotional state, the cardiovascular system has its own preferential rhythmicity in the high-frequency range while, at the same time, respiration joins the mid-frequency range. In this particular situation, there is synchronization and superposition of both rhythms and, more especially, both large and slow rhythmic heart rate variations can be seen as a result. The opposite is the case during emotional distress (better described as strain). For example, with anxiety or pain, as well as in pathophysiological states such as diabetes, renal failure, and cardiac diseases, there is a decrease in rhythmic heart rate variability. So we assume that *loss of rhythmicity is the characteristic feature of states of high physical or mental strain, such as anxiety or pain.* Although we have started to evaluate power spectra and phase diagrams of pain patients, it is yet too early to speak about differences in comparison to normal subjects. At present, our preliminary impression is that subjects suffering from chronic pain show a marked decrease in overall heart rate variability with a single but smaller peak in the high-frequency range. However, substantially more research is needed before a final determination can be made about a noninvasive tool for monitoring pain that is as important as this one.

What we can say with reference to relaxation therapy in general is that, should we try to induce a regular rhythmic heart movement by using a metronome, from a physiological viewpoint, we could obviously do great harm to these patients. And it is at this point that music as a complex and dynamic stimulus with aesthetic and emotional meaning enters the stage. For example, the variability of rhythmic stimulation through Anxioalgolytic (anxiety and pain decreasing) Music (AAM), especially through classical music, matches very well with the variability of healthy physiological, neurovegetative regulation at rest. At present, we have several studies completed or still in process. There is one with a group of 500 healthy young men as a control group. A second study includes 200 surgical patients under general anaesthesia, but in good general health (Grüning, Abel, Klüssendorf, Droh, & Koepchen, 1991; Werner, Abel, Klüssendorf, Koralewski, Droh, & Koepchen, 1992). A third study involves patients suffering from chronic musculoskeletal pain (Geier, Abel, Spintge, & Droh, this volume). And a fourth joint study with Rosalie Rebollo Pratt and her research group from Brigham Young University compares different relaxation techniques that include music for easing labor pain (Lex, Pratt, Abel & Spintge, this volume).

Preliminary results seem to substantiate our hypothesis that AAM enables the subject to develop a normal variability of vegetative parameters. This would mean that there is a significant effect of musical stimuli upon stress response in the neurovegetative nervous system that works in such a way that enhanced sympathetic nerve activity (stress response) and pain perception are decreased. There are corresponding results from earlier studies (Spintge & Droh, 1987; Spintge & Droh, 1992a; 1992b) in which stress hormone levels and cardiorespiratory parameters in similar situations were measured.

In summing up, we can say at least that the emotional content of music is now accessible to scientific analysis. It is possible to qualitatively discriminate and quantitatively monitor the somatomotor, hormonal, central nervous and vegetative manifestations and grades of intensity of different emotions (see, for example, Koepchen et al., 1993; Machleidt, 1989; Machleidt, 1992; Petsche, Lindner, Rappelsberger, Gruber, 1989; Posner & Raichle, 1994; Raichle, 1994; Sergent, 1993). Since music is the most intense means of emotional communication, these results make the emotional impact of music also accessible to scientific analysis. Furthermore, as neurovegetative rhythmicity and emotional behavior are coupled, the combination of all these approaches will open further promising fields of research in MusicMedicine.

Where is the Music?

At this point some readers may ask "Where is the music?" The answer must come from those of you who are musicians, dancers, musicologists, music psychologists, and music therapists. It is certainly only a half truth to say that music is a structured (organized) sequence of complex, dynamic acoustic stimuli over time with a specific spatio-temporal representation in the human brain. At the same time, art per se cannot be greatly quantified without destroying it. However, the need for a more qualitative approach toward music as a therapeutic means does not demean the reputation of Music Therapy and MusicMedicine and its acknowledgment by the medical and scientific communities (Spintge & Droh, 1992c). If we want to use music in medicine, we must consider the whole picture. And we must also look into Alice's mirror to be able to do so. The organization and contents of this book reflect this need.

References

Abel, H.-H., Klüssendorf, D., & Koepchen, H. P. (1989). A new approach to analyzing the neurovegetative state in man. In R. Droh, & R. Spintge (Eds.), *Innovations in physiological anaesthesia and monitoring* (pp. 21–34). Berlin-Heidelberg-New York: Springer.

Abel, H.-H, Berger, R., Conze, P., Droh, R., Klüssendorf, D., Koepchen, H. P., Koralewski, H. E., Krause, R., & Spintge, R.(1994). Kardiorespiratorische Funktionsdiagnostik und Trainingssteuerung [Diagnosis of cardiorespiratory function and exercise control]. *Deutsche Zeitschrift für Sportmedizin, 45*, 8–9.

Abel, H.-H., Geier, J., Pratt, R. R., Spintge, R., & Droh, R. (1995). Effects of music listening on cardiovascular-respiratory parameters of chronic pain patients. In Pratt & Spintge, pp. 193–205.

Aldridge, D. (1993). Artists or psychotherapists? *The Arts in Psychotherapy, 20*, 199–200.

Bohm, D., Peat, F. D. (1987). *Science, order and creativity.* New York: Wiley.

Briggs, J., Peat, F. D. (1989). *Turbulent mirror. An illustrated guide to chaos and the science of wholeness.* New York: Harper & Row.

Cramer, F. (1989). *Chaos und Ordnung [Chaos and order].* Stuttgart: Deutsche Verlags-Anstalt.

Dodge, C., & Bahn, C. R. (1986). Musical fractals. *Byte, 6*, 13.

Droh, R. (1995). Outlook. In Pratt & Spintge, pp. xiii–xv.

Gerok, W. (1989). Ordnung und Chaos in der belebten und der unbelebten Natur [Order and chaos in living and non-living nature). Stuttgart: Wissenschaftliche Verlagsgesellschaft.

Grüning, T., Abel, H.-H., Klüssendorf, D., Droh, R., & Koepchen, H. P. (1991). Perioperative cardiorespiratory relation. *Pflügers Archiv (Suppl. 1), 418*, R116.

Haken, H. (1978). *Synergetics: An introduction. Nonequilibrium phase transitions in physics, chemistry and biology.* New York: Springer.

Haken, H. (1983). *Advanced synergetics. Unstability hierarchies of self-organizing systems and devices.* Berlin-New York: Springer.

Haken, H., Kelso, J. A. S., & Bunz, H. (1985). A theoretical model of phase transitions in human hand movements. *Biological Cybernetics, 51*, 347–356.

Haken, H. (1986). *Erfolgsgeheimnisse der Natur - Synergetik, die Lehre vom Zusammenwirken [The secret of success in nature - synergetics, The science of cooperative action].* Stuttgart: Deutsche Verlagsanstalt.

Haken, H. (1991). Synergetics of physiological rhythms. In H. P. Koepchen & T. Huopaniemi (Eds.), *Cardiorespiratory rhythmicity and motor coordination. Proceedings of the 21. international congress of physiological sciences Helsinki 1989* (pp. 217–223). Heidelberg-New York: Springer.

Haken, H., & Koepchen, H. P. (1991). *Rhythms in physiological systems.* Heidelberg-New York: Springer.

Haken, H., & Wunderlin, A. (1991). *Die Selbststrukturierung der Materie [The self-structuring of matter].* Braunschweig: Vieweg.

Haken, H. (1992). *Das Konzept der Synergetik und deren Anwendung in Biologie und Medizin [The concept of synergetics and its application in biology and medicine].* Paper presented at the Medizinisch-systemtheoretisches Gespräch [Talks on medicine and system theory]. Lüdenscheid, May 28, 1992.

Hofstadter, D. R. (1979). *Gödel, Escher, Bach an Eternal Golden Braid.* Hassocks: The Harvester Press.

Holst, E.v. (1939). Die relative Koordination als Phänomen und als Methode zentralnervöser Funktionsanalyse [Relative coordination as a phenomenon and as a method for centralnervous functional analysis]. *Ergebnisse der Physio*logie, *42*, 228–306.

Kepler, J (1594). *Mysterium Cosmographicum.* Graz (Austria).

Koepchen, H. P., Droh, R., Spintge, R., Abel, H.-H., Klüssendorf, D., & Koralewski, H. E. (1992). Rhythmicity and music in medicine. In R. Spintge & R. Droh (Eds.), *MusicMedicine* (pp. 39–70). Saint Louis: MMB Music.

Kümmel, W. F. (1977). *Musik und Medizin – Ihre Wechselbeziehungen in Theorie und Praxis von 800 bis 1800 [Music and Medicine – Their interactions in theory and practice between 800 and 1800).* Freiburg: Alber.

Lex, J., Pratt, R. R., Abel, H.-H., & Spintge, R. (1995). The effects of music listening and biofeedback interventions on cardiac chronotropic control of women in childbirth. In R. R. Pratt & R. Spintge (Eds.), *MusicMedicine, Vol. 2,* pp. 182–192.

Machleidt, W., Gutjahr, L., & Mugge, A. (1989). Grundgefühle – Phänomenologie, Psychodynamik, EEG-Spektralanalytik [Basic emotions – phenomenology, psychodynamics, EEG spectral analysis]. *Monographien Gesamtgebiet Psychiatrie (Berlin), 57,* 1–251.

Machleidt, W. (1992). Basic emotions reflected in EEG-coherence. *International Journal of Psychophysiology, 13*(3), 225–232.

Mandelbrot, B. B. (1977). *The fractal geometry of nature.* New York: Freeman.

Mandelbrot, B. B. (1991). *Die fraktale Geometrie der Natur.* Basel: Birkhäuser.

Maranto, C. D. (1992). A comprehensive definition of music therapy with an integrative model for music medicine. In R. Spintge & R. Droh (Eds.), *MusicMedicine* (pp. 19–29). St. Louis, MO: MMB Music.

Petsche, H., Lindner, K., Rappelsberger, P., & Gruber, G. (1989). Die Bedeutung des EEG für die Musikpsychologie [The importance of the EEG for musicpsychology). In H. Petsche (Ed.), *Musik – Gehirn – Spiel [Music – Brain – Play]* (pp. 111–134). Basel-Boston: Birkhaeuser.

Posner, M. J., & Raichle, M. E. (1994). *Images of mind.* New York: Freeman.

Pratt, R. R. (1995). Professionalism in music therapy and MusicMedicine: Issues of the past and future. In R. R. Pratt & R. Spintge (Eds.), *MusicMedicine, Vol. 2,* pp. 301–308.

Prigogine, I., & Stengers, I. (1986). *Dialog mit der Natur (Dialog With Nature).* 5th ed. München: Piper.

Raichle, M. E. (1994). Bildliches Erfassen von kognitiven Prozessen [Imaging of cognitive processes]. *Spektrum der Wissenschaft, 6,* 58–63.

Schiek, M. (1994). *Quantifizierung und Modellierung der respiratorischen Sinusarrhythmie [Quantification And Modelling of The Sinusarrhythmia].* Jülich: Bericht 2899 Forschungszentrum Jülich.

Sergent, J. (1993). Mapping the musician's brain. *Human Brain Mapping, 1,* 20–38.

Soffer, O. (1985). *The upper paleolithic of the central Russian plain.* Orlando: Academic Press.

Spintge, R., & Droh, R. (1992a). *MusikMedizin – Physiologische Grundlagen und praktische Anwendungen [MusicMedicine – physiological basis and practical applications].* Stuttgart: Fischer.

Spintge, R., & Droh, R. (1992b). *MusicMedicine.* Saint Louis: MMB Music.

Spintge, R., & Droh, R. (1992c). Towards a research standard in MusicMedicine/music therapy: A proposal for a multimodal approach. In R. Spintge & R. Droh (Eds.), *MusicMedicine* (pp. 345–349). Saint Louis: MMB Music.

Spintge, R. (1994). Musik in der klinischen Medizin [Music in clinical medicine]. In H. Bruhn, R. Oerter, & H. Rösing (Eds.), *Musikpsychologie – Ein Handbuch [Handbook of musicpsychology]* (pp. 397–404). Hamburg: Rowohlt.

Werner, R., Abel, H.-H., Klüssendorf, D., Koralewski, H. E., Droh, R., & Koepchen, H. P. (1992). Impact of general anaesthesia on cardiac chronotropic control: Reduction in beat-to-beat variability. *Pflügers Archiv (Suppl. 1),* R89.

A METHOD FOR RESEARCH IN MUSICMEDICINE

Terry M. Mikiten

Introduction

In his 1954 story, "The Ultimate Melody", Arthur C. Clarke, to whom I am indebted for this story, told about an inventor with a "scientific theory of hit tunes". The theory said that good tunes involved a match between rhythms in music and rhythms in the brain. Using various kinds of oscillators and analyzers, he invented a device, which he named "Ludwig", that coupled brain electrical activity and patterns in music. The idea was to search for the ideal melody whose patterns perfectly matched the key rhythms of the brain. In the end, the inventor's assistant found the inventor irreversibly entranced by the music-making machine he created; the inventor had to be "taken away".

The idea that music has special divine or demonic power (Hammerstein, 1973) is a centuries-old theme. All ages of civilization have acknowledged that music has a special hold over mind and emotions. That sentiment is nicely reflected in the outcome of Clarke's story. But "The Ultimate Melody" brings an additional element to the issue, which is the prospect that an understanding of this 'power' of music can be understood in a scientific framework.

In 1954—the year of Clarke's story—Music Therapy was at least a decade old as an academic discipline (Schneider, Unkefer, & Gaston, 1968), and the idea was well-established that music somehow influenced the outcome of disease. That idea has persisted and flourished as the discipline of MusicMedicine for more than 50 years. An equally persistent idea has been the related question: What are the exact mechanisms whereby music can affect the human body? There is still little in the way of a systematic scientific approach to research in this discipline and no firm theoretical framework that the practitioner can rely on.

A systematic program for research must be based on the scientific method. But this is not enough. The scientific 'method' only assures that there will be a systematic, hypothesis-driven program of research that is shared openly with one's colleagues in a way that allows them to repeat previous experiments. Even with the operation of this powerful method, it is easy to create a webwork of ideas that links concepts to one another in satisfying ways—but that is remote from the rest of science.

Explanations that are based on hearsay abound, even in the 'scientific' literature. Many of these have only superficial explanatory value because they are not well connected to the rest of the corpus of scientific knowledge. We must guard against constructs that live in self-referential frameworks that make self-fulfilling predictions and thus have no explanatory power beyond the boundaries of those frameworks. Such ideas are typically too weak to reach into any aspect of the world—let alone Music Therapy or MusicMedicine. If MusicMedicine is to achieve its full potential, research must be done in a way that links the information gained with the rest of our understanding of physical and biological law.

Music and the Brain

It is generally agreed that the brain and nervous system are key to any theory of how we understand music or any other sound. Even Clarke's character had this notion as a part of his own thinking about music. However, the exact pathways and structures responsible for understanding music remain elusive. There are many different speculations about this issue. Some ideas come from the study of the brain itself—its anatomy and physiology. Other conjectures arise from related systems, such as the endocrine and immune systems.

Because the nervous pathways that carry information about sound are anatomically close to the brainstem structures that influence heart rate and respiration, it has been supposed that music influences these areas in a special way (Lex, Pratt, Abel, & Spintge, 1995; Koepchen, Droh, Spintge, Abel, Klüssendorf, & Koralewski, 1992). Others have observed that an important component of music is its rhythm, and that patterns in the rhythm have special significance for the operation of the brain (Boltz, 1989; Haas, Distenfeld, & Axen, 1986; Schorr, 1993). Still others suggest that the immune system is linked to these brain operations, and by this route music can affect the creation and deployment of antibodies to combat disease and various forms of stress (Ader & Cohen, 1993). Many authors give abundant reasons to suppose that the actions of music are manifested in large part through brain mechanisms. This suggests that researchers in MusicMedicine should take up the methods of workers in the neurosciences. These techniques have been productive in the past and have even more promise for the future: witness that the decade of 1990–2000 was named the Decade of the Brain by the President Bush, a gesture that is symbolic of the accepted importance of this field as a contributor to our knowledge of disease. It is also a testimonial to the power of methods that neuroscience has used to uncover nature's ways.

The Use of Animals in Music Research

A variety of methods has contributed to knowledge in neuroscience. Many of these are well-known, such as the use of electrical recording devices to detect neural activity. However, one strategy often overlooked, perhaps because it is commonplace elsewhere, is the use of animals in MusicMedicine research. The literature of neuroscience is filled with reports from investigations into the operation of the nervous systems of many different species.

The range of nervous systems that has provided important clues for *all* neuroscientists is truly enormous and includes both vertebrates and invertebrates. The frog nerve preparation taught us about the nerve impulse and how information signals are carried from place to place. The squid axon preparation of the Nobel laureates, Hodgkin and Huxley, showed that nerve impulses could be modeled by the same physical laws as electrical cables, and that they could be represented by a system of equations. The frog heart, beating outside the body, showed Otto Loewi how nerve impulses from the vagus nerve affect the heartbeat by releasing a chemical substance (acetylcholine) from the nerve endings that slows the pulse. An elegant analysis of the invertebrate sea slug, *Aplysia*, showed how its neurons communicate with one another and how that communication changes with experience and learning (Kandel, 1976; Bailey & Kandel, 1993).

The complete list of species used in neuroscience is too long to detail here. But the great success of neuroscience suggests that nature's methods for orchestrating a nervous system are similar throughout the animal kingdom. Nature has long since learned the lesson that what works well in one system can be used in another. Similarly, lessons we learn about one species can be applied—with care—to others.

MusicMedicine must broaden its vision to include members of the animal kingdom other than man. Many questions related to the action of music on mammalian physiology can be answered through carefully designed animal studies. These can explore the brain's responses to music and complex sounds just as readily as they have been used for simpler stimuli. There are enough clues to formulate an hypothesis that can serve to frame experiments in MusicMedicine.

What might be some fruitful approaches and strategies? In general, the best methods are likely to be ones that have worked before. A broad array of tools has been employed by many researchers to explore cognitive processes in both humans (Anderson, 1985; 1982) and animals (Dawkins, 1987; Krebs, 1987; Timberlake, 1993; Spear, Miller, & Jagielo, 1990; Gallistel, 1989). These can be applied to investigations that have music as their theme. Animals can be made to discriminate simple, well-controlled stimuli. It is an easy step to use sounds of increasing complexity as stimuli to determine what sound forms can be learned well enough to trigger behavior. With this information in hand, one can then seek those brain mechanisms that are involved.

Pattern Detectors

The ability of animals to detect complex patterns in sound is evident from commonly observed animal behaviors. The song of birds, the mewing of a kitten, and the undersea songs of fish and cetaceans are powerful everyday examples of animals using complex sound patterns to communicate and elicit responses from others of their kind. The ubiquity of sound-related behavior in nature suggests a fundamental theme at work throughout the animal kingdom.

One simple hypothesis to explain this theme might be that every such system has two components: the ability to create sound patterns and the ability to detect those patterns when they are created by another creature. Several lines of evidence support this idea. One is the evidence that many sensory systems seem to be designed to detect patterns and structure in the stimulus. A frequent finding in animal research is that the sensory systems consist of a set of analyzing components, arranged in tandem. The first elements in the chain serve to detect some form of energy in the world—the stimulus—and then convert it to a series of nerve impulses that are sent off to the brain. The next set of components analyzes this stream of signals for any *patterns* it might contain. Pattern-recognizing systems have been the subject of interest in neuroscience research for many years. Such pattern-recognizers have been found in all of the sensory systems, at many levels of the evolutionary tree (Merzenich, 1994; Merzenich & Sameshima, 1993; Jenkins, Merzenich, & Recanzone, 1990). While some are coarse in their resolving power, some are highly specialized. For example, neurons and neuron-circuits that specialize in pattern-detection have been documented for all levels of the visual system, from the retina to the cortex. Some have only the simple ability to discriminate edges in the visual field; others, like certain neurons in the association cortex of the monkey, respond only to the presentation of a monkey's hand; and still others respond only to a monkey's face (Merzenich & Sameshima, 1993; Damasio, Tranel, & Damasio, 1990).

Similar specializations have been found in the auditory system of many different animals (Schwartzkopff, 1977). The brains of the owl (Konishi, 1985) and the bat (Simmons, 1989) have specific neurons tuned to certain frequencies in the environment that allow these animals to develop acoustic images of the space that surrounds them. Frog brains have neurons that are specialized to detect species-specific calls (Mudry & Capranica, 1987). It has long been known that certain areas in the brainstem generate species-specific sounds. Indeed, electrical stimulation of those areas triggers the production of the sound (Ploog, 1970). In the human, collections of cortical areas collaborate to detect structure in sound (Sejnowski, 1994). It has been suggested that the brain uses these areas to construct a 'grammar' for hearing that guides detection and understanding of musical structures (Jackendoff, 1989; Jackendorff, 1994).

These examples show that throughout evolution the nervous system has developed specializations for detecting not only particular frequencies but patterns of sounds. In light of this, it seems likely that an evolutionary approach to the problem of research in MusicMedicine may have promise.

An Evolutionary Approach

A study of the evolution of the nervous system shows that systems that were evolved early are retained in later generations and later species. Thus the brainstem of the human derives from the brain of the primitive animals, such as fish, where the control for the respiratory activity of the gills was located. In humans, this ancient region still houses the neuron circuits that drive the respiratory musculature. Thus, the primitive parts of the brain, such as the reticular formation of the medulla, are found to contain neurons that respond to sound (Schwartzkopff, 1977). But in advanced animals, as successively higher levels are evolved, each creates a new, more modern system for sound processing. And so in humans we find sound-processing regions in the medulla, midbrain, diencephalon, and the cerebral cortex.

This view of the design of the brain resembles Livingston's "Triune Brain" (McLean, 1970) in which the brain of humans is said to contain a trio of nested brain structures that include the 'reptilian' brain, the 'paleomammalian' brain, and the outermost 'mammalian' brain. My own view resembles this construct since it supposes that the brain of any species contains within it brain structures that are evolutionary hold-overs. In terms of the processing of auditory signals, this idea suggests that sound patterns are extracted by *each* of the several levels of processing, in a cascade of information extraction. The more modern (in the evolutionary sense) the animal, the more steps in the cascade. And correspondingly, the more complex the brain, the more complex pattern that can be detected and processed.

The Esthetic Experience

What about the esthetic dimension of the musical experience? It is important to remember that not only the sounds of music, but also the patterns in music are very important in having an emotional impact on the listener (Hodges, 1988; Jackendoff, 1989). What parts of the brain play a role in this phenomenon, and how might they operate?

Several investigators have proposed that the hippocampus has a special role in detecting the pattern of incoming stimuli (O'Keefe, 1990). Having detected the structure in an auditory experience, the hippocampus sends that information to the neocortex for further processing and possibly consolidation into long-term memory (Squire, Knowlton, & Musen, 1993). The hippocampus has been shown to have a structure-detecting role for auditory (Brenowitz & Rose, 1994), visual (Ringo, Sobotka, Diltz, & Bunce, 1994; Callaghan, 1992), olfactory (Turro, Porter, & Picard, 1994), and tactile (Suzuki, Zola-Morgan, Squire, & Amaral, 1993) stimuli. The hippocampus appears to qualify as an all-purpose structure-detector. The limbic system is also known for its role in emotion. It is this system that gives experience an affective dimension. It is attractive to suppose that the coupling between a structured stimulus with the affective parts of the brain is the key event that gives things in the world what we ordinarily call '*meaning*', and thus can trigger appropriate behavior.

Structures in the world are detected by structures in the brain. These in turn generate cognitive structures that trigger the motor action structures we call behavior. In the case of the frogs that inhabit my backyard pond, the system may work something like this: a male frog's brain creates a sound pattern by the activation of appropriate musculature. The female frog's auditory system detects the sound. Specialized circuits detect a pattern in the sound, discriminating it from other sounds in the environment. Once the pattern is detected, a set of behaviors is triggered and there follows a series of motor acts that constitute mating.

A general rule now can be formulated as follows: A structure in the world interacts with a structure-detector. This initiates a change in some other element in the system which initiates a 'behavior', or 'action'. This rule is valid whether it is applied to an enzyme-substrate reaction or the flower-recognition by bumblebees (Laverty, 1994).

The Language of Structure

Once accepted, the idea of laboratory experimentation is reasonable except for one problem: The languages of music and neuroscience are different. How is one to equate the concepts of one realm with those of the other? How does the concept "temperament of the tuning of a piano" relate to neurons and nerve impulses? How does one create an experimental framework to attack the question? Where does one begin to look for a method that will blend powerful ideas in physics, esthetics, and the brain sciences? The task is not an easy one.

To answer all these questions we must invent a limited set of new terms that serve to bridge the two disciplines. I propose that this can be done by simply agreeing to conceptualize these issues in a new framework.

If we are to recognize that animals are capable of perceiving what humans call "music", the first question that arises is whether the backyard frog understands this idea. I suggest that this question has no value a*t the moment*. For the purposes of the moment, it is best if we agree to use words that are not loaded with species-specific implications. For example, rather than speak of music, we should speak of *sound structures,* as this terminology can apply to all beings, whether or not they have an esthetic sense.

Thus one can seriously ask the questions: "When that female frog emits a mating call, how does her mate detect that signal and differentiate it from all of the other sounds that he can detect?" Framing the question in terms of *sound structures* simplifies the issue and raises the possibility of researching the effects of frog-generated sound structures in a way that could shed light on sounds created by other species. Results could well lead to understanding the experience humans call 'music'.

The Properties of Structures

The use of this particular terminology has merit beyond being a diplomatic language that avoids conflict between disparate disciplines. For this reason, it will be helpful to review some properties of structure that will facilitate this discussion.

Structures have been the concern of scholars in many disciplines, among them psychology (Kohler, 1947; Piaget, 1968), biology (Eigen, 1974; Thompson, 1942; Weiss, 1967), architecture (Fuller, 1982; Sullivan, 1902) and literature (Rand, 1982). Each had a strong understanding of the idea of structure and how it plays a central role in the thought of the particular discipline. We will see that discussions of structure tend to be common at the meeting place of the disciplines. In our case, it is between the disciplines of Music and Medicine.

What is meant by "structure"? There are many ways to answer this question. For the sake of simplicity, think of a Tinker Toy model of 5 to 10 sticks and their joining elements. That is a structure. It meets the defining requirement that the structure be composed of a set of entities existing in some relationship to one another. A flower is also a structure, a set of components in relationship to one another. These are examples of spatial relationships involving components arranged in three-dimensional space. Events occurring in time make another class we will call temporal structures. The series of notes in a musical piece constitute such a temporal structure.

Unity of Structure

As pointed out many years ago by the Gestalt psychologists (Kohler, 1947), structures convey a sense of coherent "wholeness" or "unity". A flower is a collection of parts set in a specific relation to one another. That relationship defines the flower as a structure with wholeness and unity. Interestingly, the "wholeness" of a thing is not lost if the entity becomes a part of something else—part of a larger structure. The flower does not lose its identity in any way when it becomes part of a bouquet of many flowers. The bouquet takes on an identity with a unity—or wholeness—at the same time that the flower retains its own complete identity. In the same way, a sequence of musical notes does not lose its coherence when it becomes part of a concerto. Thus we see that a structure can contribute to the unity of a still larger structure and retain its own identity.

That we perceive the 'wholeness' of things does not mean we miss the details, or even that we, in some instances, notice the details first. The question of perceptual primacy, that is whether stimuli have a 'local' or 'global' impact on the perceiver, is still open (Pomerantz, 1983; Kimchi, 1992). But the main point here is that we do perceive whole patterns and structures in the world. The concept of structure in cognition has a long and fruitful history in cognitive science and serves as a heuristic element in that research (Callaghan, 1992; Anderson, 1985). The concept of structure—by itself—can help to frame research questions in MusicMedicine.

Elaborative Structures

Two general forms of structure, whether spatial or temporal, are evident. One is an elaborative one, reminiscent of the Tinker Toy model. It has nodes that are the basis of branches that emerge from it. This form contains many elements in complex relationships, like a fisherman's net with each knot connected to several knots around it. The other general kind of structure is linear. It is connected to no more than one or two nodes, as in a string of beads, each member with one node behind and one ahead.

Elaborative structures resemble cognitive or associational networks that characterize declarative knowledge, the knowledge we have that is embedded in language. These cognitive structures form ideas and the relationships among ideas and play a strong role in learning and the representation of knowledge (Gagné, 1985). These are radically different from linear structures that probably encode the procedural knowledge embedded in muscular activity (Gagné, 1985). Here, muscular activity is involved in orchestrating a series of muscular movements to achieve some end result.

Structures and Their Detectors

Structures can be represented by physical entities in the world or by abstract constructs. In each case, a set of identifiable elements has a unitary quality that allows it to be identified and also to be manipulated.

When structures are apprehended by some entity designed to detect them, an act of recognition takes place. In biological systems, that recognition is often the trigger for behavior. An enzyme locks into the special crevice in a protein and cleaves it in two at that location, preparing the two pieces for processing by other enzymes. By virtue of its special shape, the enzyme engages the protein. An antibody 'recognizes' an antigen, binds to it, and inactivates it. A white blood cell 'recognizes' the chemical aura of a bacterium and engulfs it. The male frog 'recognizes' the call of the female and mates with her.

This way of thinking about structure parallels the design of the sensory systems. For example, one can think of the sensory system as a collection of sensory pickup units—the sensory receptors. Each unit is 'tuned' to detect certain forms of energy more easily than others. The retina has elements that detect light, the ear detects sound, the nasal mucosa and tongue detect molecules, and so on. When the appropriate stimulus is detected by the receptors, information about the stimulus is relayed to the brain. That information is sent as nerve impulses that are coded in a way that tells the brain about the intensity and duration of the stimulus. In this discussion of structure, there are brain mechanisms that serve as structure detectors, and some of them are 'tuned' to detect structures of certain kinds. Some brain components detect chemical structures in the environment, others detect structures in visual space, and still others detect structures in auditory space.

It has been suggested that mechanisms underlying structure detectors may have common mechanisms of operation that are independent of the sensory modality involved. Indeed, some (Siegel & Read, 1993) suggest that temporal structures are mapped as spatial structures in the cortex of the brain.

Structure and Meaning

"Meaning" is a word that is hard to apply to some things, for example, enzyme reactions. However it applies perfectly well provided we use it carefully. It is easier to think about 'meaning' or 'significance' when we consider mental experiences, since that is the way these terms are conventionally defined. Thinking about 'meaning' in terms of structure works well here. In the sense that recognition of structure precedes action, the structure that triggered the event can be said to have 'meaning', or 'significance' in that system. In many biological systems, like the ones described above, nature apparently creates structures and the devices that detect them. When recognition takes place, something happens that we are inclined to call a 'functional' change. That is, it leads to other events we perceive as having 'meaning' in the context of the system under discussion. Structure and function are thus translated into recognition and action. In the case of the interaction between an enzyme and its substrate molecule, the substrate may undergo a change in its shape which has enduring significance for the cell such as triggering cell division, or some other equally permanent result.

Summary

This discussion asserts that there are three themes that should guide research in MusicMedicine. The first is that any research enterprise must seek to link the knowledge in this discipline with the rest of the body of scientific knowledge. The second says that animal research in the neurosciences can serve as a powerful starting place for MusicMedicine research since there is compelling evidence that the brain mechanisms that process sound in animals are related to those that process sound patterns in humans. Finally, there needs to be a way to link the widely disparate languages that are used in music, medicine, and the sciences. It is suggested that the idea of 'structure' and its related concepts be used as tools to engage and link these different universes of thought into hypotheses that can be tested. For example, it is hard to frame a hypothesis and conduct research into how playing a certain song makes a cancer patient 'feel' better. Further, different songs affect patients differently. However, it does make sense to hypothesize that sound structures are detected by brain structures involved in memory. The act of recognition by brain circuits triggers endorphin release that modulates the brain structures responsible for pain. This point of view facilitates the design of hypotheses for experimental verification.

References

Ader, R., & Cohen, N. (1993). Psychoneuroimmunology: Conditioning and stress. [Review]. *Annual Review of Psychology, 44,* 53–85.

Anderson, J. R. (1985). *Cognitive psychology and its implications.* New York: W. H. Freeman.

Bailey, C. H., & Kandel, E. R. (1993). Structural changes accompanying memory storage. *Annual Review of Physiology, 55,* 397–426.

Boltz, M. (1989). Perceiving the end: Effects of tonal relationships on melodic completion. *Journal of Experimental Psychology: Human Perception & Performance, 15,* 749–761.

Brenowitz, E. A., & Rose, G. J. (1994). Behavioural plasticity mediates aggression in choruses of the Pacific treefrog. *Animal Behavior, 47,* 633–641.

Callaghan, T. C. (1992). Structure in the process of seeing. In B. Burns (Ed.), *Percepts, concepts, and categories: The representation and processing of information* (pp. 149–171). Amsterdam: Elsevier Science Publishers.

Clarke, A. C. (1957). The ultimate melody. In (n.e.), *Tales from the white hart* (pp. 45–52). NY: Ballantine Books.

Damasio, A. R., Tranel, D., & Damasio, H. (1990). Face agnosia and the neural substrates of memory. [Review]. *Annual Review of Neuroscience, 13,* 89–109.

Dawkins, M. S. (1987). Minding and mattering. In C. Blakemore & S. Greenfield (Eds.), *Mindwaves* (pp. 151–162). New York: Basil Blackwell.

Eigen, M. (1974). Molecules, information, and memory: From molecular to neural networks. In F. O. Schmitt (Ed.), *The neurosciences third study program* (pp. xix–xxvi). Boston: MIT Press.

Fuller, B. (1982). *Synergertics: Explorations in the geometry of thinking.* NY: Collier Books.

Gagné, E. D. (1985). *The cognitive psychology of school learning.* Boston: Little, Brown.

Gallistel, C. R. (1989). Animal cognition: The representation of space, time and number. [Review]. *Annual Review of Psychology, 40,* 155–189.

Goldman, J. (1992). *Healing sounds: The power of harmonics.* Shaftsbury, MA: Element.

Haas, F., Distenfeld, S., & Axen, K. (1986). Effects of perceived musical rhythm on respiratory pattern. *Journal of Applied Physiology, 61,* 1185–1191.

Hammerstein, R. (1973). Music as a divine art. In P. Weiner (Ed.), *Dictionary of the history of ideas* (pp. 267–272). NY: Charles Scribner's & Sons.

Hodges, D. A. (1988). Why are we musical? Speculations on the evolutionary plausibility of musical behavior. *Journal of Research in Music Education, 36,* 7–22.

Jackendoff, R. (1989). Levels of musical structure. In R. Jackendoff (Ed.), *Consciousness and the computational mind* (pp. 213–245). Cambridge: MIT Press.

Jackendorff, R. (1994). Patterns in the mind: Language and human nature. NY: Basic Books.

Jenkins, W. M., Merzenich, M. M., & Recanzone, G. (1990). Neocortical representational dynamics in adult primates: Implications for neuropsychology. [Review]. *Neuropsychologia, 28,* 573–584.

Kandel, E. R. (1976). *Cellular basis of behavior.* San Francisco: W. H. Freeman.

Kimchi, R. (1992). Primacy of holistic processing and global/local paradigm: A critical review. *Psychology Bulletin, 112,* 24–38

Koepchen, H. P., Droh, R., Spingte, R., Abel, H. H, Klussendorf, D., & Koralewski, E. (1992). Physiological rhythmicity and music in medicine. In R. Spingte & R. Droh (Eds.), *MusicMedicine. IV International MusicMedicine Symposium* (pp. 39–70). St. Louis: MMB Music.

Kohler, W. (1947) *Gestalt psychology.* New York: New American Library.

Konishi, M. (1985). Birdsong: From behavior to neuron. [Review]. *Annual Review of Neuroscience, 8,* 125–170.

Krebs, J. (1987). The evolution of animal signals. In C. Blakemore & S. Greenfield (Eds.), *Mindwaves* (pp. 163–176). New York: Basil Blackwell.

Laverty, T. M. (1994). *Bumble bee learning and flower morphology.* Animal Behavior, 47, 531–545.

Lex, J. P., Pratt, R. R., Abel, H., & Spintge R. (1995). Effects of music listening and biofeedback interventions on cardiac chronotropic control of women in childbirth. In R. R. Pratt & R. Spintge (Eds.) *MusicMedicine, Vol. 2* (pp. 182–192). St. Louis: MMB Music.

McLean, P. (1970). The triune brain, emotion and scientific bias. In F. O. Schmitt (Ed.), *The neurosciences second study program* (pp. 336–348). NY: Rockefeller University Press.

Merzenich, M. (in press). A physiological perspective on adaptive cortical representation. Cognitive neuroscience society proceedings.

Merzenich, M. M., & Sameshima, K. (1993). Cortical Plasticity and Memory. *Current Opinion in Neurobiology, 3,* 187–196.

Mudry, K. M., & Capranica, R. R. (1987). Correlation between auditory evoked responses in the thalamus and species-specific call characteristics. I. Rana catesbeiana (Anura: Ranidae). *Journal of Comparative Physiology [A], 160,* 477–489.

O'Keefe, J. (1990). A computational theory of the hippocampal cognitive map. [Review]. *Progressive Brain Research, 83,* 301–312.

Piaget, J. (1968). *Structuralism.* NY: Harper Colophon Books.

Ploog, D. (1970). Social communication among animals. In F. O. Schmitt (Ed.), *The neurosciences second study program* (pp. 349–371). NY: Rockefeller University Press.

Pomerantz, J. R. (1983) Global and local precedence: Selective attention in form and motion perception. *Journal of Experimental Biology, 112,* 516–540.

Puff, C. R. (Ed.). (1982). *Handbook of research methods in human memory and cognition.* San Diego: Academic Press.

Rand, A. (1982) *Philosophy: Who needs it?* Indianapolis: Bobbs-Merrill.

Ringo, J. L., Sobotka, S., Diltz, M. D., & Bunce, C. M. (1994). Eye movements modulate activity in hippocampal, parahippocampal, and inferotemporal neurons. *Journal of Neurophysiology, 71,* 1285–1288.

Schneider, E. H., Unkefer, R. T., & Gaston, E. T. (1968). Introduction. In E. T. Gaston (Ed.), *Music in therapy* (pp. 1–6). NY: Macmillan.

Schorr, J. A. (1993). Music and pattern change in chronic pain. *Advances in Nursing Style, 15,* 27–36.

Schwartzkopff, J. (1977). Auditory communication in lower animals: Role of auditory physiology. [Review]. *Annual Review of Psychology, 28,* 61–84.

Sejnowski, T. (in press). Introduction: Adaptive cortical representation. *Cognitive neuroscience society proceedings.*

Shannahoff-Khalsa, D., & Bhajan, Y. (1992). The healing power of sound: Techniques from Yogic medicine. In R. Spingte & R. Droh (Eds.), *MusicMedicine* (pp. 179–193). St. Louis: MMB Music.

Siegel, R. M., & Read, H. L. (1993). Temporal processing in the visual brain. *Annals of the New York Academy of Sciences, 682,* 171–178.

Simmons, J. A. (1989). A view of the world through the bat's ear: The formation of acoustic images in echolocation. *Cognition, 33,* 155–199.

Spear, N. E., Miller, J. S., & Jagielo, J. A. (1990). Animal memory and learning. [Review]. *Annual Review of Psychology, 41,* 169–211.

Squire, L. R., Knowlton, B., & Musen, G. (1993). The structure and organization of memory. [Review]. *Annual Review of Psychology, 44,* 453–495.

Sullivan, L. (1902). *Kindergarten chats.* NY: Dover.

Suzuki, W. A., Zola-Morgan, S., Squire, L R., & Amaral, D. G.(1993) Lesions of the perirhinal and parahippocampal cortices in the monkey produce long-lasting memory impairment in the visual and tactual modalities. *Journal of Neuroscience. 13*(6). 2430–2451.

Thompson, D. W. (1942) On Growth and Form. (2nd ed.). Cambridge: Cambridge University Press.

Timberlake, W. (1993). Animal behavior: A continuing synthesis. [Review]. *Annual Review of Psychology, 44,* 675–708.

Turro, I., Porter, R. H., & Picard, M. (1994). Olfactory cues mediate food selection by young chicks. *Physiological Behavior, 55,* 761–767.

Weinberger, N. M., McGaugh, J. L., & Lynch, G. (Eds.). (1985). *Memory systems of the brain.* NY: The Guilford Press.

Weiss, P. (1967). One plus one does not equal two. In F. O. Schmitt (Ed.), *The neurosciences first study program* (pp. 801–821). NY: Rockefeller.

HUMAN BRAIN MAPPING

Justine Sergent

The understanding of the relationships between music and the brain is a legitimate goal of neuroscientific research. In spite of an already large body of experimental investigation, however, the outcome has not been as satisfactory as expected, to the point that some have voiced their incredulity at the feasibility of mapping musical functions onto cerebral structures. There are indeed considerable inconsistencies in the literature bearing on the neurobiological substrates of musical functions. Before giving in to skepticism, though, it is appropriate to examine whether such inconsistencies are unavoidable and a necessary outcome of neuroscientific investigation into musical functions. This paper, therefore, examines some of the reasons that may be responsible for the inconsistencies. Beyond the superficial similarities between language and music, these two domains are functionally distinct, yet neuropsychological research in music and its neurobiological substrates has been modeled after that in verbal language, borrowing concepts and methods that were not entirely suited to the study of musical functions. An examination of the diverse factors inherent in any study of music-brain relationships reveals a variety of potential sources of difficulties, which, if properly controlled, would guarantee higher consistency and enhance the reliability of experimental findings. It is thus suggested that progress in understanding music-brain relationships may result from 1) explicitly outlining the structural cognitive architecture of musical functions; 2) formulating the problems in terms of underlying operations rather than in terms of vague and unspecified dichotomic views of hemisphere processing; 3) designing experiments that are musically valid and coherent, and that do not lend themselves to multiple strategies; 4) setting up appropriate controls to ensure that subjects are performing as expected; 5) restricting the investigation to musically literate individuals; 6) selecting, among such individuals, a homogeneous set of subjects sharing common musical abilities; and 7) using investigatory techniques that yield reliable evidence of local cerebral involvement in realizing the tasks under study. *©1993 Wiley-Liss, Inc.*

Key words: brain damage, cerebral hemispheres, cognition, dichotic listening, experimental design, music, sight-reading, positron emission tomography

---

INTRODUCTION

Music is the art of combining discrete pitches into sequential patterns of harmonic configurations of diverse duration, intensity, and timbre. As such, it is a creation of the human mind. More correctly, it is a creation of the human brain that made use of structures it inherited from evolution, and that were designed to serve biologically relevant functions, in order to develop and sustain a domain of activity as yet unheard of and of no direct biologically adaptive value. How the brain came to devote parts of its neural tissue to the representation and processing of musical information, and which cerebral territories were recruited to sustain the diverse musical functions, are rather elusive questions because music is like nothing else the brain is called on to accomplish.

Of course, superficially, music appears to share some cognitive functions and operations with other mental activities. One sometimes refers to music as a language, with its grammar, syntax, and semantics (Meyer, 1956; Cooke, 1959; Deliège, 1984), and it is indeed a mode of expression selected by some people to transmit their thoughts and emotions. For instance, Ravel (1989) pointed out that he felt and thought in sounds; Malher indicated that he needed to express himself in music only when "indefinable emotions make themselves felt," and that, if these emotions could have been expressed in words, he would not have resorted to music to express them (Blacking, 1973). The grammar and semantics of music have, however, very little in common with their verbal counterparts. One uses the verbal language to make reference to entities in the world, and one listens to the verbal language to understand its meaning, over and above the particular sounds of the utterance. That is, one comprehends words and sentences, not sound patterns, and the linguistic message is recorded into semantic information instead of being stored verbatim. The referential symbolic system that represents knowledge of the world is stable and universal, and the verbal language is, for the most part, unambiguously tied down to specific meanings and functions.

Music, on the other hand, is nothing but organized sound. The patterns of sounds are non-referential and self-sufficient, and their combinations are governed by rules of harmony and counterpoint that are unique to the musical domain. Memories of musical pieces must retain their specific patterns of harmonic configurations to be of any subsequent use, as recalling the emotions or thoughts evoked by a musical work, or the semantics associated to it, would not stand for the actual patterns of sounds and harmonies. Music is not tied down to specific meanings and functions in the way nouns and verbs are, and it is therefore essentially ambiguous (Lerdhal & Jackendoff, 1983). This point is stressed by Henson (1977), who remarked, for instance, that the structure, style, and instrumental writing of Bach's religious and secular cantatas are in all respects similar. Music may thus possess some characteristics of a Rorschach's ink blot, and the feelings aroused in a listener, as well as the derived esthetic appreciation, are not merely a function of the properties of the musical piece but also, and essentially, a reflection of the emotional and mental state of the listener. Consequently, different individuals may feel different emotions, including none, at listening to the same musical piece and may appreciate it differently; similarly, the same individual may interpret the same piece differently on different occasions: Claudio Arrau, for instance, reported that he interpreted the fourth movement of Schubert's *Sonata (*D 958) as the expression of gaiety and free spirit at one time of his life, while it evoked feelings of forthcoming death at a later time (Horowitz, 1982).

Both language and music are constructed of perceptually discrete sounds that can be represented in a writing system, but musical notation is graphically, symbolically, and functionally different from the alphabetic writing system. In addition, although any "normal" individual has acquired the necessary skills for the production of original speech expressing his or her own thoughts, relatively few individuals possess the necessary skills for the production of original music. For most people who entertain musical interests, their experience with music is primarily of a receptive nature; when they do produce music, it essentially consists of singing or playing music originally created by a very few number of musically gifted individuals and, as such, it does not involve a true process of creation. In spite of the universality of music, musical skills and sensitivities are not homogeneously distributed among humans; music may be a universal tongue, which either speaks or does not speak to a listener, but, if it does not speak, no translating system or words will enhance a listener's sensitivity to it. Nonetheless, as noted by Blacking [1973], "there is so much music in the world that it is reasonable to suppose that music, like language and possibly religion, is a species-specific trait of man" (p. 7). One may thus assume that all human beings are biologically equipped to be musical, and, early in life, they experiment with the exploratory production of a variety of sounds with their voices. However, the degree to which human beings do become musical depends on the environment to a large extent.

The foregoing considerations suggest that music, as a form of expression and communication, serves different functions from those served by language and is governed by rules that depart from those inherent in other forms of communication. Consequently, music enjoys a large amount of functional and operational autonomy, and the processes that the brain has to perform in order to achieve receptive and expressive musical functions may therefore be distinct from, and independent of, those underlying the realization of other cognitive functions. Evidence in support of such independence comes from reports on brain-damaged individuals exhibiting selective impairment of either verbal or musical function. As early as 1745, Dalin described the case of a young man with right paresis and speech limited to the word "yes," who could nonetheless sing hymns learned before his illness. This dissociation between language and musical functions was later confirmed by Bouillaud (1865), the very year that Broca reported definitive evidence of a localization of "articulated language" in the left frontal lobe. The reverse finding, that of an isolated disruption of musical functions with spared language functions, was reported by Proust (1866); this selective impairment later led to the term "amusia" coined by Steinhals (Knoblauch, 1888) to designate an acquired impairment of music perception, performance, reading, or writing after focal brain damage, exclusive of an overall deficit of mental ability. The neurological literature is now replete with cases of aphasia without amusia and aphasia with amusia, whereas cases of amusia without aphasia seem to be less frequently encountered (see Benton, 1977; Wertheim, 1977; Brust, 1980; Marin, 1982; Wallin, 1991, for exhaustive reviews).

Another suggestion derived from these considerations concerns the difficulty inherent in studying musical functions from a cognitive standpoint. Musical expression does not enjoy the universality of verbal expression. In most cases, it consists in reproducing music composed by others rather than being an original creation. As to listening to music, it is a purely personal and hardly communicable experience that involves a subjective reaction influenced by factors such as interest, education, culture, personality, mood, etc., such that a musical piece that evokes feelings, emotions, or esthetic pleasures in some people may leave others totally indifferent. Thus, from both the expressive and receptive sides, musical abilities and functions are not of the sort that readily lend themselves to experimental inquiry. This may explain why, as noted by Sloboda (1986), "until about 10 or so years ago there was no scientific discipline which deserved the title of 'Psychology of Music' " (p. 189), a situation that may since have evolved with advances in both music theory and cognitive psychology. Nonetheless, in the current state of our knowledge and understanding of the relationships between music and the brain, very few, if any, definite conclusions about the neurofunctional organization of musical functions can be confidently suggested. Brust (1980) remarked that "the presence or absence of aphasia, or of right or left hemisphere damage, fails to predict the type or severity of amusia, including musical alexia or agraphia." In other words, it has been extremely difficult to achieve a reliable mapping of musical functions onto cerebral structures.

The reasons for this state of affairs are multifold, and it is the purpose of this paper to sort out the many variables that need to be taken into consideration and accounted for when attempting to establish relationships between music and the brain. Taking as a starting point the idea that any cognitive function is rooted in cerebral structures, the next section will examine some of the principles that govern the mapping of the former onto the latter. Thereafter, this examination will be extended to the domain of music, with particular emphasis on the various methods used to inquire about music-brain relationships. Then, some aspects of the neurofunctional organization of musical sight-reading will be presented and discussed before concluding with some current problems in this relatively new field of research. It is not the purpose of this paper to review the evidence bearing on the role of particular cerebral regions in realizing specific musical functions, an issue that will be addressed in a forthcoming paper. Instead, the present paper focuses on some of the methods currently available for the neuroscientific study of musical functions.

NEUROFUNCTIONAL MAPPING

The idea that the brain is organized into distinct areas of relative functional autonomy and specialization is a basic principle of cognitive neuroscience. This principle is supported and illustrated by the selectivity of behavioral and cognitive deficits that result from focal cerebral injury, and it governs the research aimed at understanding brain-behavior relationships. It implies that the brain realizes its functions by the conjoint activation of several of its component structures, each performing specific operations. One of the goals of cognitive neuroscience is thus to uncover what operations are performed by each of these structures and how these operations are coordinated and related to one another, within the neural network that sustains them, in order to produce adapted behavior. Because the logic of the underlying processes cannot be operationalized at a neurophysiological level, the understanding of brain-behavior relationships must rely on a clear and exhaustive description of the processes at a psychological level.

Psychological and cognitive functions are no longer viewed as made of unitary processes (e.g., reading, writing, object recognition) but rather as being composed of several subprocesses (e.g., featural analysis, structural encoding, activation of biographic memories), organized in specific ways (e.g., in parallel or in succession, independently or interactively), and the cognitive architecture of mental functions is best characterized by a compartmented organization of interactive components. It is therefore through a decomposition of a given function into its component operations (thus providing a theoretical framework specifying the nature, the goals, the logical order, and the interactive relations of the processing steps to be performed for the realization of the function under study) that a better specification of the functional organization of the cerebral cortex can be achieved. The understanding of brain-behavior relationships can then be conceived as an enterprise that aims at mapping a fractionated set of related mental operations underlying cognitive functions onto their corresponding interconnected cerebral structures.

Such an enterprise is confronted with a variety of theoretical and methodological problems. First, there is no guarantee that the brain divides its functions according to the psychological principles we apply to describe the component subprocesses that make up mental functions. A conceptual decomposition of a cognitive function does not necessarily correspond to the cerebral fractionation of its realization. What is considered as a single mental operation may in fact be implemented in the brain by the interactive recruitment of several structures. Nonetheless, such a functional-structural correspondence is an empirical question that can be answered only through experimental investigation; provided clearly defined operational criteria are specified and implemented, hypothetical functional models are the conditions for progress in understanding brain-behavior relationships and are simply meant to be subjected to verification.

On the other hand, even if there is evidence supporting a structural and functional modular organization of the brain, as indicated by the selectivity of cognitive impairments following focal brain damage, there is also considerable evidence pointing to the close interdependence of cerebral structures (e.g., Mesulam, 1990; Felleman & Van Essen, 1991). Also, the modularity of the brain is embedded within a highly interactive nervous system that is characterized by intricate forward and backward connections among its many structures (Sergent, 1984). Yet, in spite of the current state of knowledge of structures and connections of the primate brain underlying cognition—for example, 32 distinct visual areas have been identified in the monkey's brain, with more than 300 connecting pathways among these areas (Felleman & Van Essen, 1991)—the methods currently available for uncovering human brain-behavior relationships impose limitations on the level of sophistication that can be achieved. This is especially true when dealing with higher-order cognitive processes (as opposed to primary sensorimotor operations).

The main source of information about the neurobiological substrates of cognition in humans has, for a long time, come from the study of brain-damaged patients, and it is essentially obtained through two distinct but complementary approaches. One is the method, which seeks to establish correlations the site of a lesion and the patterns of successes and failures on behavioral tasks, in an attempt to identify the contribution of the damaged cerebral area to cognition (e.g., Hécaen & Albert, 1978; McCarthy & Warrington, 1990). This approach generally involves group studies, and it focuses primarily on the locus of the lesion responsible for specific impairments in broadly defined functions rather than on the nature and properties of the processes normally underlying the defective function. It is thus concerned with averages or general trends, and, by so doing, runs the risk of arriving at conclusions that do not necessarily reflect the true nature of the deficit. For instance, if performance by a group of brain-damaged patients on a given task is bimodal, then the "average" performance used to characterize the group may not be a genuine description of the actual capacities of any of these patients. Nonetheless, group studies do not preclude the examination of individual data, and, as long as interpretations take full account of its limitations, this type of study can offer valuable information.

Moreover, inquiring about which damaged cerebral area(s) is (are) responsible for the disruption of a specific cognitive function and asking which cerebral area(s) participate(s) in the normal realization of this cognitive function are two distinct questions, bearing on different issues and leading to different answers. For instance, a cerebral structure may participate in a given function, and contribute to its realization without this participation being indispensable, such that a deficit may result even when this particular structure is spared. Thus, studying patients with damage in a particular cerebral area and examining their ability to perform a given cognitive function may provide a straightforward manner of determining whether or not the integrity of this area is necessary for the optimal realization of this function, but such an approach falls short of yielding information about the actual contribution of this area.

The other approach is computationally oriented, relies essentially on single-case studies, and uses the examination of brain-damaged patients to infer the functional architecture of cognition from the pattern of disruption that characterizes the cognitive breakdown, generally irrespective of the actual site and nature of the cerebral lesion (e.g., Shallice, 1988; Caramazza & Badecker, 1989). Such an approach imposes an in-depth examination of the patient so as to achieve a detailed description of the pattern of spared and defective functions. On the other hand, this approach runs the risk of giving undue importance to idiosyncrasies, makes generalizations across patients more difficult to achieve, and may lead to the creation of as many ad hoc models as there are single patients examined, because no two patients are ever exactly alike. In spite of the current debate over the respective merits of these two approaches (e.g., Caramazza vs. Zurif, in successive issues of *Brain and Cognition*, 1989–1992), and notwithstanding their inherent limitations, both have the potential to yield relevant and complementary information. Together they may contribute to a more exhaustive and comprehensive specification of the mapping of mental functions onto cerebral structures.

A second approach to the study of brain behavior relationships has relied on techniques derived from experimental psychology to examine the respective contribution of the intact cerebral hemispheres to cognitive functions. In the auditory modality, this approach takes advantage of the anatomical arrangement of the auditory pathways whereby information received by one ear is predominantly projected to the contralateral hemisphere. By simultaneously stimulating each ear, and by observing the manner in which the speed and/or accuracy of responses to various types of stimuli and task requirements differ as a function of the stimulated ear, it is possible to make inferences about the functional asymmetry of the cerebral hemispheres (e.g., Bryden, 1982; Hellige, 1993). Although such a technique is necessarily coarse with respect to the cerebral localization of functions, it is assumed that the manipulation of task variables and the examination of the resulting interactions in the patterns of performance provide information regarding hemisphere specialization and cooperation and how the brain organizes and distributes its resources at a hemispheric level. The difficulties associated with this approach are multifold (e.g., Hellige, 1993), and they lie at the experimental, theoretical, and interpretative levels. In spite of its extensive use, the dichotic listening technique has not been subjected to a systematic evaluation of the influence of the many factors inherent in its implementation on the subjects' performance. In particular, it still cannot be unequivocally ascertained whether or not (and, if so, to what extent) an ear advantage reflects a functional superiority of the contralateral hemisphere (e.g., Mondor & Bryden, 1992; Bryden, in press). Yet this approach may provide some pertinent data about the functional organization of the normal brain (e.g., Sidtis, 1980, 1981) and yield information about dynamic factors of brain processing and hemisphere interactions (e.g., Hellige, 1993) that are not as easily obtainable with other approaches.

A more recent approach to uncovering the functional organization of the normal human brain consists of positron emission tomography (PET) measurements of local changes in regional cerebral blood flow (rCBF) during the performance of behavioral or mental tasks. With the advance in activation techniques (Raichle et al., 1983), data analyses (Mintun et al., 1989, Fox, 1991), and stereotactic mapping of physiological changes (Fox et al., 1985; Evans et al., 1989), local CBF increases underlying sensory and motor processing can be detected reliably and translated into PET images of the activated cerebral structures highlighting the areas participating in the realization of a given function (e.g., Fox et al., 1985; Lueck et al., 1989). The introduction of paired-image subtraction and intersubject averaging (Fox et al., 1988) has enhanced the sensitivity of PET measurements of rCBF and has further opened the way to the study of anatomical-functional correlations of higher-order cognitive processing whose neural substrates are more broadly distributed, and less intensively activated, than are primary sensory and motor cerebral areas. The use of short-lived isotopes (such as $^{15}0$), allowing successive tasks in the same subjects, and the application of the subtraction method, whereby measurements made in a control task are subtracted from those made in a functionally activated state (Raichle, 1990) in order to "isolate" the cerebral areas concerned with the operations that differentiate the two tasks have provided the opportunity of mapping the functional organization of the brain underlying cognition in neurologically intact subjects (e.g., Posner et al., 1988).

This approach is not immune to methodological and theoretical difficulties, however, and a large number of problems needs to be surmounted to obtain reliable data that lend themselves to unequivocal interpretations. Some of these problems are worth mentioning, such as 1) the morphological variability of cerebral structures across subjects, which makes the averaging procedure of activation data questionable, although normalization can be achieved through stereotactic mapping (Fox et al., 1988; Evans et al., 1989); 2) because of the low temporal resolution of the technique, the required scanning time (about 40 to 60 sec) implies that the actual data are an accumulation of neural activity over time during which all mental operations performed by the subject contribute to the total activation in each scanned cerebral area, whether or not these operations were relevant to the task; 3) the assumptions that underlie the use of the subtraction method to "isolate" the cerebral structures specifically involved in the component operations that differentiate two tasks violate some basic properties of cerebral processing (Sergent et al., 1992a); and 4) the choice of "control" tasks whose activation is subtracted from that of the "experimental" task is of utmost importance in the design of cognitive PET studies, because the pattern of blood flow changes resulting from the subtraction (and, therefore, considered to reflect the involvement of the activated areas in the operations specific to the "experimental" task) is dependent on, and relative to, the activation associated with the control task (see Sergent et al., 1992a).

More critically with respect to cerebral lateralization one still does not know how hemisphere superiority is manifested in terms of changes in CBF. For instance, one could assume that the higher the cerebral blood flow in a given area, the more involved this area is in the process under study, and, therefore, one may infer that it is specialized for this particular process. Alternatively, it is conceivable that the higher the cerebral blood flow in a given area, the less competent this area is, as the larger activation may reflect the greater difficulty of this area in performing the operations inherent in the task (see Sergent, 1990a, for further discussion). Each of these potential problems needs to be further examined and resolved in order to ensure that cognitive PET studies produce reliable findings. As it currently stands, the probability is high that many failures to replicate will emerge as a result of a lack of control and understanding of many parameters that have a nontrivial influence on cognitive processing and its measurement and monitoring.

When considered within the aforementioned theoretical framework and experimental approaches, the study of the structural and functional organization of cognition may proceed with fewer degrees of freedom as findings from different sources provide converging evidence and constrain one another for their interpretation.

MUSIC-BRAIN MAPPING

The study of the neurofunctional organization of musical functions has closely paralleled that of verbal functions and, by considering music as a system of communication like language, the initial concern of researchers in this area during the last century was to determine the extent to which language and music shared common neurobiological substrates. The classification of musical impairments was therefore modeled after that of verbal impairments, with their receptive and expressive aspects, and, by the turn of the century nearly every form of verbal deficit was found to have its equivalent in the musical domain (e.g., Dupr; Nathan, 1911). What was particularly debated, however, was whether aphasia and amusia could occur in isolation, and whether each deficit had a distinct anatomical basis. No general consensus emerged among the three main authors who published monographs on this issue (Henschen, 1920; Feuchtwanger, 1930; Ustvedt, 1937). For instance, although Henschen (1920) reported evidence of a dissociation between deficits in speech and music and attempted to locate the different musical functions in the brain (e.g., "center of singing," "center of musical sense," "instrumental center"; see Wertheim 19771), Feutschwanger (1930]) among 34 cases of amusia, did not find a single patient who was free from aphasic disturbances. It was therefore Feutschwanger's opinion that there is no substantial difference between amusia and aphasia, of either the expressive or receptive type. Ustvedt [1937] offered a comprehensive and more balanced evaluation of the evidence and, as noted by Benton (1977), his monograph remains the most valuable single contribution to the study of amusias (Ustvedt, in fact, considered the term "amusia" rather inappropriate as it reflects a heterogeneous collection of complicated symptom groups, in the same way that "aphasia" is too vague a term if it is not qualified by the actual nature of the disturbance). It is probably fair to say that the addition of new cases since then has not resulted in significantly enhancing our understanding of the relationships between music and the brain.

Although the only source of information for a century was the single-case study of brain damaged musically trained subjects, two additional approaches have been available since the 1960s: the group study of brain-damaged patients (e.g., Milner, 1962; Gordon & Bogen, 1974), and the group study of normal subjects through the dichotic listening technique (e.g., Kimura, 1964; Gordon, 1980). These group studies have been primarily concerned with hemisphere processing asymmetry, and they have focused on various aspects of auditory musical functions (e.g., discrimination or recognition of pitch [pure or complex tones], intensity, duration, rhythm, timbre, chord; recognition of melodies in musicians and non-musicians). The results have been particularly inconsistent regarding the respective role of the cerebral hemispheres in these functions: for nearly every finding with one parameter, one technique and one subject population, one can find another finding with the same parameter, technique, and population that points to an opposite conclusion. For instance, even though there is empirical evidence in support of the view that the right hemisphere is critically involved in various aspects of musical processing, there are, in fact, almost as many studies yielding results for or against a superiority of the right hemisphere in musical tasks.

Similarly, the suggestion that non-musicians and musicians rely on their right and their left hemisphere, respectively, to process musical information is not strongly supported by the empirical evidence. One often refers to Bever and Chiarello's (1974) study in which musicians recognized simple melodies better in their right ear and non-musicians better in their left ear, implying a different cerebral organization as a function of musical expertise and a greater role of the left hemisphere in musically sophisticated subjects; However, equally significant is Kellar and Bever's (1980) study in which non-musicians recognized chordal stimuli better when initially projected to their left hemisphere, whereas musicians showed a trend toward a right-hemisphere advantage, thus exhibiting a reverse pattern of cerebral dominance compared with Bever and Chiarello's (1974) study (see also Cook, 1973).

These few examples illustrate the inconsistencies inherent in results from the examination of music-brain relationships. One reason for these inconsistencies may lie in the fact that musical information and operations, more than in any other cognitive function, are not laid down in the brain according to a pattern of underlying cerebral structures that would be essentially stable within individuals and similar between individuals. As noted by Marin (1982):

> If neuropsychologists studying language have found it increasingly difficult to confirm the fixed anatomical locations preducted by classical neurological methods, one should anticipate that the instability of formal musical units and their combinatory rules might make such precise localizations essentially impossible (p, 471).

Although the notion of precise anatomical localization is no longer entertained in cognitive neuroscience, it remains to be determined whether a mapping of musical functions onto cerebral structures is "essentially impossible." Whatever the complexity of musical operations, they must have neurobiological substrates, and, if any "instability" of units and rules exists, it is restricted to a specific domain of mental operations with their unique cognitive processes which are unlikely to be so variable as to lack consistent cerebral representation. There may be neural plasticity within narrowly circumscribed cerebral areas (e.g., Merzenich et al., 1984), but such plasticity cannot extend to trading functions between cerebral territories (neural cells do not acquire their specific sensitivity ex nihilo and do not exchange their processing capabilities between one another). An alternative reason would then be that these inconsistencies result from the large number of factors that intricately and conjointly intervene in the realization of any musical task. This would provide for the opportunity of different combinations of such factors, across subjects, to be at play in performing a given task, implying recourse to different strategies and the recruitment of different cerebral structures. Identifying, and controlling for, such factors may then yield less variability in the findings and reveal an essentially stable pattern of cerebral organization whose variations across subjects and/or tasks are logically determined by specific and non-trivial parameters. In other words, while acknowledging that a neurofunctional mapping of musical functions may be a highly difficult and complicated endeavor, the many sources of difficulties and complexities should be identified and assessed before dismissing the feasibility of such a mapping. The next sections will therefore examine factors that can be a source of difficulty in studying the relations between music and the brain.

Sources of Difficulties

In any experimental study of human cognition, the number of factors that underlie the realization of a given function, and that must therefore be taken into account, is considerable. While such factors can be identified and listed, the main difficulty rests in finding out the actual role of each of them and in uncovering how they interact with each other during the performance of a given task. It may be relatively easy to isolate experimental factors, but, by dissecting a task into subcomponents and focusing on each one separately, one foregoes the examination of how these subcomponents interact with one another, and one thus runs the risk of losing sight of what makes the essence and originality of this task. However, reliable experimental investigation knows no other approach than such a fractionation.

Musical Representations and Operations

Music is particularly illadapted to experimental decomposition aiming at a separate examination of the underlying factors, because it is a personal and incommunicable experience, apparently hermetic to scrutiny, whose underlying processes are not clearly understood. One problem then, as rightly expressed by Marin (1982) is that "one cannot study the neuropsychology of complex behavior without a prior understanding of the cognitive structures of the systems involved" (p 454). This, in turn, implies that, without such an understanding, no explicit rule is available to guide how a musical task should be decomposed and how an experimental design should be properly set up. In the absence of a functional model of musical processing, experimental investigation can only focus on the overall performance of a given task or ability to process specific musical parameters. For instance, reading musical notation requires the implementation of a series of distinct operations from perception to execution (see below), but, without a specification of these operations, it is impossible to achieve a mapping of function onto structure because disruption of this function may result from disturbance at different stages of processing. That is, lesions in different cerebral areas may be responsible for defective musical reading, such that the same end result ("musical alexia") may have different underlying causes across subjects. A functional decomposition of a given task, specifying its cognitive architecture, is therefore necessary to ensure that each of the multiple operations underlying its realization is identified. Unfortunately, no such functional decomposition has yet been proposed, and this constitutes one major source of inconsistencies in the study of music-brain relationships.

A second problem, however, is that such a decomposition may be especially detrimental to the understanding of musical operations and functions, as a musical experience is the result of intricate interactions between a piece and the personal characteristics of the subject. As noted earlier, this can be likened to the perception of a Rorschach's ink blot, because of the ambiguity of the stimulus and the critical role of the personality of the subject in making sense of what is perceived (cf. Exner, 1978). Thus, focusing on one side or the other of the interaction separately would not provide relevant information about the particularities of this interaction. Nonetheless, sense is not assigned at random but is attributed on the basis of particular mental representations that guide the processing of the incoming musical information. These representations are a function of the subject's knowledge and experience and are therefore quite variable across individuals.

Any piece of music can indeed be represented in diverse and closely related formats, each highlighting particular aspects of the musical experience: as an auditory representation of successive pitches and harmonies as a visual representation of a notational score, as an abstract plan of performance, as a program for the patterning and tuning of limb movements on a specific instrument, as a personal experience comprising specific memories and emotions, or as an abstract representation of a musical structure and style. Each of these representations can be activated separately, but of crucial importance are the relations between them, how translations from one to the other are achieved, what is common, and what is unique to each representation in terms of relevant information and organization.

It is not yet possible to specify the functional organization and interactions of such musical representations, but it is their diversity and the variability of their contents that account for the different ways people experience music Depending on individual backgrounds, different representations may be activated, reflecting different experiences and strategies in processing musical information, and thus leading to the recruitment of different cerebral structures. For instance, Mazziotta et al. (1982), in an experiment using Seashore's (1938) tonal memory test (in which subjects must determine whether two successively presented sequences of three to five auditory tones are the same or different), reported that some subjects performed this task by forming a visual image of the sequences of tones on a score and thus making their decision on the basis of visual notations, in spite of the auditory mode of presentation. Thus, what was conceived as a specifically auditory task turned out to engage, in some subjects and unexpectedly, a series of processes requiring a translation from auditory to visual representation an elaboration of an image of a musical score, and a decision based on visually represented descriptions of the tonal sequences. Because not all subjects in the experiment of Mazziotta et al. (1982) resorted to this strategy, different cerebral areas were recruited across subjects, thus illustrating that the same task can be performed through different strategies, which entails different functional-structural relationships. This clearly reflects another important source of inconsistency in the study of music-brain mapping, and it should invite caution in designing experiments so as to prevent subjects from having the option to have recourse to different strategies to perform a given task.

The foregoing suggests that musical tasks involve the implementation of a variety of operations and can be performed by activating diverse representations of the musical information to be processed. A large number of variables, therefore, underlie the realization of such tasks. Yet, for the most part, neuropsychological studies have not focused on these representations and operations and have, instead, consisted of determining which cerebral hemisphere is the more competent at performing these tasks, with formulations of the explanations being restricted to dichotomic views of cerebral functions, such as the analytic-holistic mode of processing. This type of approach has been detrimental to progress in understanding music-brain relationships: it implies that there could only be two ways of processing music, it leads to the view that either one or the other hemisphere is exclusively competent at processing specific aspects of musical information, it dispenses with an evaluation of the actual underlying processes (how can one characterize the nature of processes that are left unspecified?), and it borrows concepts developed in the visuospatial domain and applies them to the auditory-temporal domain without preliminary examination of their appropriateness. The labels "analytic-holistic" are useless as long as the actual operations they are assumed to characterize are not spelled out, and as long as no dearly defined operational criteria are suggested to assess the nature of performance. In addition, the dichotomic view of musical processing implies that if a musical function is spared in a unilaterally brain-damaged patient, it is necessarily the opposite hemisphere that sustains it. This view is, of course, mistaken. For instance, no one would suggest that, in a patient with a left hemisphere lesion who has difficulty comprehending language but has fluent (jargonaphasic) speech, this speech is produced by the right hemisphere. Clearly, the fact that an aphasic musician, with left hemisphere lesion (e.g., Luria et al., 1965; Signoret et al., 1987), can still compose music does not tell anything about which cerebral hemisphere underlies the spared functions. The focus on hemisphere specialization in the study of music-brain relationships has thus been yet another source of inconsistencies in attempting to map musical functions onto cerebral structures.

Musicianship

As noted earlier, uncovering the relationships between a cognitive function and its neurobiological substrates requires "a prior understanding of the cognitive structures of the systems involved" (Marin, 1982). However, because of the large variability in musical abilities, sensitivities, knowledge, and experience, there is no unique functional organization of the structures that sustain musical cognition. In contrast to the verbal language, for which some underlying organization appears to be common to all humans (e.g., Hécaen & Albert, 1978), there is no basic cognitive structure underlying the processing of music that would be shared by all individuals. However, it is usually assumed (e.g., Dowling & Harwood, 1986) that, through a process of "acculturation" (implicit learning through repeated exposure to examples), cognitive structures incorporate the lawfulness of the musical system that prevails in a given culture (e.g., the tonal Western system based on the diatonic scale in our society). Thus, the basic rules of the prevailing musical system are embodied in any individual exposed to this system, and these rules must therefore be shared by everyone. Although there is definite evidence for such acculturation (e.g., Krumhansl, 1990), the actual embodiment of these musical rules is at best very coarse.

For instance, one fundamental principle of any musical system is the octave equivalence, whereby notes with fundamental frequencies standing in a 2:1 frequency ratio are perceived as equivalent (e.g., Hulse et al., 1992). Such equivalence entails that notes one or more octaves apart have the same pitch, and it allows, for example, women and men to sing together in unison the same melodies at different octaves. There is not a single musical system in the world that does not abide by this principle, which is therefore central to music. One would then expect that, by virtue of acculturation, everyone is endowed with the ability to detect such equivalence, but empirical evidence indicates otherwise. When octave equivalence is tested through similarity ratings of pairs of pitches, only subjects with musical training are able to detect it (Kallman, 1982). This also obtains when subjects rate how well different tones complete the C-major scale (Krumhansl & Shepard, 1979). Similarly, in an experiment designed to examine the ability of musically untrained subjects to identify tones an octave apart, only two of nine subjects performed significantly better than chance (Thurlow & Erchul, 1977). Together, these findings indicate that subjects without musical training lack basic cognitive structures necessary to process elementary musical information.

Such a suggestion is further supported by other findings: for instance, in the absence of musical training, subjects are unable to make a distinction between an exact transposition of a melody and a shift from major to minor key tonality of the same melody (e.g., Dowling, 1978). This may result from the inability of such subjects to code new melodies in terms of the exact interval between notes (Sloboda, 1985); instead, they rely on the contour of such melodies (the pattern of ups and downs of pitch from one note to the next, irrespective of the interval), which is a very approximate (and most often inaccurate) representation of the actual melodies. It is also the case that, compared with musicians, non-musicians do not perceive pitch categorically (Locke & Kellar, 1973); their processing of music remains at the "surface" level (cf. Schenker, 1935), as they do not possess the knowledge and expertise to access "deep" structures related to such properties as harmonic and rhythmic progression. This is not to say that lack of musical education and training precludes appreciation of, and emotional reaction to, music A vast majority of musically untrained people derive pleasure from listening to music and find it meaningful. However, such a lack of musical training implies underdeveloped cognitive structures for the processing of music and results in perceptions, processes, and interpretations that may not exploit the full potentialities conveyed in musical pieces. For instance, much of the pleasure and interest musically trained individuals derive from listening to classical music comes from unexpected progressions of harmonies, melodies, or counterpoint (e.g., Lerdhal & Jackendoff, 1983; Narmour, 1990); it is then noteworthy that the commercially most successful pieces of classical music are such pieces as Pachelbel's Ca*non* or Ravel's *Bolero*, which are conspicuous for their highly repetitive and predictible nature. Indeed, Ravel (1989), while acknowledging that the *Bolero* may have been his most appreciated composition, pointed out "but there is no music in it!"

In addition to basic differences concerned with music perception and processing, non-musicians lack the skills required to read musical notation, to play an instrument, to transpose melodies, etc., such that the representations of music they can elaborate are restricted to descriptions of auditory information that are comparatively impoverished versions of the full musical experience, which musically trained individuals can achieve.

The main conclusion to be drawn from the foregoing is that there are substantial differences between musicians and non-musicians in the nature, content, and organization of the cognitive structures underlying the processing of music. In fact, it is a priori impossible to determine what a non-musician's musical ability and knowledge are, and this implies that non-musicians cannot constitute an appropriate sample for cognitive or neurological examination of musical processing. One may in fact argue that, to understand the relations between music and the brain, one must study musicians rather than musically illiterate individuals, in the same way that one would not attempt to understand the relations between mathematical processing and the brain by studying mathematically incompetent individuals. There are at least four reasons for us to study the relations between music and the brain in musicians:

1. There is more homogeneity among literate than illiterate individuals in their knowledge and mastering of a given skill; restricting the study of music-brain relationships to musicians should reduce the amount of unexplained variance in the results, and, therefore, the likelihood of inconsistent findings.

2. It is very difficult, if not impossible, to determine the particular operations inherent in the realization of a given task by subjects who have no specific skill to perform such a task, whereas musicians have explicit access to many of the rules they apply to their processing of music, non-musicians have at best implicit knowledge of such rules, and often perform at random. In other words, there is no guarantee that the processes used by non-musicians when exposed to musical information are specific to the processing of music as such.

3. One can achieve a fuller understanding of the nature, structure, and organization of a given function by studying those who excel in it.

4. There is evidence that the cerebral organization of a given function varies considerably among individuals depending on whether they are literate or illiterate in that function. This has been demonstrated in the case of the verbal language (e.g., Lecours, 1989), and it would not make much sense to base our study of the relations between language and the brain on the examination of illiterate individuals.

Differences in musical expertise across subjects constitute yet another source of inconsistencies in neuropsychological research into music cognition. The foregoing should make it clear that there is little to learn about music-brain relationships from the study of musically illiterate individuals (which is not to say that such subjects cannot contribute to our knowledge of acoustic phenomena, musical learning, and acculturation). It must, however, be noted that restricting the study of music-brain relationships to musicians is no guarantee of group homogeneity. Important differences also occur among musically trained individuals, and such differences may result in additional inconsistencies. For instance, McFarland and Fortin (1982) reported a case of instrumental amusia due to cerebral damage in "an accomplished organist, who could neither read nor write music". The cognitive operations implemented by such a subject to play the organ must have been different from those that an organist able to read and write music would resort to. Therefore, the same instrumental amusia could result from lesion in different parts of the brain depending on musical literacy. Similarly, different musical instruments make different demands in terms of motor planning and organization (e.g., Wilson, 1986). For instance, keyboards are polyphonic instruments, whereas wind and (in most cases) string instruments are monophonic, which implies different reading, planning, and motor organization depending on the musical instrument. Moreover, although one needs one finger to play one note on a keyboard instrument, more than one finger is necessary to play one note on wind instruments in addition to the involvement of the respiratory and buccal systems; motor planning and coordination are therefore achieved through different muscles, at different levels of processing, in these two categories of instruments. Still another type of motor planning and organization is required to play string instruments, as the two hands assume different functions in the production of notes.

Many other factors may intervene in the realization of musical tasks depending on the nature of musicianship of the subjects (e.g., possession of absolute pitch, level of expertise in sight-reading as well as in music theory, breadth of knowledge of musical pieces and melodies). All these factors cannot be discussed here, but the preceding discussion should be sufficiently explicit to indicate that it is necessary to identify and control all potentially relevant factors in order to minimize inconsistencies resulting from uncontrolled, and thus unexplained, sources of variations across subjects.

Musical Tasks and Methods

In the absence of computational models of musical processing, investigations have been mainly concerned with measuring abilities and performance, thus considering a given musical function as an undivided whole. There is a large number of tests designed to assess musical abilities (Shuter-Dyson & Gabriel, 1981, describe and review 24 of them), but their validity has been questioned (see Sloboda, 1985, for a discussion). Even Seashore's test of musical talent (Seashore et al., 1960) has little predictive value, as indicated by the absence of, or very low, correlation between subjects' scores and their actual performance as musicians (see Sloboda, 1984). In addition, recourse to tests of abilities or performance to study music-brain relationships precludes any mapping of musical functions onto cerebral structures, as any function comprises a series of operations that are the critical components that must have corresponding neural substrates. For instance, there is no "musical reading center" as such, but a network of cerebral structures participating in the many operations inherent in reading (Sergent et al., 1992b), with each of these structures contributing its processing to the realization of the task. Examining whether or not a neurological patient is capable of reading musical notation will, therefore, not provide sufficient information to determine which cognitive operation, if any, is impaired by the lesion. Because most studies of brain-damaged musicians have exclusively relied on ability or performance tasks, little can be inferred from these studies about the functional organization of the brain in relation to music This may account for Brust's (1980) pessimistic statement about the understanding of music-brain relationships quoted earlier, as the investigatory tools required to make sense of the diversity of musical impairments resulting from brain damage have not yet been devised. It must be added that a large number of the difficulties associated with the study of music-brain relationships in neurological subjects are not specific to this field of research but are inherent in any investigation of brain-behavior relationships (e.g., Weiskrantz, 1968; Sergent, 1984, 1990b)

Most of the information about the respective contributions of the normal cerebral hemispheres to auditory processing comes from dichotic listening studies. As noted earlier, this technique has not been subjected to the type of scrutiny that would allow a dear understanding of the influence of procedural and methodological variables on subjects' performance, and this is particularly problematic in the study of musical processing.

Three main problems, and several minor ones, seem to limit the usefulness of this technique for understanding music-brain relationships. First is the technique itself, whereby subjects are asked to listen to two different auditory messages presented simultaneously, one to each ear, and to make subsequent responses (recognition or discrimination) based on comparisons to target stimuli. The implications of such a procedure for the processing of musical stimuli have not been examined, but the conditions prevailing in such experiments are extremely remote from normal listening conditions. The simultaneous presentation of two unrelated musical messages necessarily results in cacophony, and the actual auditory experience is that of a mixture of sounds that cannot be used to infer what musical processing normally is. Subjects are forced to base their decision on fragments of what they were able to pick up from such a mixture, and their performance cannot reflect the type of musical processing that would be at play under normal circumstances. The actual strategies that such experimental conditions impose have never been investigated, which implies that it is impossible to determine the nature of the processes underlying performance. In addition to this "competitive" situation, the dichotic listening to musical stimuli is interfered with by illusions about the source of ear stimulation and by a left-right anisotropy in the perception of tone combinations (Deutsch, 1985). As a consequence, the incoming melodies are actually distorted. The influence of such illusions and anisotropy on the pattern of results remains unexplored and, as suggested by Deutsch (1985), "further work is required to determine the extent lo which (they) may have been responsible for patterns of ear advantage" (p. 152).

A second problem is concerned with the relation between ear advantage in dichotic listening studies and hemisphere specialization. Although perceptual asymmetries are well established, it has long been known that the correlation between ear superiority and hemisphere specialization is far from perfect (e.g., Bryden, 1982). More recently, serious doubts have been cast on the validity of the dichotic listening technique as a tool to investigate functional hemispheric asymmetries, as attentional bias may override hemispheric effects in conditions under which subjects are able to develop a consistent strategy, conditions that prevail in almost all dichotic listening studies (Mondor & Bryden, 1992). In addition, because dichotic listening studies use errors as dependent variables, ear advantage can only obtain when one but not both of the simultaneously presented stimuli are incorrectly responded. Performance, therefore, is measured in terms of failures of processing when the actual source of this failure cannot be unequivocally identified and may sometimes reflect distraction, at other times genuine inability, or at other times incorrect guess as well as confusions between ears of stimulation, distortions, and so on.

A third problem is concerned with the stimuli used to examine musical processing. For the most part, dichotic listening studies test sensory and acoustic abilities, which may be a prerequisite to musical processing but which cannot be considered as representative of musical experience as such. Asking subjects to process pitch, timbre, duration, or loudness, each in isolation, has no equivalent in the musical domain. Because any musical stimulus must necessarily comprise each of these four parameters, the task requested from the subjects is not so much one of processing an isolated parameter as one of selectively attending to one parameter, which calls for specific processes unlike those normally underlying music listening. In addition, learning about performance when focusing on one parameter does not inform us about the role of this parameter, nor the processes to which it is subjected, when subjects are exposed to actual musical stimuli. A musical experience and the processes it engages are not the sum of each of the experiences and processes that one could identify when examining each parameter in isolation, but a complex of intricate interactions not only between the parameters that make up musical stimuli, but between the musical stimuli and the listener.

Even when melodies are presented, they are often restricted to three-note sequences, which an outsider musician would not consider as a relevant sample of music In addition, researchers do not always possess the musical background required to ensure appropriately constructed musical stimuli, and there are examples in the neuropsychological literature of experiments using, for instance, so. called consonant chords that are in fact dissonant.

One may, therefore, question whether the dichotic listening technique is an appropriate method of investigation into musical processes. It sets artificial listening conditions, creates musical illusions, distortions, and interferences that are not taken into consideration in the interpretation of results, uses stimuli that have little relevance for understanding musical processing, and requires processes that do not correspond to those normally involved in listening to music. More critically, almost 30 years after being first used with musical stimuli (Kimura, 1964), this technique has not yielded a single piece of unequivocal evidence regarding the respective role of the cerebral hemispheres in processing musical information, and it is still producing inconsistent findings.

Conclusions

After reviewing some of the methods and variables inherent in the study of music-brain relationships, it would appear that the conclusions are rather negative. This study is indeed confronted with a considerable number of problems, some of which are typical of any neuropsychological research, whereas others are specific to the musical domain and result from the large variability in musical abilities and sensitivities across subjects and from the difficulty in uncovering the functional organization of the cognitive operations inherent in musical processing. In addition, because neuropsychological research into music has been modeled after that into language, the experimental approaches and techniques have sometimes been borrowed indiscriminately and applied without examining their appropriateness. It may thus be that the apparent impossibility of neurofunctional mapping of musical functions (cf. Marin, 1982), and the many inconsistencies that mar this field, are essentially circumstantial and not a necessary concomitant of musical research. The identification of these problems and of some of their sources may thus suggest that the experimental investigation of the relationships between music and the brain can indeed progress, provided a series of precautions are taken to ensure that the critical variables are taken into account and controlled. It has thus been argued that advance in understanding music-brain relationships will come from the following: 1) specifically outlining the structural cognitive architecture of musical functions; 2) formulating the problems in terms of underlying operations rather than in terms of vague and unspecified dichotomic views of hemisphere processing; 3) designing experiments that are musically valid and coherent, and that do not lend themselves to multiple strategies; 4) setting up appropriate controls to ensure that the subjects are performing as expected; 5) restricting the investigation to musically literate individuals; 6) selecting among such individuals, a homogeneous set of subjects sharing common musical abilities and cognitive structures; and 7) using investigatory techniques that yield reliable evidence of local cerebral involvement in realizing the tasks under study.

Apart from the last one, these condition are not unreasonably stringent and should be met without particular difficulty. The problem of uncovering the neural substrates of musical functions is less easily resolved, however, as the anatomo-clinical method is inherently limited, especially in the case of musicians. The probability of finding musicians with focal brain damage that results in selective impairment is (fortunately) very low; even finding such subjects is not necessarily sufficient if there is no indication of their premorbid abilities; and, as noted earlier, inferences from disturbances consecutive to brain damage do not permit localization of the disrupted function. Examination of the neurofunctional organization of cognitive functions has benefited from new imaging techniques such as PET measurements of CBF. The next section will illustrate the use of this approach to one particular musical function.

SIGHT-READING

Among musical functions, some appear to be more readily amenable to experimental investigation and control than others. For instance, identifying the processes and their requirements inherent in reading a musical score is easier than identifying those underlying the arousal of emotions at listening to music. Accordingly, it may be appropriate to examine the neurofunctional organization of one such more easily controlled function, sight-reading.

Sight-reading (here defined as deciphering an unknown musical score and playing it on a musical keyboard instrument) is an extremely complex process. It is an activity that musicians perform regularly, when they learn a new piece or when they (especially pianists and organists) are called to accompany other instrumentalists or singers. Very few systematic studies of sight-reading have been carried out most of them in the 1930s and 1940s, at a time when considerations of internal representations and processes were not part of the concerns of psychologists (Ortmann, 1937; Bean, 1938; Lowery, 1940; Weaver, 1943; Van Nuys and Weaver, 1943; Lannert & Ullman, 1945). The more recent studies of sight-reading were conducted by Sloboda (1978, for a review; see also Wolf, 1976), but, as Sloboda (1985) later pointed out, we still do not understand the basic processes underlying sight-reading, nor can we explain what differentiates good from poor sight-readers and what particular skills are indispensable to achieve efficient sight reading.

Paradoxically, relatively more studies have been devoted to sight-reading from a neuropsychological perspective. Some authors have inquired whether, and in what way, verbal text reading and musical note reading differ from one another by examining the pattern of dissociations in neurological patients with musical expertise who have become alexics (e.g., Souques & Baruk, 1930; Brust, 1980; Judd et al., 1983; Signoret et al., 1987; Fasanaro et al., 1990; Stanzione et al., 1990). No consensus has emerged from such investigations, and this area of research is characterized by the same inconsistencies that are observed in the neuropsychological study of music. Some authors suggest that verbal and musical reading rely on the same processes and neural structures (e.g., Fasanaro et al., 1990; Stanzione et al., 1990) while others, on the basis of clear dissociations between verbal and musical reading, reached the opposite conclusion (e.g., Souques & Baruk, 1930; Judd et al., 1983; Signoret et al., 1987). Although these studies clarify some of the issues, they do not speak to the actual cognitive architecture of musical sight-reading that must be specified to understand functional-structural mapping. Other neuropsychological studies have examined the respective contribution of the cerebral hemispheres to the perception of single notes or chords (Oscar-Berman et al., 1976; Segalowitz et al., 1979), and the results have indicated that the left hemisphere plays a critical role in this function, although several factors that may, by themselves, have induced a left-hemisphere superiority, irrespective of the actual task demands, were not controlled in these studies. The main weakness of all these studies lies in the lack of a specific task analysis necessary to design an experimental protocol that will focus on relevant cognitive operations and that will allow the "isolation" of each component operation in order to identify the stage of processing in which a particular variable has its effect, and to infer its internal organization and the representations on which it operates.

There may be no other human activity than musical sight-reading that calls for the simultaneous and sequential processing of so much information in such a very brief time and for the immediate use of this information. A functional decomposition of this task is schematically described in Figure 1, and it illustrates the diversity of operations that must be implemented to achieve it. This task involves, in the context of prespecified clefs, key signature, tempo, meter, and dynamics (according to which the particular values of the musical notations have to be interpreted unless indicated otherwise): 1) the identification of the pitch and duration of the notes written on the two staves that comprise a piano score, implying the simultaneous processing of vertically arranged notations; 2) the identification, within a given "window" of the pitch and duration of the horizontally arranged notes on both staves, which implies detecting familiar patterns and groupings; 3) the identification of accidentals, beams, groups, rests, slurs, trills, mordents, and other ornamentations, and any indication that would modify the duration, dynamic, phrasing, or tempo; 4) the on-line uncovering of the underlying musical structure of the particular piece in order to make predictions about its harmonic progression, to determine how it should be expressed, and therefore, heard in accordance with the intentions of the composer; 5) the anticipation of what the piece should sound like, corresponding to a plan of the performance based on a structural description of the score; 6) the grouping of the visual information already processed and its storage until it is transferred for execution; 7) the generation, from the structural description of the musical score and plan of performance, of a program outlining (a) spatial codes containing information about the positioning of fingers on the keyboard and the patterning of intervals between fingers for both chordal (vertical) and sequential (horizontal) aspects of the score, (b) temporal codes for the timing of finger movements, and () "intensity" codes to specify how strong and fast each key should be hit; 8) the monitoring of the position of fingers to determine which fingers are next to be used and whether finger substitutions, displacement, or crossing of hands should be performed; 9) the actual playing; and 10) listening and feedback on performance; 11) all this taking place at a steady pace that respects the time signature of the piece.

This sketchy componential task analysis illustrates the considerable number of operations, monitoring, and quick decisions that have to be made continuously during sight-reading, and it also suggests a wide range of skills (at the perceptual, cognitive, and motor levels, the demands of speed of processing and sustained attention, along with knowledge of music notation and theory) that must underlie the realization of this function. Of particular importance is that the perceptual processes, into verbal reading, rely for a large part on spatial information, and pianists do not read the notes in terms of their absolute position on the staves but of their position relative to one another (e.g., Sloboda, 1978). That is, featural information, which is necessary to discriminate letters or words, for instance, is relatively less important than spatial information when reading musical notation. A second important aspect of sight reading is the translation from the visual structural description of a score to a representation or plan suited for motor translation, and then to a program that specifies the patterning, ù timing, and of finger movements on a particular instrument.

Using PET measurement of regional CBF in a homogeneous group of 10 professional pianists, Sergent et al. (1992b) examined the mapping of the main operations underlying musical sight-reading onto cerebral structures. Because of the large number of component operations, six control tasks were implemented in order to narrow down the interpretation of the findings obtained during the main experimental task of sight-reading The main findings of this study are shown in Figure 2, and they present the foci of activation after

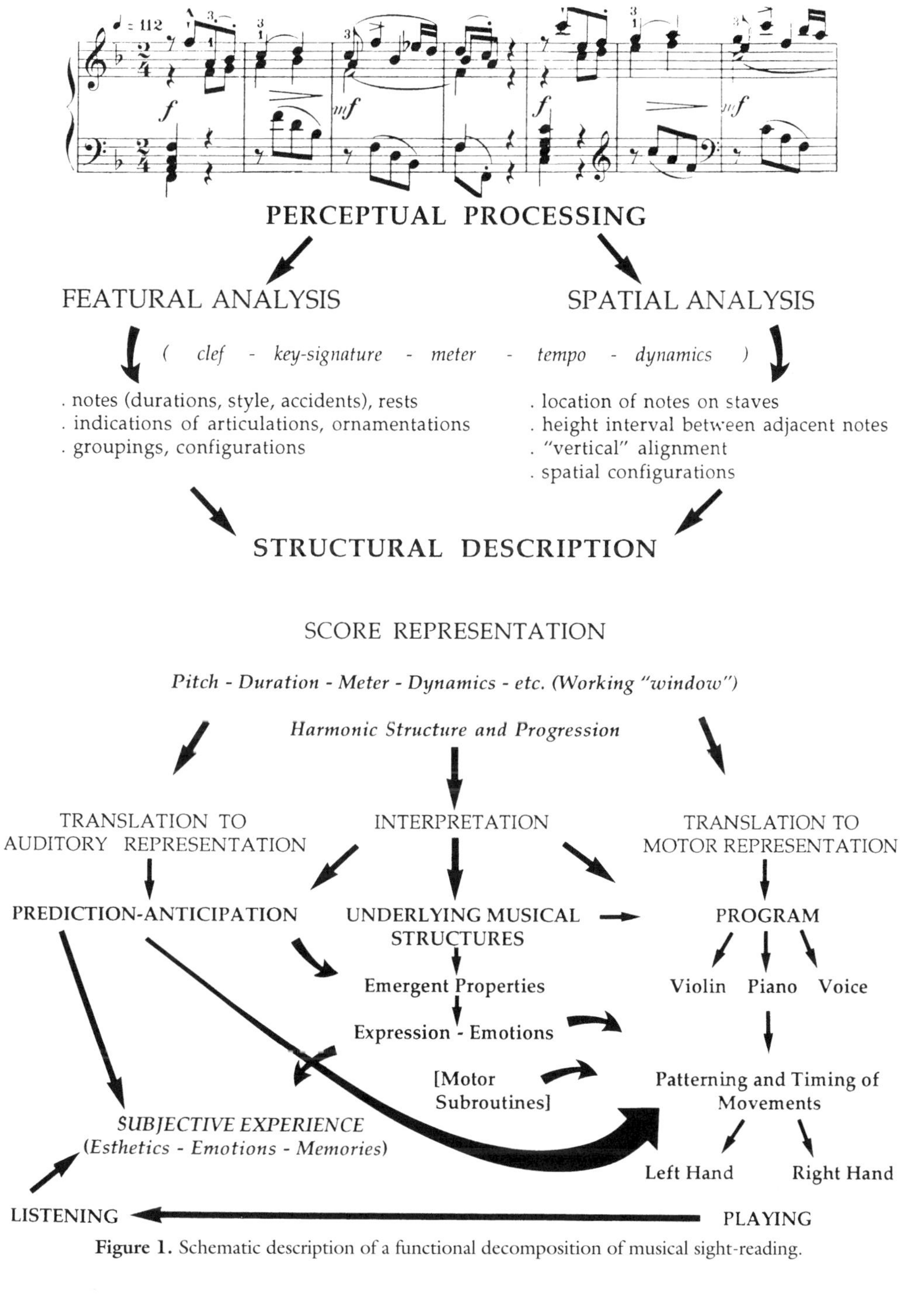

Figure 1. Schematic description of a functional decomposition of musical sight-reading.

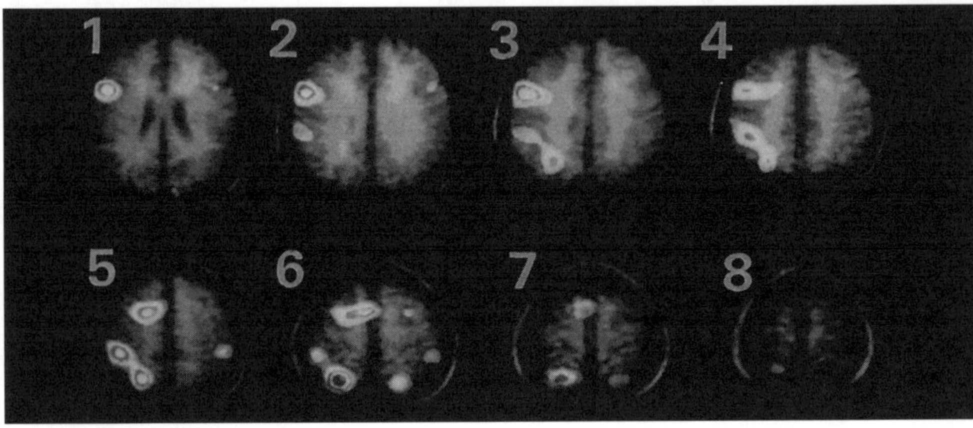

Figure 2. Cortical activation during sight-reading, listening, and right-hand piano performance obtained by PET measurements of CBF. The images were obtained after averaging over 10 professional pianists and subtracting the scale-playing condition. The PET physiological foci of activation are superimposed over horizontal magnetic resonance images of the subject's brains. The top left slice is 29 mm above the line joining the anterior and the posterior commissures, and the slices are 6 mm apart. Activation of the supramarginal gyrus (area 40) is clearly visible in slices 4–5, and it corresponds to the mapping of auditory and visual representations of musical information. Activation of the superior parietal lobule (slices 3–7) reflects the spatial processing of the musical notations and the transformation of the derived spatial information for the visually guided motor performance. The pianists used only their right hands, and the activation is essentially left-sided, but there was nonetheless significant activation in the right superior parietal lobule (shown in the second slice of the bottom row). Activation visible from slices 1–6 is located above Broca's area (area 44) and extends dorsally through area 6 to the supplementary motor area. It reflects the patterning and timing of the motor sequences required for the right manual execution of the piece.

subtracting a scale-playing condition, such that motor information related to the actual movement of the right hand does not appear in this figure. The eight slices illustrate three main foci of activation specifically associated with the sight reading condition. None of these cortical areas were activated during either scale-playing or score-reading, suggesting that the activation observed in this condition results from operations that must be implemented when both reading and playing are performed jointly. Therefore, the activated cerebral regions must reflect operations underlying transformations of musical representations from different modalities.

The activation engaged cortical regions classically called "association" areas. These areas included the supramarginal gyrus, shown in slices 4–5 Because this area was also activated during the control condition during which subjects simultaneously read and listened to a musical piece, the recruitment of the supramarginal gyrus may correspond to the mapping of visual and auditory musical information. Also activated is the superior parietal lobule, clearly apparent in slices 3–7, in the posterior part of the brain. No control condition produced activation of this area, which may therefore be mediating sensorimotor transformations from a visuospatial representation that contains descriptions of the relations between the various notes on the musical score, to information relevant for the patterning and positioning of fingers on the keyboard in order to play the musical notation. This activation is consistent with other evidence indicating a contribution of the superior parietal lobule to visually guided skilled actions and finger positioning. The recruitment of this area also illustrates the spatial nature of musical sight-reading as well as its (relative) independence from verbal reading, which is not known to require the involvement of this part of the parietal cortex for its realization (e.g., Hécaen & Albert, 1978]. A third region of the cortex recruited during the sight-reading task was the prefrontal cortex, in an area extending from just above Broca's area up to the supplementary motor area. It is noteworthy that this region was not activated when the pianists merely played the scales on the keyboard. This suggests that the activation of the prefrontal cortex must be related to motor operations based on information obtained from the score and received from the superior parietal lobule. The involvement of this region of the frontal cortex may then be related to the organization of the sequencing and timing of finger movements necessary for playing the particular score being sight-read.

These findings do not appear to be inconsistent with neurological evidence obtained from brain damaged musicians (see Judd et al., 1983, for a detailed review), even if some authors have reported no dissociation between verbal and musical reading. The requirements of sight-reading, although they differ from those of verbal reading, comprise a series of processes and transformations that are not altogether unlike those of verbal reading (mapping visual and auditory representations; translating the outcome of visual analysis into information suitable for motor production). One may, therefore, expect territories from the same cerebral region to underlie these operations. However, there are functional differences between the two types of reading (e.g., there is no direct relation between the visual shape of a word, which is arbitrary, and the motor execution of its utterance, whereas there is a direct and necessary relation between the positions and intervals of notes on a staff and the actual finger positions and intervals during motor execution on a keyboard). This suggests that functionally distinct areas of the brain may be recruited for the two types of reading, which concurs with the existence of musical and verbal reading dissociations. The contiguity of the neurobiological substrates of these two types of reading makes their conjoint disruption following brain damage highly probable, but not necessary.

CONCLUSIONS

The understanding of the relationships between music and the brain is a legitimate goal of neuroscientific research. However, in spite of an already large body of experimental investigation, the outcome has not been as satisfactory as expected, to the point that some have voiced their incredulity at the feasibility of mapping musical functions onto cerebral structures. There are indeed considerable inconsistencies in the literature bearing on the neurobiological substrates of musical functions. In large part, these inconsistencies reflect complexities inherent in studying the cognitive architecture of mental functions in general, and musical functions in particular. Until a few years ago, no explicitly defined conceptual tools had been proposed to guide the research into cognitive functions. Recent progress in this area may thus raise hopes of developing better cognitive models of the processes underlying the realization of musical tasks and setting up research programs that would enhance our understanding of these functions (e.g., Sergent, 1993).

However, some of the problems encountered in the neuroscientific study of music are specific to the musical domain. The investigation into this domain has been modeled after that into the verbal domain, thus borrowing concepts and methods developed for other fields of research, and not always realizing that these concepts and methods were not appropriately suited to the study of music. Several variables susceptible of hindering experimental investigation were identified, and suggestions were made to prevent their detrimental effects on research and to establish the necessary controls. There are, therefore, reasons to believe that the neurofunctional mapping of musical functions is achievable, and the recent PET study on musical sight-reading (Sergent et al., 1992b) seems to confirm the feasibility of such an endeavor. In addition, the results of this study, while consistent with some of the neurological evidence, provided some answers as to why so many inconsistencies have marred this field of research in the past. Nonetheless, mapping musical functions onto the brain is a considerably difficult task. Sight-reading is a relatively "peripheral" aspect of musical experience, one that lends itself more easily than most to experimental investigation. A full understanding of the neurobiological substrates of musical experience is still very remote, but not impossible. Uncovering how the brain permits some to generate musical masterpieces, and most of us to derive so much pleasure from listening to them, should prove sufficiently challenging to attract and motivate researchers interested in the neurobiological substrates of human cognition.

ACKNOWLEDGMENTS

I gratefully acknowledge the helpful and pertinent comments and suggestions of two anonymous reviewers. Preparation of this paper was supported by grants from NSERC, NIMH, and MRC.

References

Bean, K. L. (1938). An experimental approach to the reading of music. *Psychol Monogr 50,* 1–80.

Benton, A. L. (1977). The amusias. In M. Critchley & R. A. Henson (Eds.), *Music and the brain* (pp. 378–397). London: Heinemann.

Bever, T, & Chiarello, R. J. (1974). Cerebral dominance in musicians and non-musicians. *Science, 185,* 537–539.

Blacking, J (1973). *How musical is man?* Seattle, WA: University of Washington Press.

Bouillaud, J (1865): Sur la faculté du langage articule. *Bull. Acad Mede (Paris) 30,* 72–94.

Brust, J. C. M. (1980). Music and language. Musical alexia and agraphia. *Brain 103,* 367–392.

Bryden, M. P. (1982). *Laterality.* New York: Academic Press.

Bryden, M. P. (in press). Dichotic listening. In J. G. Beaumont & J. Sergent (Eds.), *Dictionary of neuropsychology.* Oxford: Basil Blackwell.

Caramazza, A., & Badecker W. (1989). Patient classification in neuropsychological research. *Brain Cogn 10,* 256–295.

Cook, R. B. (1973). Left-right differences in the perception of dichotically presented musical stimuli. *J Mus Ther 10,* 59–63.

Cooke, D. (1959). *The language of music.* London: Oxford University Press.

Deliège, C. (1984). *Les fondements de la musique tonale.* Paris: Lattes.

Deutsch, D. (1985). Dichotic listening to melodic patterns and its relationship to hemispheric specialization of function. *Mus Percept 3,* 127–154.

Dowling, W. J. (1978). Scale and contour: Two components of a theory of memory for melody. *Psychol Rev 85,* 341–354.

Dowling, W. J., & Harwood, D. L. (1986). *Music cognition.* New York: Academic Press.

Dupre, F., & Nathan, M. (1911). *Le langage musical: Étude médicopsychologique.* Paris: Alcan.

Evans, A., Marett, S., Collins, L., & Peters, T. M. (1989). Anatomical-functional correlative analysis of the human brain using three-dimensional imaging systems. *Proc. Soc. Photogr Optic Instrum Eng 1092,* 264–274.

Exner, J. E. (1978). *The Rorschach: A comprehensive system. Vol 2: Current research and advanced interpretation,* New York: Wiley.

Fasanaro, A. M., Spitaleri, D. L. A., Valiani, R., & Grossi, D. (1990). Dissociation in musical reading: A musician affected by alexia without agraphia. *Mus percept 7,* 259–272.

Felleman, D. J., & Van Essen, D. C. (1991). Distributed hierarchical processing in the primate cerebral cortex. *Cereb Cortex, 1,* 1–47.

Feutschwanger, E. (1930). *Amusie. Studien zur pathologischen Psychologie der akustischen Wahrnehmung und Vorstellung und ihrer Strukturgebiete besonders in Musik und Sprache.* Berlin: Springer.

Fox, P. T. (1991). Physiological ROI definition by image subtraction. *J Cereb Blood Flow Metab. 11,* A79–A82.

Fox, P. T., Perimutter, J. S., & Raichle, M. E. (1985). A stereotactic method of anatomical localization for positron emission tomography. *J Comput Assist Tomogr 9,* 141–153.

Fox, P. T., Mintun, M. A., Reinman, E. M., & Raichle, M. E. (1988). Enhanced detection of focal brain responses using intersubject averaging and change-distribution analysis of subtracted PET images. *J Cereb Blood Flow Metab 8,* 642–653.

Gordon, H. W. (1980). Degree of ear asymmetry for perception of dichotic chords and for illusory chord localization in musicians of different levels of competence. *JEP:HPP 6,* 516–529.

Hécaen, H, Albert, M. L. (1978). *Human neuropsychology.* New York: Wiley.

Hellige, J. B. (1993). *Hemisphere asymmetry: What is left and what is right?* Cambridge, MA: Harvard University Press.

Henschen, S. E. (1920). *Aphasie, Amusie und Akalkulie. Klinische und anatomische Beirage zur Pathologie des Gehirns.* Stockholm: Nordiska Bokhandeln.

Henson, R. A. (1977). The language of music. In M. Critchley & R. A. Henson (Eds.), *Music and the brain* (pp. 233–254). London: Heinemann.

Horowitz, J. (1982). *Conversations with Arrau.* New York: Knopf.

Hulse, S. H., Takeuchi, A. H., & Braaten, R. F. (1992). Perceptual invariances in the comparative psychology of music. *Mus Percept 9,* 151–184.

Judd, T., Gardner, H., & Geschwind, N. (1983). Alexia without agraphia in a composer. *Brain 106,* 435–457.

Kallman, H. J. (1982). Octave equivalence as measured by similarity ratings. *Percept Psychoph 32,* 37–49.

Kellar, L. A., & Bever, T. G. (1980). Hemispheric asymmetry in the perception of musical intervals as a function of musical experience and family handedness background. *Brain Lang 11,* 24–38.

Kimura, D. (1964). Left-right differences in the perception of melodies. *QJ Exp Psychol 16,* 355–358.

Knoblauch, A. (1888). Über Storungen der musikalischen Leistungs-fahigkeit infolge von Gehirnlat. *Dtsch Arch Klin Med 4,* 331–352.

Krumhansl, C. L. (1990). *Cognitive foundations of musical pitch.* New York: Oxford University Press.

Krumhansl, C. L., & Shephard, R. N. (1979). Quantification of the hierarchy of tonal functions within a diatonic context. *JEP:HPP 5,* 579–594.

Lannert, V., & Ullman, M. (1945). Factors in the reading of piano music. *Am J Psychol 5,* 91–99.

Lecours, A. R. (1989). Literacy and acquired aphasia. In A. Galaburda (Ed.), *From reading to neurons* (pp. 27–41). Cambridge, MA: MIT Press.

Lerdhal, F., & Jackendoff, R. (1983). *A generative theory of tonal music.* Cambridge MA: MIT Press.

Locke, S., & Kellar, L. A. (1973). Categorical perception in a non-linguistic mode. *Cortex 9,* 355–369.

Lowery, H. (1940). On reading music. *Br J Physiol Opt 1,* 78–88.

Lueck, C. J., Zeki, S, Friston, K. J. Deiber, M. P., Cope, P., Cunningham, V. J., Lammertsma, A. A., Kennard, C., & Frackowiak, R. S. J. (1989). The colour center in the cerebral cortex of man. *Nature 3*, 386–389.

Luria, A. R., Tsvetkova, L. S., & Futer, D. S. (1965). Aphasia in a composer. *J Neurol Sci 2*, 288–292.

Marin, O. S. M. (1982). Neurological aspects of music perception and performance, In D. Deutsch (Ed.), *The psychology of music* (pp. 453–477). New York: Academic Press.

Mazziotta, J. C., Phelps, M. E., Carson, R. E., & Kuhl, D. E. (1982). Tomographic mapping of human cerebral metabolism: Auditory stimulation. *Neurology 3*, 921–937.

McCarthy, R. A., & Warrington, E. K. (1990). *Cognitive neuropsychology. A clinical introduction*. London: Academic Press.

McFarland, H. R., & Fortin, D. (1982). Amusia due to right temporoparietal infarct. *Arch Neurol 3*, 725–727.

Merzenich, M. M., Nelson, R. J., Stryker, J. P., Cynader, M. S., Schoeppman, A., & Zook, J. M. (1984). Somatosensory cortical map changes following amputation in adult monkeys. *J Comp Neuol 2*, 591–605.

Mesulam, M. M. (1990). Large-scale neurocognitive networks and distributed processing for attention, language, and memory. *Ann Neurol 28*, 597–613.

Meyer, L. B. (1956). *Emotion and meaning in music*. Chicago: University of Chicago Press.

Milner, B. (1962). Laterality effects in audition. In V. B. Mountcastle (Ed.), *Interhemispheric relations and cerebral dominance* (pp. 177–195). Baltimore: The Johns Hopkins Press.

Mintun M., Fox P. T., & Raichle, M. E. (1989). A highly accurate method of localizing neuronal activity in the human brain with positron emmision tomography. *J Cereb Blood Flow Metab 9*, 96–103.

Mondor, T. A., & Bryden, M. P. (1992). On the relation between auditory spatial attention and auditory perceptual asymmetries. *Percept Psychoph 52*, 393–402.

Narmour, E. (1990). *The analysis and cognition of basic melodic structures*. Chicago: University of Chicago.

Ortmann, O. (1937). Span of vision in note reading. In *Music Educators National Conference Yearbook* (pp. 88–93). Reston, VA: MENC

Oscar-Berman, M., Blumstein, S., & DeLuca, D. (1976). Iconic recognition of musical symbols in the lateral visual fields. *Cortex 12*, 41–248.

Posner, M. I., & Peterson, S. E., Fox, P. T., & Raichle, M. E. (1988). Localization of cognitive functions in the brain. *Science, 240*, 1627–1631.

Proust, M. (1866). L'aphasie. *Arch Gen Med 1*, 64–98.

Raichle, M. E. (1990). Images of the functioning human brain. In H. Barlow, C. Blakemore, & M. Westion-Smith (Eds.), *Images and understanding*. Cambridge: Cambridge University Press.

Raichle, M. E., Martin, W. R. W., Herscovitch, P., Mintun, M. A., & Marham, J. (1983). Brain blood flow measured with intravenous H_2O. Il. Implementation and validation. *J Nucl Med 24*, 790–798.

Ravel, M. (1989). *Lettres, Écrits et Entretiens* (présentés et annotés par Arbie Orenstein). Paris: Flammarion.

Schenker, H. (1935). *Neue Musikalische Theorien und Phantasien. Vol III. Die Freie Satz.* Universal Edition, E. Oster (Ed.). 1956. London: Longman.

Seashore, C. E. (1938). *Psychology of music*. New York: McGraw-Hill.

Seashore, C. E., Lewis, D, & Saetvit, J. G. (1960). *Seashore's measures of musical talent*. New York: The Psychological Corporation of New York.

Segalowitz, S., Bebout, L. J., & Lederman, S. J. (1979). Lateralization for reading musical chords: Disentangling symbolic, analytic, and phonological aspects of reading. *Brain Lang 8*, 315–323.

Sergent, J. (1984). Inferences from unilateral brain damage about normal hemispheric functions in visual pattern recognition. *Psychol Bull 96*, 99–115.

Sergent, J. (1990a). The neuropsychology of image generation: Data, method and theory. *Brain Cogn 13*, 98–129.

Sergent, J. (1990b). Les dilemmes de la gauche et de la droite: Confrontation, cohabitation ou coopération? In X. Seron (Ed.), *Psychologie et Cerveau* (pp. 121–151). Paris: Presses Universitaires de France.

Sergent, J. (1993). Music, the brain and Ravel. *TINS 16*, 168–172.

Sergent, J., Zuck, E., Levesque, M., & MacDonald, B. (1992a). Positron emission tomography study of letter and object processing: Empirical findings and methodological condiderations. *Cereb Cortex 2*, 68–80.

Sergent, J., Zuck, E., Terriah, S., & MacDonald, B. (1992b). Distributed neural netowrk underlying musical sight-reading and keyboard performance. *Science 257*, 106–109.

Shallice, T. (1988). *From neuropsychology to mental structure.* Cambridge, UK: Cambridge University Press.

Shuter-Dyson, R, & Gabriel, C. (1981). *The psychology of musical ability.* London: Methuen.

Sidtis, J. (1980). On the nature of the cortical function underlying right hemisphere auditory perception. *Neuropsychologia 18*, 321–330.

Sidtis, J. (1981). The complex tone test: Implications for the assessment of auditory laterality effects. *Neuropsychologia 19*, 103–112.

Signoret, J. L., Van Eeckhout, P., Poncet, M., & Castaigne, P. (1987). Aphasie sans amusie chez un organiste aveugle. Alexie-agraphie verbale sans alexie-agraphie musicale en braille. *Rev Neurol (Paris) 143*, 172–181.

Sloboda, J. A. (1978). The psychology of music reading. *Pychol Mus 6*, 3–20.

Sloboda, J. A. (1984). Review of Wing and Seashore tests. In H. Goldstein & P. Levy (Eds.), *Tests in education: A book of critical reviews.* London: Academic Press.

Sloboda, J. A. (1985). *The musical mind.* Oxford: Oxford University Press.

Sloboda, J. A. (1986). Cognition and real music: The psychology of music comes of age. *Psychol Belg 26*, 199–219.

Souques, A., & Baruk, H. (1930). Autopsie d'un cas d'amusie (avec aphasie) chez un professeur de piano. *Rev Neurol (Paris) 34*, 545–556.

Stanzione, M., Grossi, D., & Roberto, L. (1990). Note-by-note music reading: A musician with letter-by-letter reading. *Mus Percept 7*, 273–284.

Thurlow, W. R., & Erchul, W. P. (1977). Judged similarity in pitch of octave multiples. *Percept Psychoph 22*, 177–182.

Ustvedt, H. I. (1937). Über die Untersuchung der musikalischen Functionen bei Patienten mit Gehirnleiden, besonders bei Patienten mit Aphasie. *Acta Med Scand Suppl 86*, 7–737.

Van Nuys, K., & Weaver, H. E. (1943). Memory span and visual pauses in reading rhythms and melodies. *Psychol Monogr 5*, 33–50.

Wallin, N. L. (1991). *Biomusicology.* Stuyvesant, NY: Pendragon Press.

Weaver, H. E. (1943). Studies of ocular behavior in music reading. *Psychol Monogr 55*, 1–30.

Weiskrantz, L. (1968). Some traps and pontifications. In L. Weiskrantz (Ed.), *Analysis of behavioral change* (pp. 415–429). New York: Harper & Row.

Wertheim, N. (1977). Is there an anatomical localisation for musical faculties? In M. Critchley, & R. A. Henson (Eds.), *Music and the brain* (pp. 282–297). London: Heinemann.

Wilson, F. R. (1986). *Tone deaf and all thumbs?* New York: Viking Penguin.

Wolf, T. (1976). A cognitive model of musical sight-reading. *J Psychol Res 5*, 143–171.

INFANTS' HEMISPHERIC COMPUTATION OF MUSIC AND SPEECH

Giuseppe Cossu, Carmine Faienza, and Carlo Capone

Introduction

Current neurological theory honors the computation of language by the left hemisphere as an axiomatic proposition. Even those scholars who dispute the strict dichotomy model and favor a nonmarginal role of the right hemisphere in language processing (Zaidel, 1985) recognize that most core-linguistic functions are left lateralized. In the last decade, however, the recognition of individual variability in cerebral dominance (Segalowitz, 1987) and recovery from aphasia (Basso, 1989; Martins & Ferro, 1990) has sparked some theoretical rethinking that has shifted the paradigm from a simple "black and white" model to a multifactorial and "graded" model of cerebral specialization (Baynes, 1990; Geshwind & Galaburda, 1987; Schneiderman, 1986). What still remains hopelessly unclear (and also a neglected issue) is "the metric over which degrees of lateralization should be computed" (Marshall, 1987, p. 51). Not surprisingly, the matter becomes more controversial when the issue turns to developmental age, where the factors of emerging structure, hierarchical reorganizations and brain plasticity inevitably overlap.

Two opposing views have characterized the approach to the initial state of hemispheric lateralization:

1. The equipotentiality theory, and
2. The antiequipotentiality theory.

In his classic work on the biology of language acquisition, Lenneberg (1967) concluded that "for some time in infancy, both hemispheres still retain a potential identity [and] at least in the right hemisphere, the acquisition of language can take place [only] between the ages of 2–12 years" (p. 173). A few years earlier, in a seminal work, Basser (1962) had indeed shown that brain lesions within that age range were unlikely to produce permanent language disorders.

Other scholars such as Dennis and Kohn (1975), Dennis and Whitaker (1976), and Aram and Whitaker (1988) have claimed that the left hemisphere is genetically predisposed to syntax; hence, early left hemisphere damage would result in syntactic deficit. This position has recently been questioned by Bishop (1983; 1988), who has shown that children who have had an early left hemispherectomy do not perform differently on syntactic tasks from normal children of the same age.

This paper will provide a critical survey of both experimental evidence and theoretical accounts pertaining to the emergence of functional hemispheric asymmetries. It will also include some preliminary experimental results from a research project currently in progress in the Neuropsychiatric Infants' Unit, University of Parma. Our analysis will scan the territory from the unique observatory of the infant's computation of music and speech, since these two functions provide a challenging testing ground. Though located within an identical perceptual (auditory) domain, the two functions (at least, in adults) appear to be subserved by distinct mechanisms and to have distinct neural representations. The final observations resulting from this investigation may be explained by two contrasting hypotheses:

1. The distinction of music and speech processes may be the outcome of ontogenetically distinct architectures; or

2. The distinction of music and speech processes may have emerged from common primitive components, whose different trajectories were induced by epigenetic pressure.

We will then examine how these two contrasting views are reflected in current neurophysiological evidence.

Biological Frames

Initial State(s) and Steady State

A definitive neuropsychological description of the state of cognitive architecture will not appear in the near future. Even if this point had been reached, it would still be necessary to cover a long distance, that is, to bridge the gap between description and explanation. Description of a final state, per se, does not spontaneously become an account of the internal architecture of the function, nor does it elucidate the developmental steps that may have generated that architecture from an initial state. In order to explain the final result of cognitive architecture, it is necessary to be equipped with a structural description of the functions of, and a principled hypothesis about, its growth, be it a stage-timed metamorphosis model (Piaget, 1967), or an additive architecture model (Marshall, 1989).

In developmental neuropsychology, the issue of cerebral dominance has usually been reasoned from two opposite views:

1. Functional hemispheric asymmetries are genetically predetermined; or

2. The two hemispheres are functionally equipotential at birth; the hemispheric asymmetries progressively grow, being completed by the time of puberty (Lenneberg, 1967).

More elaborate explanations have recently suggested that whereas hemisphere specialization remains constant throughout life, brain plasticity decreases with age (Witelson, 1985).

Theoretical divergencies reflect the difficulty of obtaining clearcut evidence for a black or white picture. It has been shown, for example, that an infant's left hemisphere is peculiarly sensitive to (some) linguistic subcomponents (Molfese & Betz, 1988; Bertoncini, Bijeljac-Babic, McAdams, Peretz, & Mehler, 1989). Hemispheric asymmetries for phonological input thus appear to be established long before the child is actively engaged in full language performance. Are Kinsbourne and Hiscock (1977) correct when they claim that the brain is specialized for a function before the actual performance of it? The evidence is controversial. For example, clinicians have reported that recovery from acquired aphasia in children is largely unpredictable from the side and size of the brain lesion (Geschwind, 1972). The overall picture seems to be that language recovery is remarkable even after extensive damage around the age of 12 to language areas of the left hemisphere (Cossu, Da Prati, & Marshall, 1994). The problem remains to reconcile these seemingly conflicting results.

It may be that the developmental brain/language relationship cannot be productively examined until the boundaries between distinct analysis levels are clarified (Marr & Poggio, 1976), that is, until we specify the level at which an algorithm is committed to a particular mechanism. It is therefore a fundamental task to outline comparable maps of the brain's formal structure and its neurodynamic representations. Once this is accomplished, studying a function that emerges from the processes of brain growth may be productive.

Brain Growth and the Epigenetic Frame

The nervous system originates from the ectodermic plate and each ontogenetic step is modulated by a species-specific genetic program. The rate and time of growth processes (cell differentiation and neuronal migration) are strictly constrained by genetic code (Cowan, 1984). However, "it is the state of the cytoplasm that decides which particular gene locus will be active" (Waddington, 1966, p. 63). In this respect, every molecular step in embryonic growth is epigenetic in nature.

The early stages of embryonic growth are predominantly governed by the internal environment (Johnson & Morton, 1991), that is, they are confined within the molecular dimension of the cell (and cell populations) biology. As the embryo becomes an increasingly complex organism, new variables begin to regulate the neurodevelopmental processes. At this stage, the embryo's activity becomes a major factor in determining the neurodynamic architecture. For example, the functional refinement of the neuromotor system arises from progressive neuronal death. Hamburger (1975) has calculated that the lateral motor column of the chick embryo contains some 20,000 neurons, while the adult chicken has no more than 12,000. Some 40% of the original neuronal population dies during the transition from embryo to adulthood, due to pruning of the functionally redundant connectivity.

Another example is the adult opossum in whose brain certain cerebral motor areas are organized in columns (or barrels) corresponding to the digits of its forelimbs. If one of the neonate opossum's limbs is amputated, the corresponding cortical columns do not differentiate (Johnson, Hamilton, Hsung, & Ulinsky, 1972). The same phenomenon occurs with chimpanzees. When one finger is amputated, a radical reorganization of the corresponding cortical topography occurs due to the functional recruitment of cortical representation of the two contiguous fingers into the area of the amputated finger (Merzenich, Nelson, Kaas, Stryker, Jenkins, Zook, Cynader, & Schoppman, 1987). Similar results are also obtained by tactile stimulation of an owl monkey's finger (Jenkins, Merzenich, Ochs, Allard, & Guic-Robies, 1990).

Effects of neural plasticity can be detected in the auditory and visual domains as well. Tonotopic organization and cortical topographic representation of auditory space in the brain are modified by experience during normal development in several animal species (King & Moore, 1991). Likewise, visual stimulation, within a critical period, regulates the cortical architecture of the visual system (Hubel, 1991).

In sum, in the early stages of development, two interacting mechanisms are at work:

1. The genetically constrained processes of assembling the neuronal structures.
2. The functional (and structural) refinement of those neuronal architectures induced by ontogenetic adaptive processes (Changeux, 1985; Prechtl, 1994).

Selection Processes

There are limits, however, both to the effects of ontogenetic adaptation and to the power of genetic forces. We can best appreciate the role of selection processes in regulating the emergence of functional architectures by analyzing those consequences some exceptional (external) environmental circumstances bring to bear on the architecture of cognitive systems.

This point is well illustrated by the motor and cognitive development of those children reared in exceptional circumstances (i.e., in a nonhuman environment). These so-called "wild" boys and girls manifest an inability to stand on their own legs and walk efficiently; and none of them ever developed language (Itard, 1801, 1807; Lodovico, 1978). During the first weeks following their rescue, these children were unable to sustain a standard walking posture, although they could run at high speed in a four-legged position. The acquisition of a standard walking posture required intense and systematic training that eventually resulted in good control of the walking posture. Similarly, in spite of their excellent motility, these children were unable to use their hands for bringing food to the mouth. Proper use of the hands for daily activities likewise required long training.

These children never developed expressive language in spite of systematic training, even in cases where they survived for several decades. Oral comprehension as well was severely impaired in terms of significant practical context or routine events. Language achievements for these children were limited to a few vocabulary items. The usually cited case of Kaspar Houser (who even attended high school) is not prototypical. The boy was reared (although in subhuman conditions) by human beings who may have spoken to him in one way or another.

These data suggest that there is no predetermined fate for the growth of cognitive functions. The chance for genetic information to be actually implemented depends on the availability of proper external conditions. When adverse environmental conditions persist throughout the early stages of development, the developmental trajectory of a functional system can be distorted and its structural components rearranged in alternative ways.

Environmental pressure, however, has its own limitations. It can only induce the emergence (or distort the original trajectory) of the function; it cannot determine its primary neurodynamic architecture. Likewise, external stimulation can hardly rebuild a damaged system; at best, it can recruit some cortical areas and thus approximate (or restore) functional efficiency.

Cognitive Architecture

The Vertical Faculties

Thus far we have analyzed the interaction of the internal and external environments in determining the architecture of functional systems during brain growth. We now need to explore the external boundaries and the internal architecture of the cognitive systems.

Within the traditional compartmentalizing of the mind, the faculties of memory, reasoning, perception, and attention were individuated with respect to their effects rather than their subject matter (Marshall, 1983). Over the past 10 years this age-old position has been subverted by a theoretical approach that postulates the domain specificity of the vertical faculties (Fodor, 1983). The modularity theory revives at least some of the theoretical postulates of phrenology advanced in the 18th century by Franz Joseph Gall. Phrenological theory claimed that faculties are inborn in animals and man and, since they are independent from each other, they must be localized in different areas of the brain (Gall, 1798). All of these fundamental points have been endorsed by the modular theory that further specified other crucial features of the system. The interface systems in particular play a key role in the theoretical system. They are located at the interface between the transducers (sense organs) and the central system (concerned with the fixation of beliefs), and their function is to decode the distal objects that correspond with particular proximal stimulation (Liberman & Mattingly, 1985). In Fodor's analysis, the modularity of these input systems consists in their possession of several properties, some of which are of crucial relevance to our analysis and will be briefly considered here.

Input systems are domain-specific. The specialization of these systems provides rigid constraints to the range of information they can access. Current neurophysiological research has revealed the existence of vertical boundaries within a given perceptual mode. For instance, in the visual domain, independent neurodynamic systems control the perception of shape, movement, and color (Zeki, 1993). In the auditory domain, speech perception appears to be distinct from other auditory nonverbal computations (Mann & Liberman, 1983).

Input systems are computationally encapsulated. Contrary to what top-down models claim, this property of modular systems holds that at least some perceptual mechanisms compute the structure of a percept largely, perhaps solely, in isolation from background information (Fodor, 1983). The same subject who knows that two horizontal segments in the are alike, still finds the two segments of asymmetrical length when their boundaries are marked by inverted arrows, as in the Müller-Lyer optic illusion.

The ontogeny of input systems exhibits a characteristic pace and sequencing. In accordance with Franz Joseph Gall's phrenological program (1798), Fodor (1983) claims that "a great deal of the developmental course of the input systems is endogenously determined" (p. 100).

The theory of modularity has direct implications for pursuing a study of cognitive development because it is based on the following points:

1. Each neuropsychological system can be internally fractionated
2. The external boundaries of function are discrete.

The overall picture resembles a collection of vertically positioned faculties, a view strongly supported by clinical evidence.

In spite of congenital motor impairment, a high degree of cognitive and linguistic development can be achieved (Fourcin, 1975; Cossu, Urbinati, & Marshall, 1987). In the case of mirror dissociation, however, language can be severely impaired even if the child has normal intelligence and motor skills. In addition, even children with severe developmental disabilities can achieve a high degree of linguistic and orthographic skills (Cossu & Marshall, 1990; O'Connor & Hermelin, 1994). It appears, therefore, that all of these functions and related subcomponents are independently implemented by distinct neurodynamic architectures.

The Functional Architecture of Language

A detailed description of the functional architecture of language is beyond the scope of this paper. Therefore, a brief outline will be presented of the basic components of a formal language model and some of the fractionations that language pathology reveals.

Language architecture can be accurately described in the Universal Grammar model (UG) of Chomsky (1981, 1986). UG comprises a set of distinct components and subtheories embodying different principles and parameters. The UG model includes sentence structure in terms of the simultaneous limitations of the X-bar theory that accounts for deep structure, and both movement and boundary principles that link surface and deep structures. Theta theory accounts for the possible semantic roles that can be assigned to sentence elements and the like. Linguistic information emanating from the interplay of these structural components is converted into phonological and logical forms. The former provides the interface transcription for the phonetic implementation of the message, and the latter conveys the semantic representation of the sentence. In sum, UG gives us a principled description and explanation of components of natural language.

Somehow, formal language architecture must be represented in the brain and reflected in actual processing by different brain structures. In approaching the neurobiology of language, much can be learned from developmental language pathology, where an asymmetrical growth of the linguistic system may emerge because of selective impairment of one single subcomponent. Clinical analysis of these dissociations may prove enlightening and even pave the way for a principled reconstruction of the neurodynamic architecture of language growth. Several such dissociations have already been reported, although not with hard data and objective research methods.

Practical competence, for example, can be selectively dissociated from the entire language system (Rapin & Allen, 1985), thus indicating that phonology, morphology, and syntax per se do not guarantee effective verbal communication. Congenital anarthria may sometimes camouflage that part of the linguistic system that has actually developed. In one such case, the orthographic skills of F. M., a child of 16 years, demonstrated that a perfect linguistic system was in place (Cossu, Urbinati, & Marshall, 1985). Equally striking linguistic anomalies are seen in developmental disorder cases where selective impairment of expressive phonology persists in the face of phonological, morphological, and syntactical functions that have not been affected. The picture is reversed in the case of developmental agrammatism where syntactic impairment persists—long after the phonological impairment has disappeared—in spite of intact pragmatic and communicative competence (Rapin & Allen, 1983). Therefore, there is preliminary evidence that different language components can be selectively impaired in children.

The Functional Architecture of Music

Though the literature on the neurobiology of music is still in its infancy, several significant discoveries have already surfaced. As Peretz and Morais (1994) have shown in their excellent paper on music-specific brain function, we are now beginning to grasp a more detailed picture of this usually overlooked research area. Current neuropsychological analysis clearly documents the external boundaries and some aspects of the internal structure of music function. These two very general traits clarify the deep architectural similarities between music and language. In both, the external boundaries are marked by computational independence within a common auditory domain; the compositional nature of the internal architecture of each function is documented by the fractionabilty of distinct subcomponents. In short, music and language share a common modular taxonomy.

The next task is to examine some aspects of the architecture of music function that may bear a direct relevance to the emergence of hemispheric lateralization. The first issue relates to the independence of musical skills from those of general cognitive development. A growing body of experimental evidence indicates that implicit musical knowledge is part of each individual's biological endowment. Davidson (1994) notes that musically untrained persons have remarkably sophisticated musical abilities that can be detected in a number of musical tasks. What is of interest to us here is that individual differences in musical abilities are not necessarily related to corresponding levels of overall cognitive development. Most importantly of all, exceptional musical talents can be dichotomized from general cognitive development. Miller (1989) provides an excellent example in his detailed description of a 5-year-old musical savant, Eddie. The musical performance of the young boy revealed keen sensitivity to the tonal structure of a melody line as well as the ability to reproduce the melody in any key or range of the piano. The literature reports that all musical savants have an impressive degree of absolute pitch; their musical talent seems to have emerged without any systematic formal training. Chomsky's remarks here are pertinent:

> The child quite effortlessly makes use of an intricate structure of specific rules and guiding principles to convey his thoughts and feelings to others, arousing in them novel ideas and subtle perception and judgments.... Thus language is a mirror of the mind in a deep and significant sense. (Chomsky, 1975, p. 6)

In a deep and significant sense, music can also be seen as a mirror of the mind, and it can reflect what the human mind as a biological structure is apt to generate. The nature of musical skills may thus be highly specific and deeply rooted in the biology of the human species. Experimental phonetics, for example, documents that speech perception is selectively computed by a dedicated module that cannot be turned on by any other auditory stimuli (Libermann, Cooper, Shankweiler, & Studdert-Kennedy, 1967; Mann & Liberman, 1983). Furthermore, the nonspeech auditory domain appears to be under control of more than just one general purpose system. Clinical cases of pure word deafness (Albert & Bear, 1974; Tanaka, Yamadori, & Mori, 1987) have been reported in which recognition of music and other environmental sounds were untouched by the disorder. Spreen, Benton, and Fincham (1965) have also described the specular condition of auditory agnosia without aphasia. These double dissociations strongly suggest that speech, music, and other environmental sounds may be processed by independent computational systems.

Sloboda (1985) and Jackendoff (1987) have recently produced theoretical studies that present a plausible account of the internal architecture of musical function. Two components are particularly preeminent: the sequential variations in pitch (melodic structure) and the sequential variations in duration (temporal structure). Although melody and rhythm must be integrated at some point by the listener, the two components may be processed independently at an early stage. Neuropsychological experiments with brain-damaged patients show that focal hemisphere lesions may produce a selective loss for either melody alone or for rhythm alone (Peretz, 1990). In patients with left hemisphere lesion, the recognition of melodic contour was left undisturbed, although they were unable to retrieve internal information. Patients with right hemisphere lesions failed to recognize both dimensions. These recent discoveries provide further support for the theories advanced in the classic work by Bever and Chiarello (1974), who had shown that trained musicians and nonmusicians used different parameters in the recognition of pitch sequences. Musicians used an interval-based route to recognize a melody and had a right ear advantage, whereas nonmusicians mostly relied on melodic contour and showed a left ear advantage. It remains an unsettled issue whether the same contour and rhythmic discrimination processes are involved in speech recognition.

Converging Points in Development

The Growth of Hemispheric Specialization

Experimental evidence is now available that shows some computational processes in the language domain are already left lateralized a few days after birth. By using the nonnutritive sucking response, Bertoncini, Bijeljac-Babic, McAdams, Peretz, and Mehler (1989) found that 4-day-old infants show a greater recovery of sucking when a linguistic change occurred in the right ear, and a musical change in the left ear. Best, Hoffman, and Glanville (1982) obtained analogous results by means of the orienting response. They showed that left ear advantage for music (timbre) is clearly established at around 2 months of age, but a right ear advantage for speech (syllable) appears only after 2 months. Likewise, Molfese and Betz (1988) found asymmetrical ERP responses on the two hemispheres for music and speech stimuli.

Overall, these data suggest that the left hemisphere is primarily involved in the computation of language, whereas the right hemisphere plays a leading role in the analysis of music. The usually accepted conclusion from this set of data is that the left hemisphere dominance for language must be genetically prespecified, or, put another way, language is more extensively represented in the left hemisphere.

Clinical evidence, however, appears to conflict with both data and interpretation. In many instances of severe left hemisphere damage, the pediatric neurologist witnesses in younger and older children an astonishingly rapid recovery from acquired aphasia (Martins & Ferro, 1990; Cossu, Da Prati, & Marshall, 1994). Furthermore, full language acquisition by the right hemisphere is possible when the left hemisphere has been removed for clinical reasons at an early age (Dennis & Whitaker, 1976). This evidence clearly yields conflicting conclusions by showing that linguistic computations are left lateralized at birth, and yet, extensive left hemisphere damage does not prevent language recovery.

It seems reasonable to assume that language recovery from acquired aphasia in children involves different variables, most notably the site and size of the brain lesion. This raises the possibility that both inter- and intrahemispheric differences may be crucial in shaping language architecture in the brain. Furthermore, the possibility should be considered that distinct subcomponents of language architecture are implemented through multiple and asymmetrical cortical representations. Language activity may involve more than just one restricted area and the left hemisphere. Language architecture suggests the possibility that the metric over which the cortical representations of language should be computed might be tailored for each specific linguistic component.

Finally, it should be considered that hemispheric asymmetries can best be uncovered by focal and circumscribed computational processes. Previous studies of hemispheric asymmetries in infants have used single syllables and individual notes (or a chord) as linguistic and musical input, respectively. The question remains as to what would be the result of presenting an infant with a short piece that was a genuine musical example, or with a fragment of a full language monologue. The problem of hemispheric lateralization was addressed by analyzing the electrophysiological responses of 4-day-old infants to complex musical and linguistic stimuli.

Work in Progress

Hemispheric Computation of Language and Music in Infants

Seven fullterm 4-day-old infants (four males and three females) were involved in a project study conducted by the authors. These infants had experienced no pathological events in utero, and their deliveries were free of complications. Their neurological profiles were therefore within normal range, and they were therefore at a low neurological risk (following the criteria of Prechtl's optimality scores).

Parents were informed about the scope of the investigation and each infant was included in the project only after parental consent and the agreement of the mother to play an active role in the experiment.

In this study, neurophysiological investigation of language and music perception in the two hemispheres was based on a spectral analysis of EEG data from 14 electrodes positioned on the scalp. The EEG power spectra for theta and delta frequency bands was calculated from each electrode's spatial function and then converted into a topographical plot of the energy distribution in each spectral range. The methodology involved in mapping brain electrical activity (BEAM) allowed an automatic spatial analysis (Duffy, Mc Anulty, & Schachter, 1984).

EEG recording was collected in a soundproof room during the period between the second and third morning feedings, while the infant was in an awakened condition (state 3 or 4, following the Prechtl protocol). Three experimental conditions were considered: (a) silence, (b) music, and (c) language. Each recording session lasted 3 minutes and the infant's awake state was constantly monitored so as to avoid data confounding through inclusion of EEG samples from sleep states. The following conditions were present for each infant:

1. In condition (a), an EEG baseline was recorded for the analysis of variance induced by music and speech perception, respectively.

2. In condition (b), the infant heard a 3-minute tape of the *Nocturne no. 97* from the *Mikrokosmos* of Bela Bartok.

3. In condition (c), the infant's mother quietly spoke to her child in an extemporaneous monologue.

From each of these three conditions, a 50-second artifact-free segment was selected. Tables 1 and 2 show the mean scores of EEG power spectra in the theta and delta frequency bands, respectively. It is clear that there is a wide variability within the sample.

Table 1. *Mean Score and sd of Power Spectra for Delta Frequency Band*

S	MUSIC				SPEECH			
	LEFT		RIGHT		LEFT		RIGHT	
	m	sd	m	sd	m	sd	m	sd
01	855.4	208.5	612.6	349.9	901.8	236.1	832.6	518.1
02	394.4	49.1	336.4	146.2	505.1	54.7	559.7	276.7
03	201.1	24.7	189.4	25.7	193.1	25.5	198.9	17.5
04	389.7	27.7	489.5	344.6	585.2	70.7	592.0	400.1
05	200.8	36.9	177.5	11.3	430.6	64.0	402.2	126.9
06	288.8	56.7	361.8	177.9	392.4	52.3	439.2	272.8
07	391.8	42.9	324.8	34.3	360.0	86.9	333.1	14.3

Table 2. *Mean Score and sd of Power Spectra for Theta Frequency Band*

S	MUSIC				SPEECH			
	LEFT		RIGHT		LEFT		RIGHT	
	m	sd	m	sd	m	sd	m	sd
01	826.1	226.2	1105.5	576.7	971.0	230.0	1213.1	608.1
02	314.1	70.6	524.4	91.1	619.0	109.0	444.7	175.3
03	347.8	18.0	322.3	46.9	316.0	25.2	311.2	24.7
04	521.5	117.1	440.6	100.7	621.8	102.0	606.6	211.1
05	301.6	45.4	268.9	28.8	465.1	96.3	483.7	95.5
06	285.5	65.5	360.4	224.2	338.1	52.7	428.1	343.5
07	769.1	102.2	816.8	80.4	744.4	104.4	683.1	63.7

The spectral analysis of data for each subject shows that right/left asymmetries are not homogeneous and that discrepancy values are low for both language and music. A two-way ANOVA was run for each subject, with music and language examined as the *within* factors and right/left hemisphere as the *between* factor. When hemispheric location was not considered, highly significant computational differences in the spectral values for the theta frequency band were found in six out of seven cases between the two conditions of music and language. (See Table 3.)

Table 3. *ANOVA for Differences between Music and Speech Irrespective of Hemispheric Location*

S	TASK			
	DELTA		THETA	
01		n.s.	$F = 7.51$	$p = 0.021$
02	$F = 33.21$	$p < 0.001$	$F = 113.03$	$p < 0.001$
03		n.s.	$F = 5.86$	$p = 0.036$
04	$F = 30.96$	$p < 0.001$	$F = 15.70$	$p = 0.003$
05	$F = 73.08$	$p < 0.001$	$F = 79.45$	$p < 0.001$
06	$F = 16.02$	$p = 0.003$		n.s.
07		n.s.	$F = 14.00$	$p = 0.004$

These data suggest that music and language induce different computational processes, although the difference does not correspond to an asymmetrical hemispheric activation. In some infants, language and music may actually induce a striking discrepancy in the distribution of spectral patterns across the two hemispheres. In most cases, however, the picture is more likely to resemble the foreign language perception of the kind reported by Petsche, Richter, Etlinger, and Filz (1994). Overall, the data from this study reveal that, unlike the phoneme or the pure tone stimulus conditions, when infants compute structurally complex linguistic or musical information, the computational discrepancies between the two hemispheres may be masked.

From a developmental perspective, although these data might appear to push the pendulum swing toward equipotentiality, the temptation to do so should be resisted. The experimental evidence supporting a selective involvement of left and right hemispheres in speech and music perception, respectively, is too compelling to be ignored. On the other hand, as noted previously, evidence of massive reorganization of language function (following extensive left hemisphere lesions in older children) indicates that the linguistically minor hemisphere can take over the major linguistic job when exceptional circumstances require it.

A Componentially Distributed Architecture

Our data on infants' hemispheric asymmetries are, at present, quantitatively too limited to draw any conclusions. The data, however, suggest some trends. Language acquisition first requires a selective ability to differentiate phonetic events from other surrounding environmental sounds. The Haskins' group has shown that a specific, built-in modular system does the job efficiently and automatically. Two- or 3-day old infants, for example, can differentiate their mother language from other tongues, although they are unable to tell the difference between two foreign languages. Intonational contours (i.e., melodic and rhythmic components) that characterize a clause or a sentence appear then to be major players in coping with the task of specific language recognition. These parameters might also provide a cue to mark syntactic boundaries, although not to decode the structural syntactic relationships.

Components of language structure can be selectively impaired either by developmental disorders or by acquired brain lesions. These conditions further support the hypothesis of an internal fractionability of the linguistic system. The semantic system, for example, can be selectively impaired in adults (McCarthy & Warrington, 1989). In developmental pathology, morphological features can be selectively impaired (Gopnik & Crago, 1991). Similarly, in developmental agrammatism, there can be a selective deficit of syntax (Rapin & Allen, 1985). The fractionability of the linguistic system therefore implies a corresponding neurological architecture in which distinct functional subcomponents are specifically dedicated to compute independent linguistic components.

Current knowledge about the neurophysiology of cognitive functions does not allow for reliable correlations among cognitive systems and brain structures. However, it would not be far fetched to suspect that each distinct processing component of a corresponding functional system may have more than just one cortical representation and be asymmetrically distributed both inter- and intrahemispherically (Kass, 1989; Ojeman, 1990). These converging characteristics outline a rather complex neuropsychological architecture, far different from what the dichotomy model implicitly suggests.

We consider it to be a plausible hypothesis that the topographical architectures of language and musical functions are genetically prespecified. However, adverse environmental conditions may lead to substantial reorganization of the standard architecture and yet end up with normal function. The resulting picture that we suggest is akin to a componentially distributed architecture, where the different processing components may come into play at different maturational times. The hypothesis of additive architecture (Marshall, 1991) implies that some components (of any functional system) may already be present and active at birth or soon after, whereas other components become active subsequently.

Conclusions

Analysis of hemispheric computation in infants suggests that discrete and highly specific processing components may already be active and efficient at birth or soon after. Other components may come into play subsequently. The task of these modular units is to select and automatically process their target subcomponent, which usually comes interspersed with many diverse components that constitute a structurally complex system. Complex information is likely to be dealt with only through simultaneous activity of several computational units. The neurophysiological outcome of this integrated process may correspond to the simultaneous activation of distinct topographical areas.

Each processing component may have multiple, though asymmetrical representations in each hemisphere, and the processes it subserves may be shifted toward the intact hemisphere in pathological conditions.

Acknowledgments

This paper and research were supported by grants no. 9200085PF41 and no. 9300651PF41 from the National Research Council (CNR), Targeted Project FATMA "Prevention and Control of Disease Factors", Subproject no. 7, research area no. 3.

This paper is a revised version of one previously published in: *Music speech and the developing brain: The case of modularity of the mind*, C. Faienza, (Ed.), 1994, through the kind permission of Guerrini Associati, Milan, Italy, and the authors.

References

Albert, M. L., & Bear, D. (1974). Time to understand. A case study of word deafness with reference to the role of time in auditory comprehension. *Brain, 97,* 373–384.

Aram, D., & Whitaker, H. A. (1988). Cognitive sequelae of unilateral lesions acquired in early childhood. In D. L. Molfese & S. J. Segalowitz (Eds.), *Brain lateralization in children: Developmental implications* (pp. 417–436). New York: Plenum Press.

Basser, L. S. (1962). Hemiplegia of early onset and the faculty of speech with special reference to the effects of hemispherectomy. *Brain, 85,* 427–460.

Basso, A. (1989). Spontaneous recovery and language rehabilitation. In X. Seron & G. Deloche (Eds.), *Cognitive approaches to neuropsychological rehabilitation* (pp. 17–37). Hillsdale: L.E.A.

Baynes, K. (1990). Language and reading in the right hemisphere: Highways or byways of the brain? *Journal of Cognitive Neuroscience, 2,* 159–179.

Bertoncini, J., Bijeljac-Babic, R., McAdams, S., Peretz, I., & Mehler, J. (1989). Dichotic perception of laterality in neonates. *Brain and Language, 37,* 591–605.

Best, C., Hoffman, H., & Glanville, B. B. (1982). Development of infant ear asymmetries for speech and music. *Perception and Psychophysics, 31,* 75–85.

Bever, T., & Chiarello, R. (1974). Cerebral dominance in musicians and nonmusicians. *Science, 185,* 537–539.

Bishop, D. V. M. (1983). Linguistic impairment after left hemidecortication for infantile hemiplegia? A reappraisal. *Quarterly Journal of Experimental Psychology, 35a,* 199–207.

Bishop, D. V. M. (1988). Can the right hemisphere mediate language as well as the left? A critical review of recent research. *Cognitive Neuropsychology, 5,* 353–367.

Changeux, J. P. (1983). *L'uomo neuronale.* Milano: Feltrinelli.

Chomsky, N. A. (1975). *Reflections on language.* New York: Plenum.

Chomsky, N. A. (1981). *Lectures on government and binding.* Dordrecht: Foris Publications.

Chomsky, N. A. (1986). *Knowledge of language.* New York: Praeger.

Cossu, G., Da Prati, E, & Marshall, J. C. (in press). Deep dyslexia and the right hemisphere hypothesis: Spoken and written language after extensive left hemisphere lesion in a 12 year old boy. *Cognitive Neuropsychology.*

Cossu, G., & Marshall, J. C. (1990). Are cognitive skills a prerequisite for learning to read and write? *Cognitive Neuropsychology, 7,* 21–40.

Cossu, G., Urbinati, M. L., & Marshall, J. C. (1987) *Reading without speech and writing without arm movements.* Paper presented at the 5th European Workshop on Cognitive Neuropsychology, Bressanone.

Cowan, M. W. (1979). The development of the brain. *Scientific American, 241,* 112–133.

Davidson, L. (1994) Songsinging by young and old: A developmental approach to music. In R. Aiello (Ed.), *Musical perceptions* (pp. 99–130). Oxford: Oxford University Press.

Dennis, M., & Kohn, B. (1975) Comprehension of syntax in infantile hemiplegics after cerebral hemidecortication: Left hemisphere superiority. *Brain and Language, 2,* 472–482.

Dennis, M., & Whitaker, H. A. (1976) Language acquisition following hemidecortication: Linguistic superiority of the left over the right hemisphere. *Brain and Language, 3,* 404–433.

Duffy, F. H., Mc Anulty, G. B., & Schachter, S. C. (1984). Brain electrical activity mapping. In N. Geschwind & A. M. Galaburda (Eds.). *Cerebral dominance* (pp. 53–74). Cambridge, MA: Harvard University Press.

Eimas, P. D. (1974). Auditory and linguistic processing of cues for place of articulation by infants. *Perception and Psychophysics, 16,* 513–521.

Fodor, J. (1983). *The modularity of mind.* Cambridge, MA: MIT Press/Bradford Books.

Fourcin, A. J. (1975). Speech perception in the absence of productive ability. In N. O'Connor (Ed.), *Language, cognitive deficits and retardation* (pp. 33–43). London: Buttherworths.

Gall, F. J. (1798). Lettera aperta sul programma organologico. In F. J. Gall (Ed.), (1985). L'organo dell'anima (pp. 41–52). Venezia: Marsilio Editori.

Geschwind, N. (1972). Disorders of higher cortical function in children. *Clinical proceedings, Children's Hospital National Medical Center, 28,* 261–272.

Geschwind, N.,& Galaburda, A. M. (1987). *Cerebral lateralization.* Cambridge, MA: MIT Press.

Gopnik, M., & Crago, M. (1991). Familial aggregation of a developmental language disorder. *Cognition, 39,* 1–50.

Hamburger, V. (1975). Cell death in the development of the lateral motor column of the chick embryo. *Journal of Comparative Neurology, 160,* 535–546.

Hubel, D. H. (1988). *Eye, brain and vision.* New York: Scientific American Books.

Itard, J. (1801) Rapport sur les premiers développements de Victor de l'Aveyron. In G. Mariotti (Translator), *J. Itard, Il giovane selvatico* (pp. 21–83). Parma: F. M. Ricci.

Itard, J. (1807). Rapport sur les nouveaux développements de Victor de l'Aveyron. In G. Mariotti (Translator), *J. Itard, Il giovane selvatico* (pp. 85–146). Parma: F. M. Ricci.

Jackendoff, R. (1987). *Consciousness and the computational mind.* Cambridge, MA: MIT Press /Bradford Books.

Jenkins, W. M., Merzenich, M. M., Ochs, M. T., Allard, T.,& Guic-Robies, E. (1990). Functional reorganization of primary somatosensory cortex in adult owl monkeys after behaviourally controlled tactile stimulation. *Journal of Neurophysiology, 63,* 82–104.

Johnson, M. H., & Morton, J. (1991). *Biology and cognitive development.* Oxford: Blackwell.

Johnson, J. I., Hamilton, T. C., Hsung, J. C., & Ulinsky, P. S. (1972). Gracile nucleus absent in adult opossum after leg removal in infancy. *Brain Research, 38,* 421–424.

Kaas, J. H. (1989). Why does the brain have so many visual areas? *Journal of Cognitive Neuroscience, 1,* 121–135.

King, A. J., & Moore, D. R. (1991). Plasticity of auditory maps in the brain. *Trends in Neuroscience, 14,* 31–37.

Kinsbourne, M., & Hiscock, M. (1977). Does cerebral dominance develop? In S. J. Segalowitz & F. A. Gruber (Eds.), *Language development and neurological theory* (pp. 171–191). New York: Academic Press.

Lenneberg, E. H. (1967). *Biological foundations of language*. New York: Wiley & Sons.

Liberman, A. M., & Mattingly, I. G. (1985). The motor theory of speech perception revised. *Cognition, 21,* 1–36.

Liberman, A., Cooper, F., Shankweiler, D., & Studdert-Kennedy, M. (1967). Perception of the speech code. *Psychological Review, 74,* 431–461.

Ludovico, A. (1979). *La scimmia vestita*. Roma: Armando Armando.

Mann, V., & Liberman, A. M. (1983). Some differences between phonetic and auditory modes of perception. *Cognition, 14,* 211–235.

Marr, D., & Poggio, T. (1976, May). From understanding computation to understanding neural circuitry. *MIT A. I. Memo,* 357.

Marshall, J. C. (1983). Phrenology revived. *Nature, 306,* 137–138.

Marshall, J. C. (1987). Cerebral lateralization: A graded or a discrete characteristic? In A. Glass (Ed.), *Individual differences in hemispheric specialization* (pp. 51–53). New York: Plenum Press.

Marshall, J. C. (1989). The description and interpretation of acquired and developmental reading disorders. In A. M. Galaburda (Ed.), *From reading to neurons* (pp. 69–86). Cambridge, MA, MIT Press.

Martins, I. P., & Ferro, J. M. (1991). Recovery from aphasia and lesion size in the temporal lobe. In I. P. Martins, A. Castro-Caldas, H. R. van Dongen, & A. van Hut (Eds.), *Acquired aphasia in children* (pp. 171–184). Dordrecht: Kluver Academic Publishers.

McCarthy, R. A., & Warrington, E. K. (Eds.) (1990). *Cognitive neuropsychology* (pp. 152–170). San Diego, Academic Press.

Merzenich, M. M., Nelson, R. J., Kaas, J. H., Stryker, M. P., Jenkins, W. M., Zook, J. M., Cynader, S., & Schoppmann, A. (1987). Variability in hand surface representations in areas 3b and 1 in adult owl and squirrel monkeys. *Journal of Comparative Neurology, 258,* 281–296.

Miller, L. K. (1989). *Musical savants*. Hillsdale: L.E.A.

Molfese, D. L., & Betz, J. C. (1988). Electrophysiological indices of the early development of lateralization for language and cognition, and their implications for predicting later development. In D. L. Molfese, & S. J. Segalowitz (Eds.), *Brain lateralization in children. Developmental implications* (pp. 171–190). New York: Plenum Press.

O'Connor, N., & Hermelin, B. (1994). The idiot-savant: Talent, intelligence and cognition. In C. Faienza (Ed.), Music, speech and the developing brain (pp. 91–109). Milano: Guerrini Associati.

Ojemann, G. A. (1990). Organization of language cortex derived from investigations during neurosurgery. *Seminars in Neurosciences, 2,* 297–305.

Peretz, I. (1990). Processing of local and global musical information in unilateral brain-damaged patients. *Brain, 113,* 1185–1205.

Peretz, I., & Morais, J. (1993). Specificity for music. In Boller, F., & Grafman, J. (Eds.), *Handbook of neuropsychology, Vol.8* (pp. 373–390). Amsterdam: Elsevier.

Petsche, H., Richter, P., Etlinger, S. C., & Filz, O. (1994). EEG facilities for the study of brain processes elicited by music and language. In C. Faienza (Ed.), *Music, speech and the developing brain* (pp. 157–180). Milano: Guerrini Associati.

Piaget, J. (1967). *Biologie et connaissance*. Paris: Gallimard.

Prechtl, H. F. R. (1994). Principles of early motor behaviour. In C. Faienza (Ed.), *Music, speech and the developing brain* (pp. 19–26). Milano: Guerrini Associati.

Rapin, I., & Allen, D. (1983). Developmental language disorders: Nosologic considerations. In V. Kirk (Ed.), *Neuropsychology of language, reading and spelling* (pp. 155–184). New York: Academic Press.

Schneiderman, E. I. (1986). Learning to the right: Some thoughts on hemisphere involvement in language acquisition. In J. Vaid (Ed.), *Language processing in bilinguals: Psycholinguistic and neuropsychological perspectives* (pp. 233–251). Hillsdale: L.E.A.

Segalowitz, S. J. (1987). Individual differences in hemispheric specialization: Sources and measurement. In A. Glass (Ed.), *Individual differences in hemispheric specialization* (pp. 17–30). New York: Plenum Press.

Sloboda, J. (1985). *The musical mind: The cognitive psychology of music.* London: Oxford University Press.

Spreen, O., Benton, A., & Fincham, R. (1965). Auditory agnosia without aphasia. *Archiv. Neurol., 13,* 84–92.

Tanaka, Y., Yamadori, A., & Mori, E. (1987). Pure word deafness following bilateral lesions. A psychophysical analysis. *Brain, 110,* 381–403.

Waddington, C. H. (1966). *Principles of development and differentiation.* New York: Macmillan.

Witelson, S. (1985). On hemisphere specialization and cerebral plasticity from birth: Mark II. In C. T. Best (Ed.), *Hemispheric function and collaboration in the child* (pp. 33–85). London, Academic Press.

Zaidel, E. (1985). Language in the right hemisphere. In D. F. Benson & E. Zaidel (Eds.), T*he dual brain: Hemispheric specialization in humans* (pp. 205–232). New York: The Guilford Press.

Zeki, S. (1993). *A vision of the brain.* Oxford: Blackwell.

THE EFFECTS OF COHERENCE ESTIMATES OF EEG AT REST ON DIFFERENCES BETWEEN SUBJECTS WITH AND WITHOUT MUSIC TRAINING

Julene K. Johnson, Hellmuth Petsche, Peter Richter,
Astrid von Stein, and Oliver Filz

Abstract

The present study examined differences in spontaneous EEG in terms of music training. Coherence estimates obtained by spectral analysis provided an efficacious method to study these differences. Differences in the spontaneous EEG between subjects with and without music training were observed. Subjects with music training exhibited significantly higher coherence values both intra- and interhemispherically when compared to subjects without music training. The most striking differences were observed in the two lowest (delta and theta) and two highest (beta 1 and beta 2) bands, with differences in the temporo-parietal regions of both hemispheres being most prominent. The findings are discussed in terms of specialized organization of brain activity that influences cortical connectivity.

Introduction

Prior to the 1970s, the electroencephalogram (EEG) was generally regarded as representing electrical noise of metabolic brain processes. Evoked potentials research provided convincing evidence that information is contained in the EEG signal. However, this method only allows for the application of restricted questions concerning brain functioning. Questions include how the brain may react to specific sensory stimulation such as repeated auditory tones or clicks or other sensory events. Such reactions represent the interactions of the neural system with its environment. However, whether or not intrinsic information is contained in the EEG is a question that remains unanswered.

To address this question, the nature of the spontaneous electrical activity of the brain must be investigated. The spontaneous EEG signal (i.e., EEG at rest) represents the steadily ongoing activity of the brain. It is, therefore, present at times when no tasks are being performed. Traditional EEG studies in cognition are designed so that periods of EEG during tasks (e.g., listening to music or doing mental arithmetic) can be compared with periods while at rest. However, the spontaneous EEG exhibits large inter-individual variability with respect to topography, amplitude, and frequency. The aim of the current study is to address the possible differences in the spontaneous EEG among subjects with regard to the degree of their music training.

Differences in the spontaneous EEG of subjects with and without music training have not yet been investigated. We were interested in determining whether or not our method of studying coherence could also provide information about this issue. Concerning the question of how music training may influence EEG patterns during music listening, Petsche, Lindner, Rappelsberger, and Gruber (1988a) found differences in the EEG between musically trained and untrained subjects while listening to music. In addition, some coherence differences in the spontaneous EEG were also found. This previous study, however, was restricted to the analysis of the relationships between adjacent electrodes only. Therefore this question was reinvestigated with improved methods for coherence analysis and with a larger subject pool.

Spectral analysis is one efficacious method for the analysis of spontaneous EEG. Its aim is to transform potential time diagrams into potential frequency diagrams. In the past, EEG and evoked responses were only evaluated in the time domain. The transformation from the time into the frequency domain can be achieved through Fourier analysis. The fast Fourier transformation (FFT), one of several types of Fourier transformations, is the most common method used to analyze EEG data (Regan, 1989; Zappulla, 1991). This method offers the advantage that long epochs of EEG can be investigated and represented as spectra. Spectral analysis provides information about power, or amplitude, at a certain frequency. If applied to two different signals, information about cross-correlation and phase can be obtained. Coherence, the normalized cross-correlation, provides information about the cooperation between various brain areas.

Coherence is frequency-dependent. It represents the degree of similarity between EEG signals and ranges between 0 and 1, indicating no synchrony to maximum synchrony respectively. Applied to the EEG, coherence provides information about the electrical relatedness of brain areas. It has been shown that electrical relatedness in some way reflects the functional relationships among brain areas (Petsche, Pockberger, & Rappelsberger, 1986; Sheppard, 1990).

The application of coherence in studying mental processes has been helpful in investigating the cooperation of different brain regions. Rappelsberger and Petsche (1988) previously developed a method to systematically study such processes. The principle of this method consists of comparing long EEG epochs during mental tasks with at least equally long epochs of EEG at rest. These results showed changes in the EEG due to various mental tasks, such as listening to speech and music, reading, doing mental arithmetic, visual imaging, or others (Janata & Petsche, 1992; Petsche, Lacroix, Lindner, Rappelsberger, & Schmidt-Heinrich, 1992a; Petsche & Rappelsberger, 1992; Petsche, Etlinger, & Filz, 1993a; Petsche, Richter, von Stein, & Etlinger, 1993b). This method not only allows for the comparison of EEG during a task and at rest, but also for the comparison of groups with different characteristics, such as the amount of training in a certain field.

Method

Subjects

The study consisted of 49 right-handed, male subjects. Twenty-four subjects were musically trained (mean age 26.7 years, SD = 9.5), and 25 of them had no music training (mean age 21.2 years, SD = 8.0). Music training was operationally defined as having at least 5 years of music training (i.e., 5 years of private voice or instrument lessons) beginning before puberty. All subjects were clinically healthy, had not sustained any head injuries, and were not presently taking medication. All subjects had at least 12 years of formal education. The subjects were volunteers and were paid for their participation.

Experimental Design

Subjects were selected from several EEG studies in which various cognitive tasks (e.g., verbal, musical, and visual) were investigated. In all of these experiments, the task conditions were alternated with periods of rest at least 1 minute in duration. These at rest EEG periods were later merged, yielding an average of at least 5 minutes of EEG data per subject. The subject data were assigned to two groups: subjects with music training and subjects without music training.

The subjects sat with eyes closed in a reclined armchair in a dimly lit, sound attenuated room with 19 gold electrodes attached with electrode conducting gel onto the head (international 10/20 system). The EEG were recorded from the 19 electrodes with reference to averaged recordings from both ear lobes and were monitored by an ink-writer system (Nihon Kohden electroencephalograph) and stored on hard disk (using a "Papierloses EEG" package from Walter Graphtek GmbH). The EEG were filtered with a bandpass filter between 0.3–35 Hz and digitized on-line with a sampling rate of 128/second. Technical details are found in Rappelsberger and Petsche (1988). The EEG were segmented into 1-second segments, and artifacts (including eye and muscle movements or electrode popping) were later excluded by off-line visual inspection and eliminated from analysis. Electrode sites on the figures correspond to the international 10–20 system.

Spectral analysis (fast Fourier transformation) was performed using artifact-free epochs of 2 seconds each. Averaged power and cross-power spectra were computed. Coherence was estimated between all pairs of electrodes (i.e., 171 values per frequency band) both intra- and interhemispherically. To further reduce the number of data, the spectrum of the EEG between 1.5–31.5 Hz was divided into six frequency bands: delta (1.5–3.5 Hz), theta (4.0–6.5 Hz), alpha 1 (7.0–9.0 Hz), alpha 2 (9.5–12.5 Hz), beta 1 (13.0–18.0 Hz), and beta 2 (18.5–31.5 Hz). See Figure 1 for a summary of this process.

The next step consisted of statistical comparisons between the two groups. The Wilcoxon rank-sum test was utilized to evaluate possible group differences in the param-

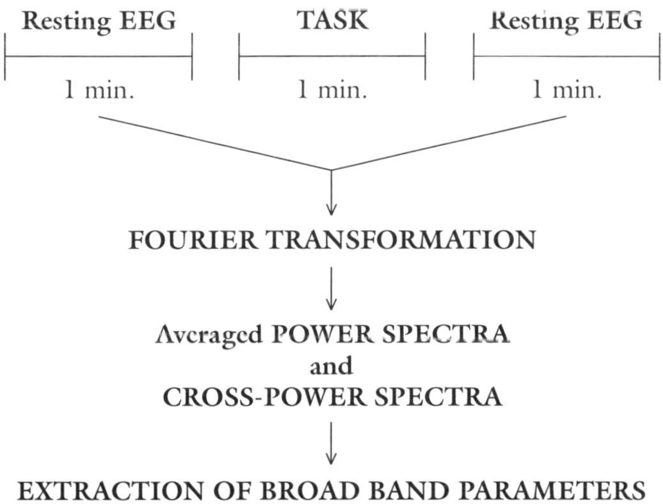

Figure 1. Flowchart depicting the extraction of EEG parameters. (Adapted from Pockberger, Rappelsberger, & Petsche, 1988.)

eters *amplitude* and *coherence.* In this study, the statistical approach is only descriptive; statistical application is not used to confirm or reject a null hypothesis, but rather to yield tendencies about various comparisons for which possible differences exist.

Significant coherence differences between the spontaneous EEG of the two respective groups are presented topographically by schematic drawings of the brain with electrode positions as seen from both sides and from the top for both intra- and interhemispheric coherence differences respectively. Note that electrodes O1 and O2 actually refer to posterior parietal and not to occipital brain areas. Significant increases of coherence are depicted by solid lines and decreases by broken lines connecting the respective electrode sites. The width of the lines corresponds to $p <= 0.01$, 0.02, and 0.05, with the highest level of significance represented by the thickest line. Thus, the significant differences between the two groups of subjects are plotted as topographic probability maps.

Results

In terms of *amplitude,* the Wilcoxon rank-sum test showed that the subjects with music training had significantly lower amplitudes ($p <= 0.01$) across all frequency bands and all electrodes when compared to subjects without music training. These results are not represented as a figure.

In terms of *intrahemispheric coherence,* the Wilcoxon rank-sum test yielded numerous significant differences between the groups. Column A of Figure 2 represents the significant differences ($p <= 0.01, 0.02, 0.05$) between groups seen in the left hemisphere. Column C of Figure 2 represents the right hemisphere differences between groups ($p <= 0.01, 0.02, 0.05$). Overall, the subjects with music training had significantly higher coherence values than subjects without music training.

The most striking differences were found in the two lowest (delta and theta) and the two highest (beta) frequency bands, with theta being the most prominent. Both hemispheres were almost equally involved, however, with a predominance of left hemisphere differences in the alpha 1 and alpha 2 frequency ranges. Generally, the posterior regions of both hemispheres were more involved than the anterior parts. Significantly lower coherence values in musically trained subjects were found only between a few electrode sites and were limited to one frequency band (alpha 1).

Many *interhemispheric coherence* values among multiple electrodes were also significantly higher (Wilcoxon rank-sum test, $p <= 0.01, 0.02, 0.05$) in subjects with music training (row A of Figure 3). Again, these differences primarily concerned the two lowest and two highest frequency bands in the temporal and parietal regions. However, subjects trained in music also exhibited a few lower coherence values between the temporal and frontal-basal electrodes in beta 1 and between the right posterior temporal region (T6) and the left frontal regions in alpha 1.

Because of the fact that numerous coherence differences were found, we applied two additional strategies to elucidate the most prominent findings. The first strategy consisted of increasing the level of significance to the $p <= 0.001$ level so that only the most significant differences could be seen. The second approach addressed the consistency of changes across frequency bands. In addition, information about the nodal points of connectivity is provided.

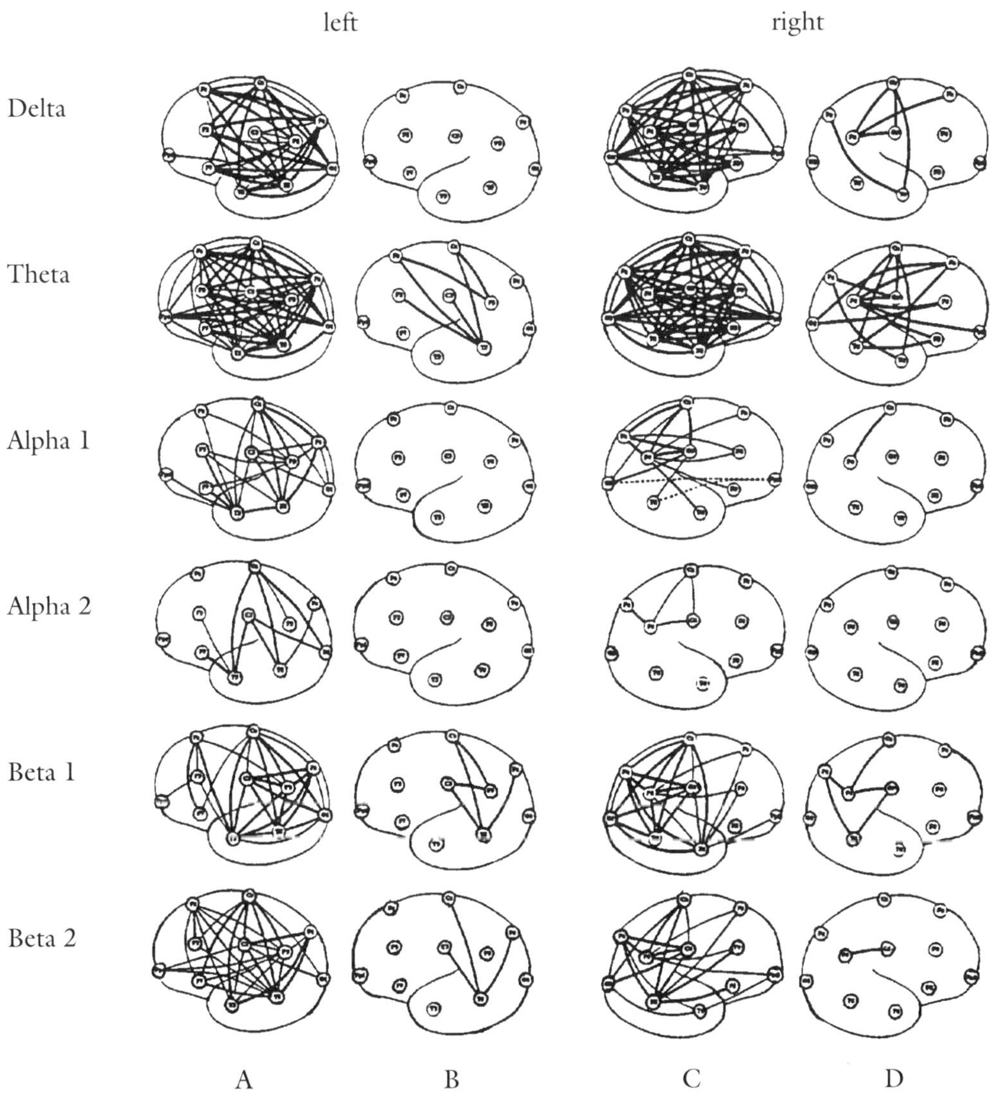

Figure 2. Group comparison of the differences of coherence in the spontaneous EEG between subjects with and without music training. Wilcoxon Rank-sum test. From the top to bottom, the six frequency bands for left and right hemispheres are represented. Significantly higher coherences in trained subjects are marked by full lines, lower coherences by dashed lines. Columns A and C represent $p = < 0.05, 0.02, \& 0.01$ indicated by different thickness of lines, with the highest level of significance represented by the thickest line. Columns B and D represent $p = < 0.001$.

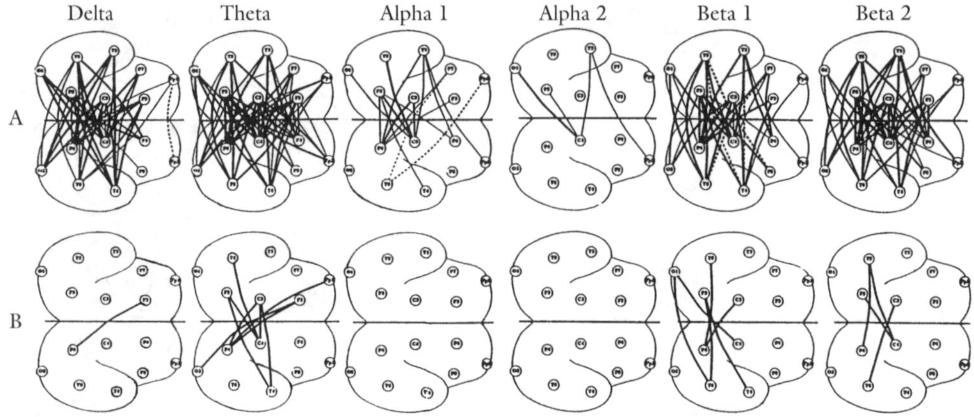

Figure 3. Group comparison representing interhemispheric differences in coherence. Frequency bands are illustrated from left to right. Row A represents $p <= 0.05, 0.02, 0.01$. Row B represents $p =< 0.001$.

Level of Significance

In terms of *intrahemispheric coherence,* subjects with music training have significantly higher coherence values (Wilcoxon rank-sum test, $p <= 0.001$) in both hemispheres than subjects without training. This is shown in Figure 2 (columns B and D) and in Figure 3 (row B). The lower frequency ranges are clearly more involved in the right than in the left hemisphere. In contrast to the lower frequency bands, the beta bands did not show as many intrahemispheric differences. Generally, most coherence differences concentrated around P4 and T6 in the right hemisphere and T5 in the left.

Significant differences in *interhemispheric coherence* values (Wilcoxon rank-sum test, $p <= 0.001$) primarily concern the posterior temporal and parietal regions as seen in row B of Figure 3. In theta, the coherence values among the right temporal and parietal regions and the left frontal regions were higher in subjects with music training than in subjects without training.

Consistency Across Frequency Bands

The second analytic strategy addressed the consistency of changes across frequency bands. The traditional way of describing EEG data consists of dividing the frequency spectrum into various bands primarily for convenience. There is, however, minimal knowledge about the functional significance of these divisions, with the exception of alpha rhythm (Klimesch, Schimke, Ladurner, & Pfurtscheller, 1990). If any differences in coherence are seen across multiple frequency bands, they may be thought to be of more significance than if found in only a few bands. This idea motivated us to look for the abundance of significant differences across frequency bands. This is shown in Figure 3 where those connections occurring in at least five of the six frequency bands are illustrated.

As can be seen in Figure 4, most of the consistent *intrahemispheric coherence* differences concerned the parietal and temporal regions of both hemispheres with an involvement of the midline electrodes. Numerous differences between subjects with and without music training, therefore, exist across the range of the EEG signal. Another feature worth noting is the lack of consistent frontal differences across all frequency bands.

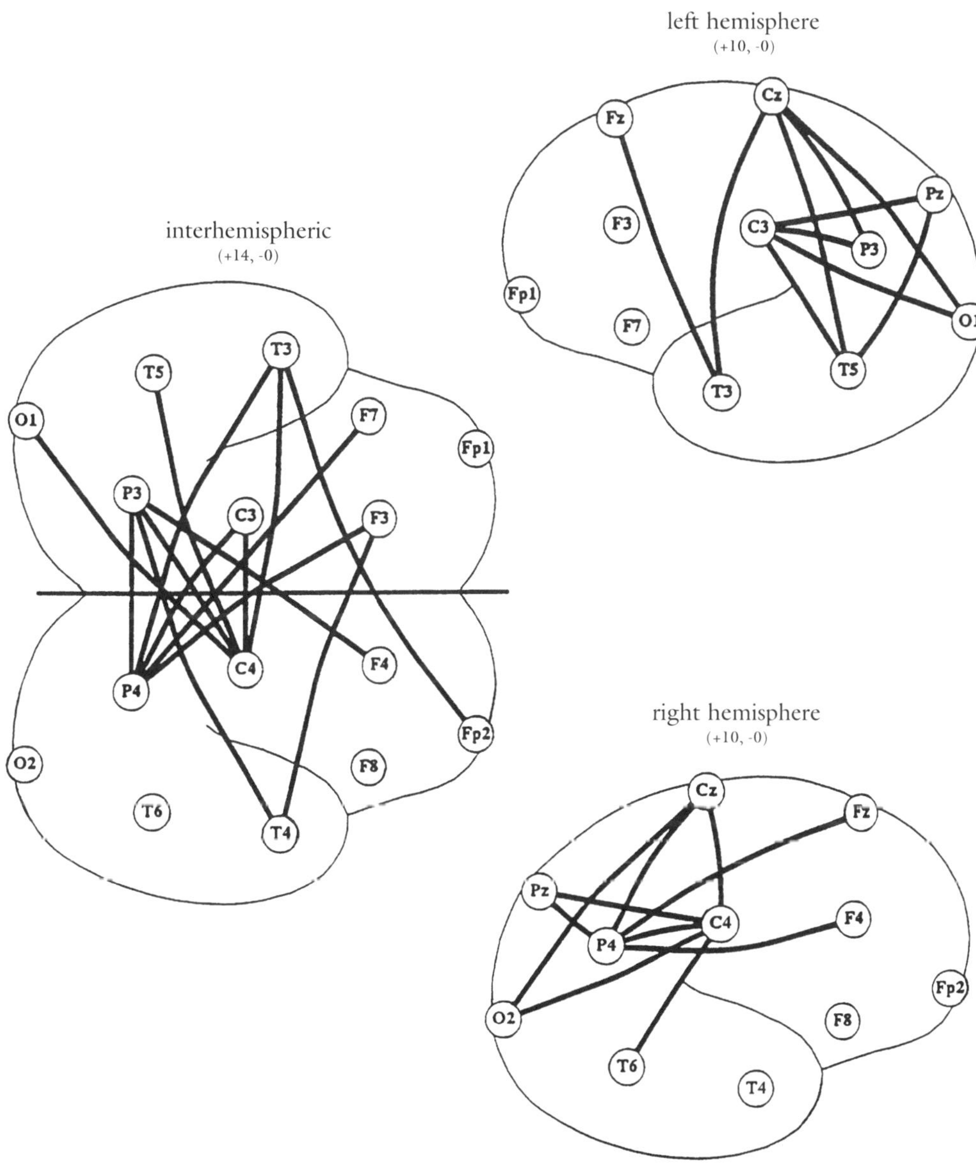

Figure 4. Group comparison with consistent connections across at least five of the six frequency bands ($p = < 0.05$).

Also as seen in Figure 3, the *interhemispheric coherence* pattern demonstrated that the degree of functional coupling between the two hemispheres was much greater for the subjects with music training. More coupling was found between the parietal than between the temporal areas.

Nodal Points of Connectivity

Additional information about laterality is addressed when taking into account the number of connections arising from each electrode site. Previous research concerning the effects of tasks on the EEG supported the idea that the number of coherence changes arising at one electrode site provides information about the functional significance of the respective region. Petsche, Etlinger, and Filz (1993a) refer to these as "nodal points of connectivity".

Applied to the present study, one may speculate that the large number of significantly higher coherence values at certain electrodes in the group of musically trained subjects indicates that these subjects may be equipped with a higher level of connectivity. Therefore, we calculated the number of coherence differences at each electrode and mapped them topographically as seen in Figure 4. The number of significantly higher coherence values are represented in a probability map with squares of different sizes depicted at the respective electrode sites of a head schema as seen from the top. The black squares indicate significant increases of power with the size of the squares corresponding to $p <= 0.01, 0.02$, and 0.05, respectively. This figure further shows that the maximum coherence differences between the two groups were seen at the right central and parietal regions. This is additional support for the prominence of the right hemisphere in the processing of music.

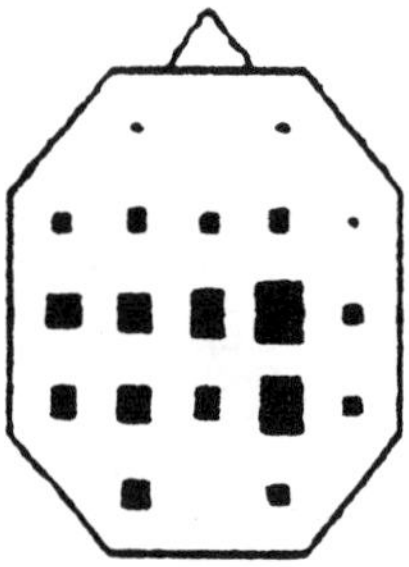

Figure 5. Topographical plotting of the number of coherence differences found at each electrode site.

Discussion

Before interpreting the data reported above, the two parameters amplitude and coherence must be discussed in terms of brain functioning. Concerning *amplitude,* the functional significance of the different frequency ranges is not yet known, particularly not while the brain is at rest. In addition, our knowledge about the significance of individual frequency bands during task conditions is sparse, with the exception of the alpha rhythm. However, even within this field, there is no general agreement.

In the present study, significant differences in *amplitude* between subjects with and without music training were found. In all frequency bands and across all recording sites, subjects with music training exhibited significantly lower amplitude values than the subjects with no training. These results suggest a reliable association with music training. Because EEG artifacts were excluded and minimal differences in age exist between the two groups, these confounds can be excluded. Therefore, it is possible that music training over several years influences the cortical organization. Further research with subjects having different types of specialized cognitive training should address the possible reasons for this most likely training-dependent lower amplitude values.

Differences in *coherence,* however, provide much information about the differences between these two groups. As was discussed earlier, differences in coherence values can provide information about the functional connectivity within brains of individuals with various levels of training. Because coherence has been shown in previous studies to be an appropriate tool for studying the cooperation of signals, one must ask how coherence analysis could be used for studying the differences in the spontaneous EEG. The applicability of this type of analysis is fostered by the fact that neuronal messages are mainly transported in the form of cooperative processes. That is, messages do not travel through the brain mediated by discharges of single neurons but as statistically distributed clouds of neuronal activity (Singer, 1990). Synchronization probably depends on cortico-cortical association and/or subcortical connections adaptive for learning. This idea has been supported by human and animal experimental data (Abeles, 1991; Sheppard, 1990; Villa, 1992).

In the present study, it was shown that there exist considerable differences in the coherence pattern between subjects with and without music training. This pattern reveals a network of connections between electrode sites in which coherence values are higher in subjects with music training than in subjects without music training. A point worth emphasizing is the fact that in both lower and higher frequency bands, there is more intra- and interhemispheric coupling in subjects with music training. This increased degree of coupling of cooperative processes in terms of brain activity suggests that, even at rest, more efficient data transfer may exist between these areas in subjects with music training. This facilitation could be associated with the utilization of these connections over and over during music training.

It is not difficult to imagine that the study of music could exert influences on the nervous system of an individual when considering the complex nature of music abilities. Much evidence supports that basic music skills in children are acquired without music-specific training (Shuter-Dyson & Gabriel, 1981). Music training adds specific skills through instruction or study. These skills include, among others, the development of an understanding of pitch structures, acoustical structures in time, rhythmic patterns, reading of nonverbal symbols, motor control, etc. However, we have minimal knowledge about the specific combination of skills required to be successful in music. Recent research by Gardner and Wolf (1983), Hassler (1990), and Rauscher, Shaw, and Ky (1993) shows that, in addition to training specifically music skills, general cognitive skills can also be influenced.

Next, the coherence pattern is considered in more detail to determine whether or not its topography may also provide information about the regions of the brain that are influenced by music training. For this purpose, the discussion will begin with the data representing the most significant group differences (see Figure 2). Significant differences in the low and high frequency bands are found. The involvement of these frequency ranges, however, occurs in different ways. In the lower frequency range where more differences in the right hemisphere (particularly in the temporal and parietal areas) are seen, there is a tendency for a coupling of the right posterior with the left frontal areas in subjects with music training. In the upper frequency bands the findings are more symmetrical, and the increased coupling in the trained subjects involves only the posterior parts of the two hemispheres without any considerable connection to frontal regions. As for the alpha bands, there are fewer differences as may be expected because no task was required from the subjects.

In the context of spontaneous EEG, coherence differences between two groups, therefore, could be possibly be interpreted as reflections of trained patterns used to interact with specific demands from the environment. For the processing of music, a special presupposition seems to be required. These changes, however, cannot yet be considered as music-specific and may relate to a more general strategy of cognitive functioning as was discussed above. It is striking that, in addition to task dependent changes in the EEG as were previously reported, differences in the resting EEG may be influenced by training. In this context, it is difficult to determine how much of the results are due to music training or innate abilities in those who choose to study music. These findings are preliminary, and further research must be conducted.

Summary

In summary, the present study provides evidence for differences in spontaneous EEG between subjects with and without music training. Coherence estimates obtained by spectral analysis provided a method to study these differences. Subjects with music training exhibit significantly higher coherence values both intra- and interhemispherically when compared to subjects without music training. These coherence patterns may reflect a specialized organization of brain activity in subjects with music training. In addition, music training may influence the cortical connectivity that is observable even in the spontaneous EEG. These findings, therefore, demonstrate distinctive coherence patterns that differentiate subjects with and without music training.

Acknowledgment

This work was supported by the Austrian Academy of Sciences and the Herbert von Karajan Stiftung der Gesellschaft der Musikfreunde in Wien. We would also express our appreciation of Betinna Bolzer and Anni Schneider for their contributions and Dr. Don Hodges for comments on an earlier version.

References

Abeles, M. (1991). *Corticonics: Neural circuits of the cerebral cortex.* Cambridge: University Press.

Freeman, W. J., & Skarda, C. A. (1985). Spatial EEG patterns: Non-linear dynamics and perception: The neo-Sherrington view. *Brain Research Review, 10,* 147–175.

Gardner, H., & Wolf, D. (1983). The waves and streams of symbolization. In D. Rogers & J. A. Sloboda (Eds.), *Acquisition of symbolic skills* (pp. 19–42). New York: Plenum Press.

Hassler, M. (1990). Functional cerebral asymmetries and cognitive abilities in musicians, painters, and controls. *Brain and Cognition, 13,* 1–17.

Janata, P., & Petsche, H. (1993). Spectral analysis of the EEG as a tool for evaluating expectancy violations of musical contexts. *Music Perception, 10,* 281–304.

Klimesch, W., Schimke, H., Ladurner, G., & Pfurtscheller, G. (1990). Alpha frequency and memory performance, *Journal of Psychophysiology, 4,* 381–390.

Petsche, H., Etlinger, S. C., & Filz, O. (1993a). Brain electrical mechanisms of bilingual speech administration: An initial investigation. *Electroencephalography and Clinical Neurophysiology, 86,* 385–394.

Petsche, H., Lacroix, D., Lindner, K., Rappelsberger, P., & Schmidt-Heinrich, E. (1992). Thinking with images or thinking with language: A pilot EEG probability study. *International Journal of Psychophysiology, 12,* 31–39.

Petsche, Lindner, K., Rappelsberger, P., & Gruber, G. (1988a). The EEG: An adequate method to concretize brain processes elicited by music. *Music Perception, 6,* 133–159.

Petsche, H., Pockberger, H., & Rappelsberger, P. (1986). EEG topography and mental performance. In F. H. Duffy (Ed.), *Topographic mapping of brain electrical activity* (pp. 63–98). Boston: Butterworth.

Petsche, H., & Rappelsberger, P. (1992). Is there any message hidden in the EEG? In E. Basar and T. Bullock (Eds.), *Induced rhythms of the brain* (pp. 65–87). Boston: Birkhaeuser.

Petsche, H., Richter, P., von Stein, A., Etlinger, S. C., & Filz, O. (1993b). EEG coherence and musical thinking. *Music Perception, 11,* 117–152.

Pockberger, H., Rappelsberger, P., & Petsche, H. (1988). Cognitive processing in the EEG. In E. Basar (Ed.), *Dynamics of sensory and cognitive processing by the brain* (pp. 266–274). Berlin: Springer-Verlag.

Rappelsberger, P., & Petsche, H. (1988). Probability mapping: Power and coherence analysis of cognitive processes. *Brain Topography, 1,* 46–54.

Rauscher, F. H., Shaw, G. L., & Ky, K. N. (1993). Music and spatial task performance. *Nature, 365,* 611.

Regan, D. (1989). *Human brain electrophysiology.* New York: Elsevier.

Sheppard, W. D. (1990). Parietal EEG coherence as a predictor of semantic priming effects. *Brain and Language, 39,* 57–68.

Shuter-Dyson, R., & Gabriel, C. (1981). *The psychology of musical ability* (2nd ed.). London: Metheun.

Singer, W. (1990). Search for coherence: A basic principle of cortical self-organization. *Concepts in Neuroscience, 1,* 1–26.

Villa, A. E. P. (1992). Temporal aspects of information processing in the central nervous system. *Swiss Federal Institute of Technology LAMI-EPFL, Annales du groupe CARNAC, 5,* 1–28.

Zappulla, R. A. (1991). Fundamentals and applications of quantified electrophysiology. In R. A. Zappulla, F. F. LeFever, J. Jaeger, & R. Bilder (Eds.), *Windows on the brain: Neuropsychology's technological frontiers* (pp. 1–21). New York: New York Academy of Sciences.

EVENT RELATED BRAIN WAVE POTENTIALS IN AN AUDITORY-MOTOR SYNCHRONIZATION TASK

Robert A. Miller, Michael H. Thaut and Jorge I. Auñón

ABSTRACT

This study sought to investigate event-related brain potentials (ERPs) as indicators of the neural correlates of the process of translating rhythmic acoustic stimulus pat terns into synchronized rhythmic movement responses. Motor timing and brain-wave patterns were studied in healthy young musicians while performing self-paced and metronome cued finger-tapping tasks at 2-second intervals. The brain-wave character found while performing rhythmic tasks, negative pre-motor activity and positive late potentials, was not observed in the nonrhythmic tasks. A larger amplitude in the early phase of the late ERP is associated with cued versus self-paced tasks, indicating that this activity is associated with auditory-motor synchronization. Comparison of the cued and self-paced rhythmic tasks shows no difference in the motor-response interval variance. Since the motor performance is not improved with cueing, monitoring of SE does not appear to be a factor in motor-timing adjustments. Significant improvement in motor-timing stability was observed when texture was placed in the metronome sequence by addition of an evenly spaced second tone. The brain-wave character, however, remained unchanged. This indicates that mechanisms other than feedback of synchronization errors are responsible for coordinating rhythmic-motor function to rhythmic-external stimuli and a more continuous textured stimuli enhances the stability in matching the external rhythm.

INTRODUCTION

Little is known about how the nervous system produces temporal sequences that result in coordinated motor function. Scientific investigation in this area normally requires a stimulus that can be controlled. Auditory cueing of motor-function is a good choice since these sensorimotor transformation processes are important, particularly in music and dance performance, as well as in auditory cueing of motor responses found in music therapy applications. It has been shown that rhythmic auditory stimulation has a strong facilitating effect on gait parameters in normal subjects and in stroke patients (Thaut, McIntosh, Prassas, & Rice, 1992 & 1993). The mechanisms behind this facilitation are still largely unknown, and research into the interaction between motor activity and auditory cueing will not only provide credibility to the field of music therapy, but may lead to better application of music therapy techniques. Two areas of research that have dealt with auditory-motor interaction are the development of motor-timing models and auditory-motor brain-wave research. This investigation is an effort to combine these areas of study.

Motor timing has been studied in rhythmic synchronization with auditory cueing through mathematical analysis of the series of synchronization errors (SEs) and inter-response intervals (IRIs). Wing and Kristofferson (1973a,1973b) propose a motor-timing model consisting of a central clock generator and peripheral motor delay. Most of the variability in the SEs and IRIs is due to random variability in the peripheral motor delay. Hary and Moore (1987) have investigated the stability of motor-timing models based on reset of the central clock generator and feedback of SE to adjust the interval duration. They have developed a model (Hary & Moore, 1985) that mathematically mimics real data by using a random reset on the metronome or tapping event along with a very poor SE estimation and a very small feedback of the SE information. These models are limited in that only SEs are used to maintain rhythmic motor function. There is evidence that a more complex system exists. In continuation tasks where the auditory stimulus is terminated, subjects are able to maintain the rhythm with a high degree of accuracy (Collyer, Broadbent & Church, 1992). At high tapping rates, 180 ms intervals or less, subjects generate a stable IRI that nearly match the metronome rate, even though the drift causes large synchronization errors (Peters, 1989). With small step changes in interstimulus interval (ISI), subjects respond to the change by quickly shifting their IRI to the new ISI, without correcting the SE that has been altered due to the slight delay in matching the new ISI (Thaut & Miller, 1994). In each of these examples, synchronization errors appear to play little or no part in the matching of response to stimulus intervals.

Movement related brain potentials were originally reported by Kornhuber and Deecke (1965). Since that time, several papers have been published, most dealing with the negative potentials over the premotor, motor, and somatosensory cortices preceding voluntary movement. Up to three negative-shifts in scalp recorded potentials preceding motor activity have been linked to readiness and preparation of motion (Barrett, Shibasake, & Neshige, 1986). Additional negative waves have been identified in warned reaction time experiments (Walter, Cooper, Aldridge, McCallum & Winter, 1964). This so-called "contingent negative variation" (CNV) occurs between the warning and response stimuli. Also of interest are slow positive potentials, that is, P300 and Slow Waves, which occur after the stimulus and reflect some cognitive process (Ruchkin, Sutton, & Stega, 1980). The presence of these waveforms may reflect some motor-timing adjustments made as part of synchronization with auditory cueing.

In the current study, motor timing and ERPs were investigated in rhythmic motor tasks that are paced internally (self) and externally with metronome sequences of 1-to-1 and 2-to-1 stimulus to motor-response ratios. To date, there has been little ERP research involved with rhythmic tapping, since most brain-wave responses are reduced by adaptation to rhythmic stimuli (Squires, Wickens, Squires, & Donchin, 1976). However, analysis of the late positive potentials in rhythmic tasks may provide insight into the mechanisms of auditory-motor synchronization. The 2-to-1 metronome sequence allows for the investigation of the effects of additional auditory information on motor timing stability and brain wave activity, in particular, whether the additional cueing behaves as a CNV warning stimulus or is integrated as texture in the rhythmic auditory stimuli.

METHOD

Five adult male subjects, musicians, aged 22–25, with no known neurological disorders, volunteered to participate in the study. EEG and EMG signals were recorded while performing a motor task, using the preferred hand to depress a key on a muted electronic keyboard. The arm was supported above the keyboard in a position that minimized extraneous EMG activity. Subjects were seated in a soundproof isolation booth. The task was performed rhythmically, both self-paced and in synchronization with an auditory stimulus. Additional control conditions were monitored that involved a stimulus-response and a "listen-only" task sequence. The following task sequences, each 2 minutes long, were performed in the order listed. Task 1 had the subjects listen to the tone delivered at 2008 ms intervals. Task 2 had the subjects perform the motor task without auditory cueing (self-paced) at an IRI interval of approximately 2 seconds. Task 3 had the subjects perform the motor task in synchronization with the 2008 ms interval tone. In task 4, the subjects performed the motor task in synchronization with every other tone delivered at 1004 ms intervals. In task 5, the subjects performed the motor task in response to a tone given at random intervals ranging from 1 to 3 seconds.

The electronic keyboard output (Roland D-5 Multi Timbral Linear Synthesizer) was digitized and recorded to obtain motor-response timing information. Motor activity was monitored by bipolar silver/silver chloride surface EMG electrodes attached to the extensor and flexor digitorum of the tapping arm. The electrode unit contained an on-site preamplifier (gain = 35) with further amplification (2000) and high-pass filtering (at 40 Hz) provided by an EMG amplifier (Therapeutics Unlimited model 544). The EEG signals were measured at the P3, P4, C3, C4, F3, F4, T3, T4 locations of the 10/20 configuration with the reference voltage at the left earlobe. Electrode placement was achieved by use of an ECI Electro-Cap. Ocular activity was monitored by recording the EOG to check for eye-blink contaminated data. The EEG signals were amplified using a Grass Model-12 Neurodata acquisition system with a bandwidth of 0.1 to 100 Hz and a gain of 50,000 v/v. The stimulus tone bursts, 40 ms duration with 5 cycle rise and fall times, were delivered to the subjects through earphones at a level of 50 dB above threshold using a Grass Audio Click-Tone Module, model S10CTCMB.

Software was written (in C language) to perform the experiments and collect and analyze data on an IBM compatible personal computer. Data acquisition was achieved using Scientific Solutions Labmaster A-D hardware and LabPac software subroutines. The EEG signal was sampled at a rate of 250 per second and recorded digitally on a personal computer. The average evoked potentials were computed by ensemble averaging over the 60 events occurring in each task sequence. The events were aligned using the tone stimulus except for the second task sequence where the keyboard signal was used. The EMG signal was sampled at 500 Hz and full-wave rectified with an RMS processor. The onset and termination of EMG activity was measured in relation to the cueing stimulus. A computer algorithm was developed to detect EMG onset and termination times that were later checked by visual inspection of the graphical record.

RESULTS

Motor and Response Timing

The timing of EMG and keyboard response to rhythmic auditory stimuli, performed in task sequences 3 and 4, is illustrated in Figures 1 and 2 respectively. The basic pattern, as expected, was for the keyboard response to occur between the onset and termination of EMG activity. The keyboard response was close to, but preceded slightly, the auditory cueing. There was large intersubject variability in the EMG onset time (task 3: -150 to -697 ms, task 4: -110 to -636 ms), with less intersubject variability in keyboard response times (task 3: -15 to -158 ms, task 4: 5 to -59 ms). The synchronization errors between keyboard response and cueing tone are listed in Table 1 for each of the subjects, with a negative value indicating a response preceding cueing. With the added auditory information in task 4, the

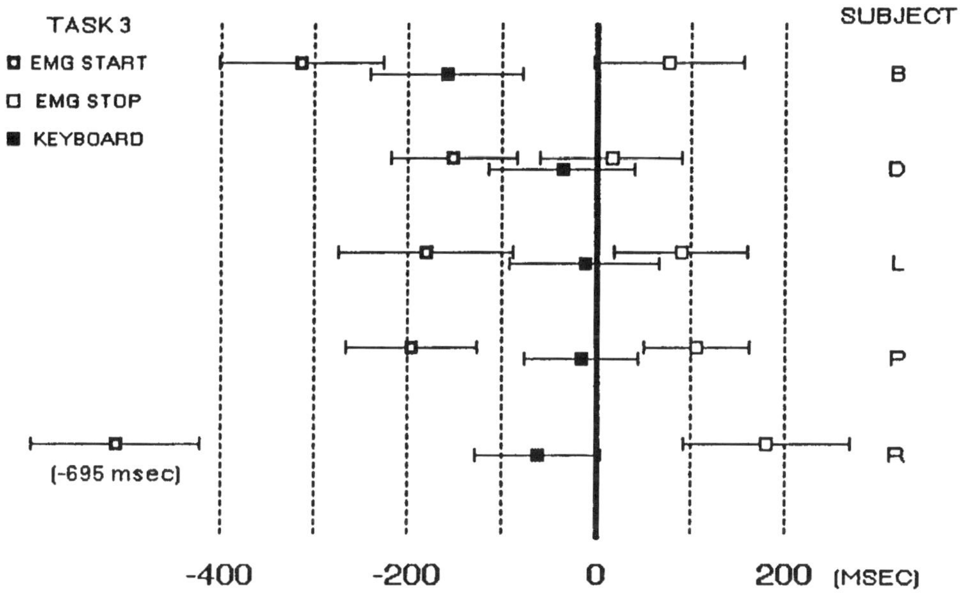

Figure 1. Motor-timing data for each subject in task 3, the 1-to-1 metronome to motor-response sequence. The temporal relationship of EMG onset, termination, and keyboard response is shown relative to the stimulus delivered at time zero. The mean and standard deviation were computed over 60 trials.

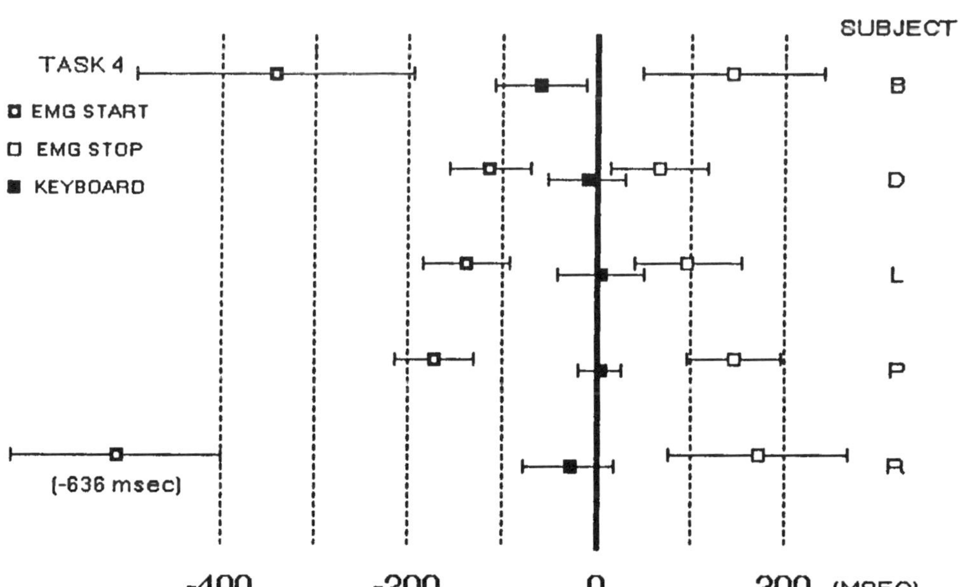

Figure 2. Same as Figure 1 except data is from task 4, the 2-to-1 metronome to motor-response task sequence.

response became more synchronous with the cueing, shifting temporally from 57 to 18 ms before the tone.

Table 1. *Synchronization Errors*

	TASK 3		TASK 4	
subject	mean	sd	mean	sd
B	-158	81	-59	48
D	-36	76	-10	42
L	-12	80	4	46
P	-15	60	5	23
R	-62	65	-28	48
average	-57	72	-18	41

values in milliseconds

The rhythmic stability of the motor response was examined in both auditory synchronization tasks and compared with the self-paced activity in task sequence 2. Table 2 shows the means and standard deviations of the response intervals during the self-paced task. The coefficient of variation (COV) was computed as the ratio of standard deviation to mean. To remove the effects of drift in the self-paced response intervals, the linear trend was removed from the data; results are presented in column 2(t). Based on the COV, there is no statistical difference in rhythmic stability between the self-paced and externally paced task sequences, 4.9% versus 4.8% group averages. With the presence of an additional tone, the rhythmic stability increased significantly ($p < 0.01$, paired t-test analysis) with a COV average of 2.6%.

Table 2. *Response Interval Variation*

	TASK 2		COEFFICIENT OF VARIABILITY			
subject	Tap Interval		Task			
	mean	sd	2	2(t)	3	4
B	2.978	0.178	6.0%	5.6%	5.9%	2.7%
D	2.208	0.104	5.1%	4.3%	4.4%	3.6%
L	1.787	0.121	6.8%	4.5%	4.9%	2.5%
P	2.585	0.212	8.2%	4.8%	4.4%	1.6%
R	2.344	0.134	5.7%	5.2%	4.6%	2.8%
			average	4.9%	4.8%	2.6%

Event-Related Brain Potentials

In order to examine gross ERP characteristics of brain wave activity during rhythmic auditory-motor synchronization, combined subject average were computed and compared among the various task sequences (Figure 3). During all three rhythmic-motor tasks, the brain-wave character consisted of negative pre-motor activity along with late positive ERPs. The positive ERPs began at the time of the stimulus and ended 500–1000 ms later. The two

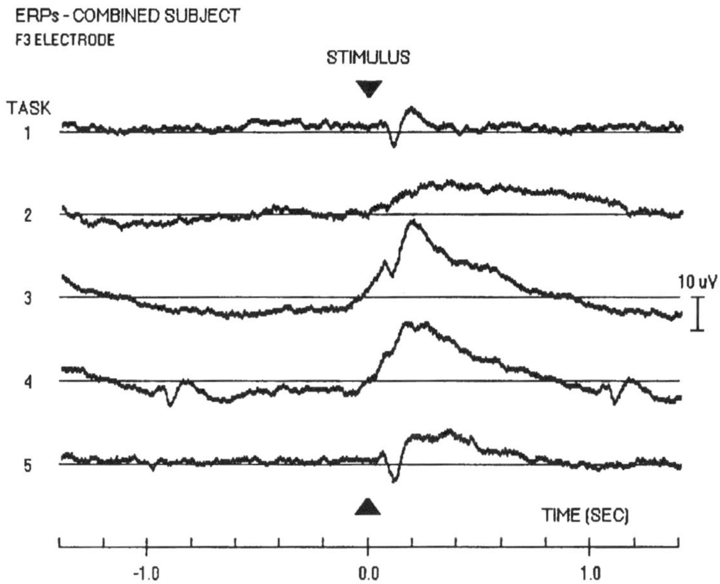

Figure 3. ERPs for the five experimental tasks. The data is from the frontal (F3) electrode and is the combined ensemble average of all five subjects. Data was aligned with the stimulus tone given at time zero, except in task 2 (no tone), where the keyboard response is aligned to time zero.

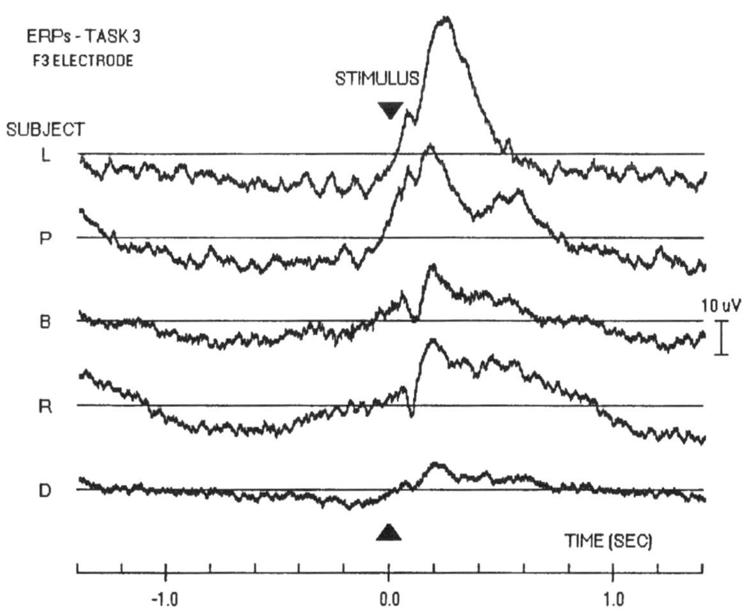

Figure 4. Task 3 (1-to-1 metronome to motor-response) ERP ensemble averages from each subject. The data is from the frontal (F3) electrode and aligned with the stimulus tone given at time zero.

task sequences without rhythmic motor activity, 1 and 5, both had ERPs characterized by little baseline fluctuation. There were no negative potentials preceding motor function in the stimulus-response task (5), with positive late potentials, lasting 100–400 ms after the stimulus, present in only some of the subjects.

Auditory ERP responses consisting of N1 and P2 peaks were observed in subjects listening to the stimulus tone with little baseline drift. Key tapping without auditory cueing generated a prolonged positive ERP field, 3–10 μV, lasting until 500–1000 ms after the tap along with slight negative potentials preceding motor activity. In general, synchronous tapping with the auditory cueing combined the activity seen in the first two tasks. The individual subject responses (Figure 4) were largest in the frontal position, 30% and 50% larger than at the central and parietal locations respectively.

Both rhythmic synchronization tasks exhibited a late positive potential that began shortly after the tone, sometimes masking the N1 auditory peak, with an amplitude of 10–30 μV and duration of 600–800 ms. Synchronous tapping with alternate tones produced similar results as seen in the standard metronome sequence, but with the extra auditory ERP embedded in the response. In synchronization tasks, the late positive potential was shorter in duration and had a different morphology than seen in the self-paced task sequence. During self-paced activity the late potential field had a relatively constant positive amplitude. With synchronization tasks a much larger amplitude occurred in the early phase (200–300 ms after stimulus), which decreased steadily throughout the later phase of the late ERP. In both rhythmic synchronization sequences, a negative pre-motor potential was present with a positive slope deflection, 10–40 μV per second, occurring prior to the tone that was correlated with the beginning of EMG activity.

DISCUSSION

During synchronized tapping, EMG activity began prior to the tone. A feedforward time decision process must then exist, such as a neural oscillator, that triggers the start of motor activity. This neural mechanism is still unknown but it must have ways of modifying temporal sequences. As a cardiac pacemaker adjusts its interval rate through changes in threshold potential and membrane potential decay rate, a neural temporal oscillator could adapt through changes in the perceived time interval and the rate of time passage. We have recorded brain-wave activity in synchronized and self-paced rhythmic tapping tasks, as well as in nonrhythmic stimulus-response tasks. By comparing the ERPs in these trials, we can associate features in the brain-wave activity with the rhythm generating mechanism.

The prominent feature in the brain-wave potentials found in the rhythmic synchronization tasks were the slow potential shifts that, in general, were negative preceding the motor response and positive afterwards. The same brain-wave activity was present in the self-paced motor tasks but was often absent in the stimulus-response tasks. This suggests that these ERPs are associated with basic temporal perception needed in rhythmic-motor function. The positive ERP potentials appear to be similar to P300 or Slow Waves but were strongest frontally rather than parietally as found with typical cognitive processes. This frontal dominance may reflect the involvement of the premotor cortex, which is known to be involved in motor responses to external sensory information.

Motor-timing data indicates that self-paced activity was as stable as cueing with the 1-to-1 metronome sequence, at least with our subject pool of musicians. These results suggest that adjustments based on synchronization error are not necessary to generate a stable train of motor response intervals. The character of the late positive ERPs was slightly different in the self-paced tapping compared to the synchronization tapping. There was less activity in the early phase of the ERP during the self-paced tapping. The increase in early activity in the synchronization tasks likely reflects processes associated with auditory-motor synchronization. If the self-paced and external-cueing performance is similar, why was there more activity in the early phase of the late positive potentials during auditory cueing? The activity may reflect the perception and comparison of stimulus and response intervals. It also may reflect the monitoring of SE, even though this information may not be used to adjust motor timing as long as the SE is within a tolerance range. Evidence for multiple synchronization strategies based on the magnitude of SE has been found in experiments with perturbed metronome sequences (Thaut & Miller, 1994).

The overall character of the slow potential shifts was not changed by the presence of an additional rhythmic cue in task sequence 4. The extra cueing did not elicit a sudden negative potential shift usually found with warning stimuli in "contingent negative variation" paradigms. Rhythmic synchronization may thus constitute a different temporal process than a motor response cued by a warning stimulus. Since the extra cueing improved motor performance, the added stimulus must be processed by the brain, but no changes in brain-wave character occurred other than typical auditory ERPs. If motor-timing adjustments based on SEs are the primary mechanism of auditory-motor coordination, the presence of an additional cue that significantly improves performance would be expected to elicit a change in the brain-wave response. This suggests that the additional tone is integrated as texture in the rhythmic stimuli and the basic auditory-motor synchronization strategies are unchanged from the standard metronome sequence. Since added texture in rhythmic stimuli enhances the stability of motor-timing, a strong case can be made for the benefit of musical rhythms over simple metronome sequences in coordinating motor activity.

References

Barret, G., Shibasaki, H., & Neshige, R. (1986). Cortical potentials preceding voluntary movement: Evidence for three periods of preparation in man. *Electroencephalography and Clinical Neurophysiology, 63*, 327–339.

Collyer, C. E., Broadbent, H. A., & Church, R. M. (1992). Categorical time production: Evidence for discrete timing in motor control. *Perception & Psychophysics, 51*(2), 134–144.

Hary, D., & Moore, G. P. (1985). Temporal tracking and synchronization strategies. *Human Neurobiology, 4*, 73–77.

Hary, D., & Moore, G. P. (1987). On the performance and stability of human metronome-synchronization strategies. *British Journal of Mathematical and Statistical Psychology, 40*, 109–124.

Kornhuber, H. H., & Deecke, L. (1965). Hirnpotentialänderungen bei Willkürbewegungen und passiven Bewegungen des Menschen: Bereitschaftspotential und reafferente Potentiale. Peters, M. (1989). The relationship between variability of intertap intervals and interval duration. *Psychological Research, 51*, 38–42.

Ruchkin, D. S., Sutton, S., & Stega, M. (1980). Emitted P300 and slow wave event related potentials in guessing and detection tasks. *Electroencephalography and Clinical Neurophysiology, 49*, 1–14.

Squires, K. C., Wickens, C., Squires, N. K., & Donchin, E. (1976). The effect of stimulus sequence on the waveform of the cortical event-related potential. *Science, 193*, 1142–1146.

Thaut, M. H., McIntosh, G. C., Prassas, S. G., & Rice, R. R. (1992). Effect of rhythmic auditory cueing on temporal stride parameters and EMG patterns in normal gait. *Journal of Neurologic Rehabilitation, 6,* 185–190.

Thaut, M. H., McIntosh, G. C., Prassas, S, G., & Rice, R. R. (1993). Effect of rhythmic auditory cueing on temporal stride parameters and EMG patterns in hemiparetic gait of stroke patients. *Journal of Neurologic Rehabilitation, 7,* 9–16.

Thaut, M. H., & Miller, R. A. (1994). Multiple synchronization strategies in tracking of rhythmic auditory stimulation. *Society for Neuroscience Abstracts, 24th annual meeting, Miami Florida, 20*(1), 336.

Walter, W. G., Cooper, R., Aldridge, V. J., McCallum, W. C., & Winter, A. L. (1964). Contingent negative variation: An electrical sign of sensorimotor association and expectancy in the human brain. *Nature (London), 203,* 380–384.

Wing, A. M., & Kristofferson, A. B. (1973a). The timing of interresponse intervals. *Perception & Psychophysics, 13,* 455–460.

Wing, A. M., & Kristofferson, A. B. (1973b). Response delays and the timing of discrete motor responses. *Perception & Psychophysics, 14,* 5–12.

PERCEPTION OF INHARMONIC SOUNDS: THEORETICAL IMPLICATIONS, EMPIRICAL FINDINGS

Albrecht Schneider

Introduction

The theory of hearing has been a topic of constant interest since the days of Helmholtz who died on 9 August, 1894, more than 100 years ago. Especially in the last few decades, a multitude of new empirical discoveries and theoretical works about nearly all aspects of tone sensation has been published (Plomp, 1976; Tobias, 1970; Keidel & Neff, 1974–1976; Keidel, David, Finkenzeller, Kallert, Plattig, Rinsdorf, & Spreng, 1975; Evans & Wilson, 1977; Moore, 1982, 1986; Warren, 1982). Among the points at issue are the approaches directed either to frequency or time domain of signals and signal processing, and the role of "place" versus "period". In addition, cochlear functions, mechanisms and stages of neural transduction, interplay of subcortical and cortical regions, tonotopic organization of the auditory cortex, hemispheric specialization, and other problems have been a matter of much debate (Zatorre, 1984; Petsche, 1989; Keidel, 1992).

Although there have been attempts to integrate new information as well as to develop advanced models of hearing, there are many difficulties to surmount as evidence from physiological studies and clinical reports must be related to data and hypotheses derived from psychoacoustic experiments. Moreover, much of the new information so far has been obtained from stimuli such as pure tones, clicks, or other sources suited to laboratory testing, yet quite different from the complex musical or speech signals that contextualize organized elements. It is clear that grouping elements into a context is highly relevant to the analysis and cognitive structuring of auditory events (Handel, 1989; Bregman, 1990).

This paper will consider the perception of certain inharmonic sounds within and out of a musical context with respect to pitch formation theories, on the one hand, and some features of the signals involved, on the other.

Auditory Pathways

Inner ear mechanisms, principles of neural coding, and sections as well as performance of the auditory pathways from the cochlea to areas understood as the primary auditory cortex have been investigated for many years in mammals such as the cat and also in humans (Whitfield, 1967; Keidel & Neff, 1975; Keidel et al., 1975; Merzenich, Roth, Anderson, Knight, & Colwell, 1977; Merzenich, 1981; Pickles, 1988). From these studies can be derived a scheme of main auditory pathways that contains major afferent stages as well as a few efferent and contralateral interconnections.

Since approximately 70% of the nerve fibers in one ear are connected to the contralateral auditory cortex, while only 30% are linked to the ipsilateral, the result is a crossover network that is obviously suited to signal processing with information input that differs in the time domain. The network thereby accounts for onset differences between right and left ear and permits localization in "auditory space" (Whitfield, 1977). The great number of interconnections and transformations of the original signal structure on higher stages of pathways above the cochlear nuclei indicate that processing is complex, although tonotopic organization can be followed up to the inferior colliculus, whereas the medial geniculate

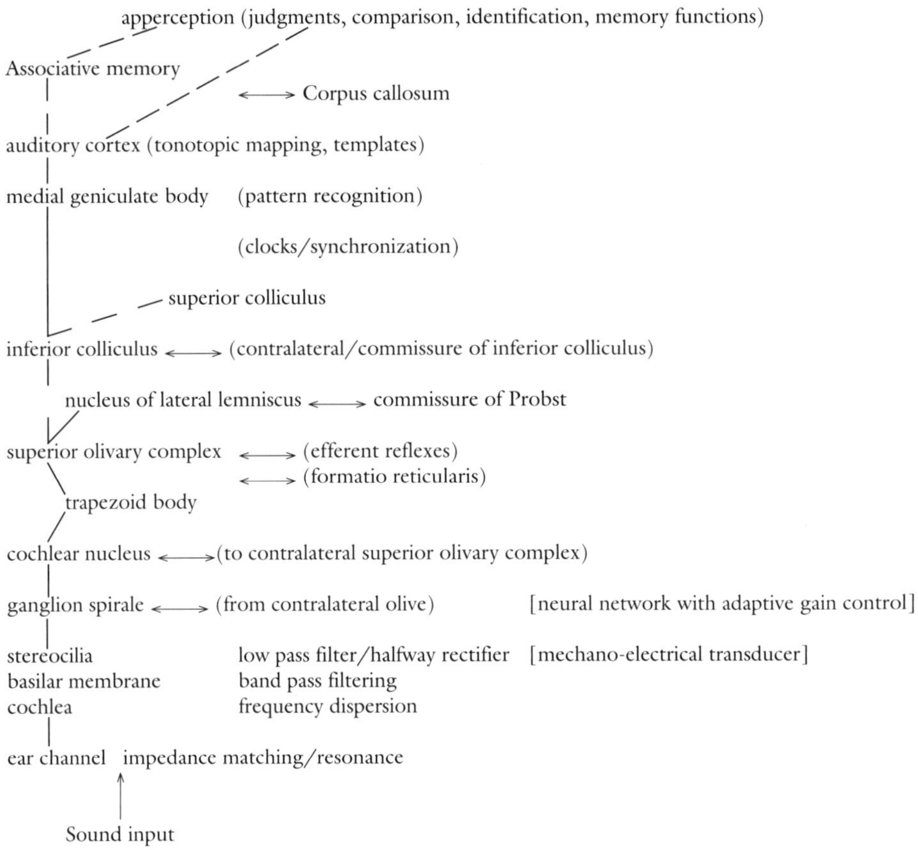

Figure 1. Main auditory pathways and auditory functions.

body (corpus geniculatum mediale [cgm]) seems to operate as a major relay with units that respond in various ways to original input signals and also with units that exhibit spontaneous periodic activity (Keidel et al., 1975; Keidel & Kallert, 1979). According to neuromagnetic studies, tonotopic organization is either maintained at the level of the human auditory cortex (Romani, Williamson, & Kaufman, 1982; Pantev, Hoke, Lehnertz, Lütkenhöner, Anogianakis, & Wittkowski, 1988) or, through signal representation and transduction in the cgm, is regained. Because of integration of stimulus patterns, complex signals such as musical chords are not represented as discrete elements at the cortical level (Keidel, 1992, pp. 349, 351). It is common knowledge that exact boundaries of the primary auditory cortex are even more difficult to define than those of nuclei at lower stages. Moreover, in the cat, no less than four auditory cortical fields have been identified, all of which are topographically organized to allow for highly ordered representation of sound frequencies (Merzenich, 1981).

In order to approach processing in real-time complex stimuli, which constitute a quasi-continuous auditory stream of sound events, the neural network can be expected to reduce overall input and to eliminate nonessential information (e.g., background noise) as well as to sharpen contrasts of signal features, previously discussed with respect to tuning curves, best frequencies, and other mechanisms observed in the functional organization and performance of the auditory neural system (Keidel & Kallert, 1979; Pickles, 1988). Especially from the aspect of the multitude of excitation and inhibitory responses found in cells of the dorsal cochlear nucleus (Shofer & Young, 1985), it has been argued, however, that the incoming signal most likely is retained as completely as possible and transmitted in both an unprocessed form as well as in variants that underwent transformations, with little probability that information reduction and sharpening of signals occurs as far up as the cortex (Handel, 1989).

As far as registrations of neural activity are concerned, coding and decoding of the signal at various stages and locations has been investigated. As a result, one of the principles that has been formulated has to do with phase-locking of firings to signal features. Synchronicity of firing seems to play a role in the perception of "place" pitch (Merzenich, 1981). There are also indications for synchronization of firings to both amplitude and frequency modulated signals, with an optimal modulation frequency of $\tilde{=}$ 10 Hz in units of the mammalian auditory cortex (Gaese & Ostwald, 1990). In several nuclei, especially in the thalamic brain regions, clock units have been identified, which appear to generate reference signals for specific time measurements and synchronization processes that are particularly useful in the auditory modality, although they are not restricted to this field (Keidel et al., 1975). It hardly needs to be emphasized that periodicity is a central feature in most of musically relevant sounds, and periodicity detection (Ritsma 1970) is one of the principal approaches discussed in the theory of hearing (see below).

Clock units seem to be essential in the demultiplication processes that cause a frequency reduction in the area of the corpus geniculatum mediale and inferior colliculus. Frequency response of the neural network here is such that it produces maximal excitation patterns for a given stimulus frequency f_i and its integer multiples ($n \times f_i$). From this discovery, first recorded in the cat, it has been concluded that there is a neural harmonic analyzer found in the cgm and adjacent areas that is relevant to the perception of small integer ratio intervals (Keidel et al., 1975). As these are neurally distinguished from random patterns of stimuli, the subcortical analyzer would also account for the fact that, in psychoacoustic experiments, subjects typically "detect" simple ratio intervals against mere tonal distances of arbitrary size $d(f_i, f_k) > 0$ (Reinecke, 1964). Moreover, the analyzer would support the preference of harmonic sounds that are therefore understood to have a physiological basis in neural signal processing itself and are not just the result of cultural selection (Keidel, 1975, 1992; Hesse, 1972).

Remarkably, the neural harmonic analyzer is located in that part of the brain that is old in terms of evolution, namely, the thalamus, which is said to involve emotions because of interconnections with the limbic system. What might therefore be assumed is that the feeling of pleasantness and relaxation usually assigned to harmonic intervals and chords also has foundations in the brain structures and processes actually involved in auditory signal processing.

The thesis of a neural harmonic analyzer working as a template for small integer frequency ratios is entirely in accordance with recent studies on the performance of single hair cells of the organ of Corti, which showed that both Hensen's cells and outer hair cells mechanically driven to resonance are much better "tuned" to specific excitation frequencies than has been previously assumed. The vibratory response measured by Khanna, Ulfendahl, & Flock (1989) as velocity waveform is actually Fourier transformed into spectra that plot frequency ./. vibration amplitude (which is a conversion of velocity). The experiments of the *International Team for Ear Research* (ITER) are described in detail in some 30 contributions that make up Supplement 467 of Acta Otolaryngologica Stockholm (1989).

As can be seen from the spectra, outer hair cells especially produce a number of harmonics with a maximum between 170–220 Hz, where up to 10 odd and even harmonic components have been registered. From the velocity waveforms and their spectra, it can be inferred that "harmony" is already produced in the inner ear, and basically within single outer hair cells. As to their performance, it should be added that quite sharp frequency

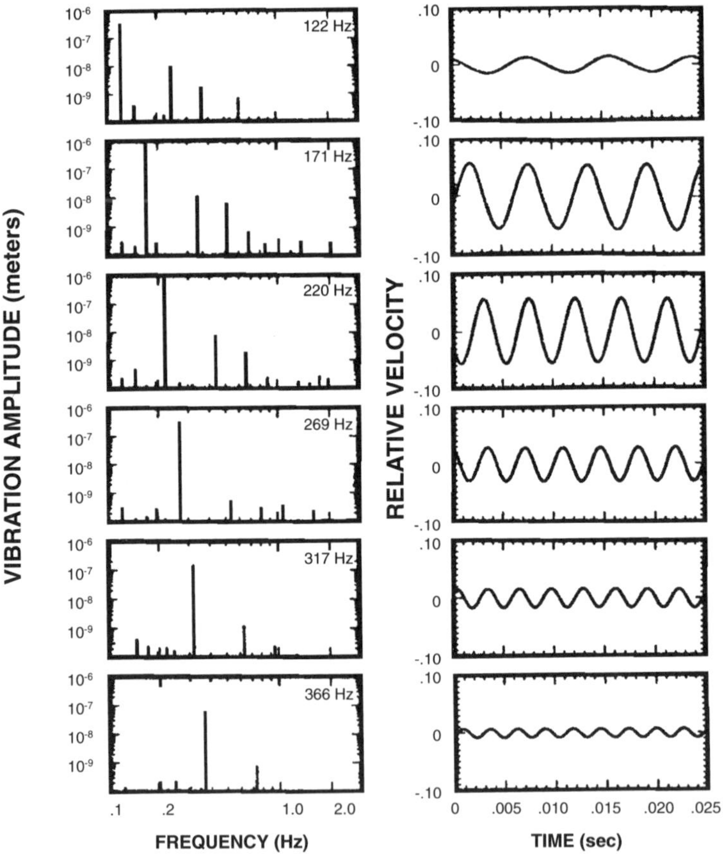

Figure 2a (Khanna et al. 1989, 191). Waveforms of the vibratory responses of a single Hensen's cell in the apical turn of a guinea pig cochlea. Relative velocity of the cell vibration is shown on the right as a function of time. The absolute velocity magnitude (in meters/sec.) can be obtained by multiplying the relative velocity by 1.9×10^{-2}. The spectrum corresponding to the waveforms on the right is shown on the left. At each of the test frequencies the vibration amplitude of the spectral component is plotted as a function of frequency.

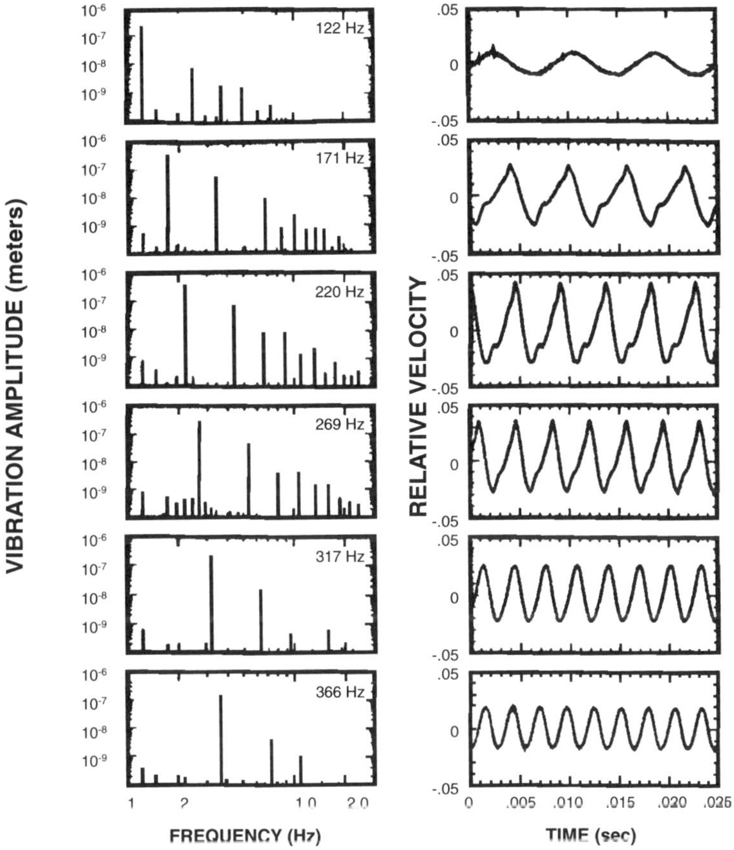

Figure 2b (Khanna et al. 1989, 191). Waveforms and spectra of vibratory responses of a first row outer hair cell in the apical turn of a guinea pig cochlea. The relative velocity amplitude is shown on the right as a function of time for six test frequencies, below, at, and above the frequency of maximum response. The spectrum corresponding to the velocity waveforms is shown on the left. The spectrum is calculated to show the absolute vibration amplitude at the signal frequency and its harmonics.

discrimination as observed in hair-cell receptor potentials, as well as in basilar membrane motion patterns, has led to considerations of active mechanisms involving efferent stimulation and probably some kind of feedback control (Khanna & Leonard, 1982; Hudspeth, 1985).

Models of Pitch Extraction

With respect to their central aspects and main thesis, most pitch theories can generally be classified as such directed to "place", while some others emphasize "period". Both have a long history from Ohm and Seebeck to the present day and account for certain phenomena very well, but not so well for others (Nordmark, 1970; de Boer, 1975; Plomp, 1976). For place theories, the basic point is that the cochlea and, in particular, the basilar membrane can be regarded as a mechanical spectrum analyzer capable of performing a Fourier analysis of complex sounds within certain limits (Plomp, 1976; Zwicker, 1980; Pickles, 1988). As to the limits of frequency resolution, it has often been pointed out that what is involved is the critical bandwidth and the plain experience of roughness caused by two simultaneous pure tones too close in their respective frequencies to be perceived as individual components. In the light of research on the basilar membrane as well as on the performance of the hair cells, the multitude of findings related to the concept of critical bands probably needs to be reconciled, however, with more recent reports pointing to "improved" filter characteristics of the organ of Corti (Keidel, 1992).

One of the main arguments that refutes the place theory of pitch has been that it is not possible to mask the (pseudo-) fundamental of a residue-type complex tone (higher harmonics [4, 5, 6] that are sufficient to produce the sensation of a "fundamental") by means of low-pass noise in the same frequency range. The (pseudo-) fundamental thus perceived cannot be a product of peripheral stimulation yet must be attributed to "higher" stages of processing. The consequence of a variety of phenomena usually discussed under the heading of residue pitch (de Boer, 1975) seems to be that distinct pitch perception is not totally dependent on the information that is obtained from the output of the chain of cochlearic bandpass filters, yet related to the time domain of the signal. As can be easily demonstrated, periodicity is maintained in harmonic complex sounds that lack the fundamental component.

Of course, the wave shape has changed what accounts for a slight yet noticeable difference in timbre. If the auditory system indeed comprises phase-locking and capability to recognize zero crossings, it should be suited to periodicity detection as well as the detection of frequency modulation, as in fact it does, above certain threshold levels (Ritsma, 1970; Coninx, 1977).

It was mainly with respect to the phenomena discussed in the realm of Schouten's (1970) by then famous work on the acoustical residue that several advanced theories of pitch perception were published in the 70s, including algorithms for the prediction of pitch most likely to be attributed to classes of complex tones. Theories and models that gained widespread interest include that of the optimum processor of Goldstein (1973), the pattern-transformation approach of Wightman (1973), and the virtual-pitch approach of Terhardt (1972, 1982). The first, in brief, hypothesizes a central pitch processor working on spectral components that have been resolved by the ear. From the information thereby made available, the central processor makes an optimum estimate of the fundamental frequency of complex sounds. The model that contains a mathematical formulation for the maximum likelihood estimation does not consider the relative amplitude and phase of components. Wightman's model is directed to pattern recognition and is based on the Fourier transform of the signal as well as the autocorrelation function. In a three-step processing system, pitch first yields a power spectrum that is then neurally transformed into another pattern of neural activity that roughly represents the autocorrelation function of the original signal. Finally, pitch is derived from the position and relative power of certain components. Typically, lower spectral components are of greater pitch importance than are higher ones. From the virtual pitch approach, Terhardt also evaluates spectral energy distribution and salience of components, while pitch, in the main, is derived from a process of subharmonic matching (previously discussed by Walliser, 1969).

In(1): =

Plot {[Sin(x) + Sin(2x) + Sin(3x) + Sin(4x) + Sin(5x) + Sin(6x)], [x, 0, 15]}

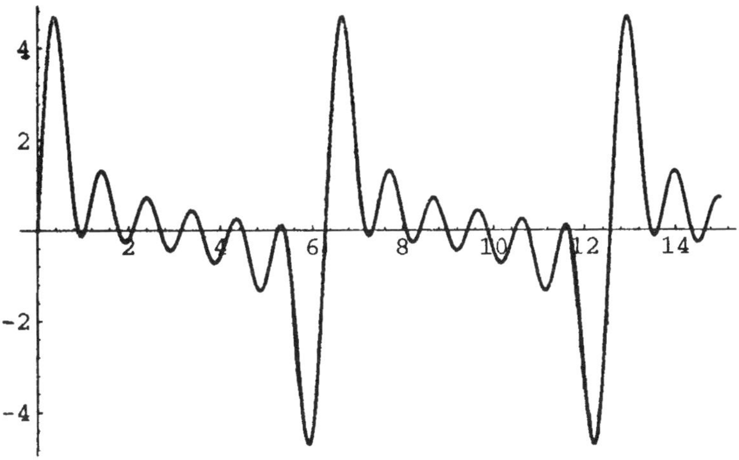

Out(1): =

-Graphics-

In(2): =

Plot {[Sin(3x) + Sin(4x) + Sin(5x) + Sin(6x)], [x, 0, 15]}

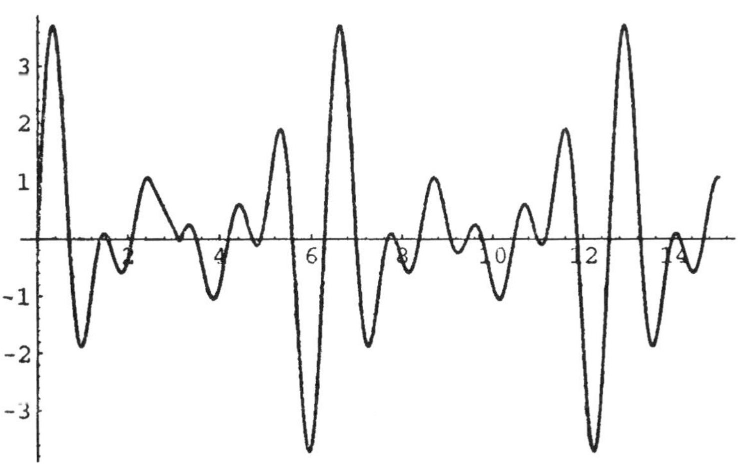

Out(2): =

-Graphics-

Figure 3. Period of sound with six harmonics (top) and same sound after harmonics 1 and 2 have been removed (bottom).

All three approaches, which have some commonalities (Patterson & Wightman, 1976; de Boer, 1977), regard the ear as a spectrum analyzer of limited resolution capability, and pitch perception as a pattern recognition task based on the output of spectrum analysis. Final pitch calculation or estimation is usually conceived of as evaluation of harmonic or inharmonic components, whereby number, spacing, relative amplitude, and phase of components form the parameters that can have an influence on actual pitch or pitches perceived (Schouten, 1970; Patterson, 1973; Patterson & Wightman, 1976; Terhardt, Stoll, & Seewann, 1982a/b).

In the investigation of number, spacing, and phase of components (Patterson, 1973; Patterson & Wightman, 1976), phase was found to be almost irrelevant as was the absolute number of components in most experiments, which, however, established predictable relations between spacing and pitch shift.

Spectral Content and Periodicity

As previously discussed, pitch extraction models are usually phase insensitive and tied mainly to spectral features of stimuli, namely, those tones and/or components that can be resolved in the cochlea (Houtsma & Goldstein, 1972). In musical practice, however, there are, on the one hand, sounds with high spectral density (e.g., African lamellophones), while, on the other hand, constant time envelopes are rare because of vibrato as it is used in playing wind and string instruments, in singing, etc. Moreover, in contemporary rock/pop, a variety of devices, in addition to pitch bending, is used to produce all kinds of time-axis manipulation (phasing, flanging, chorus). It is well known that pitch perception of frequency modulated sounds can be difficult since it has long been evident that the temporal envelope of sounds contains prime information relevant to pitch (and especially residue) perception. If sounds with a constant temporal envelope evoke a clear pitch, and sounds that undergo frequency modulation tend to cause ambiguity, the resultant correlation of time function and pitch of a signal can be taken as an argument in favor of periodicity detection. As far as perception of complex sounds is concerned, spectral content of course is as important as is periodicity because inharmonic sounds especially will not only produce complex waveshapes, but also extended periodicities that often are not easily recognized. Moreover, concerning the natural inharmonic sounds from, for example, idiophones of the Indonesian gamelan, following the attack (which itself is nonperiodic), both amplitude modulation and shifts in spectral energy distribution are found along with high spectral density (Schneider & Beurmann, 1991, 1993).

Consequently, the pitch of these sounds is often perceived as ambiguous and consisting of several components, some of which can be identified by subjects matching the signal of a tone generator to spectral frequency components that are "real" in that they can be measured as partials. Besides, a "residue effect" similar to the strike note in bells does occur; that is, perception of a "pitch" that is not caused by a single spectral component but by spectral content as a pattern of partials that can interact because of their relative frequencies, amplitudes, etc.

Results of Experimental Studies

Earlier experiments carried out in our institute with sampled sounds from African xylophones and Javanese gamelan led to further research with respect to pitch perception and the factors that were causing ambiguity in judgments of pitch. As stimuli for the experiments herein described, two basic sounds were used, namely, (a) the "ideal xylophone", based on the first eight partials typically found in a bar with free-free boundary conditions, and (b) two hammers clashing and forming a not very ideal "metallophone". The first of these is the xylophone, which was generated by means of Fourier synthesis both in analog form on a multitrack tape recorder, and digitally, by means of a computer with dsp (Mathematica© running on a NeXT©).

In(16): =

Plot {[Sin(x) + Sin(2.76x) + Sin(5.4x) + Sin(8.93x) + Sin(13.34x) + Sin(18.63x) + Sin(24.81x) + Sin(31.87x)], [x, 0, 60]}

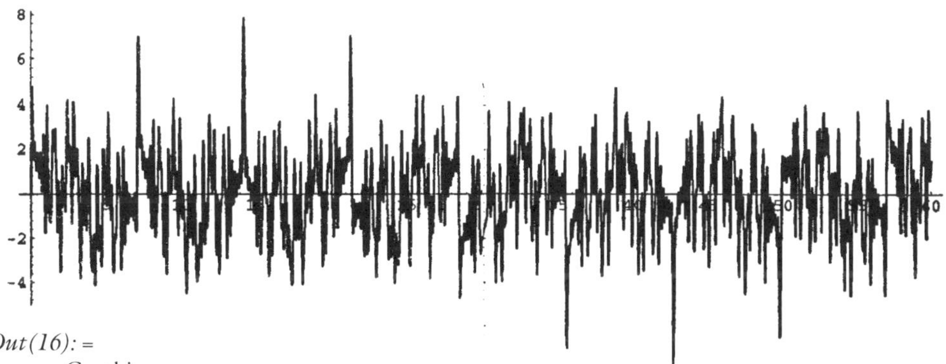

Out(16): =

-Graphics-

Figure 4a. Time function/Waveshape: "ideal xylophone"

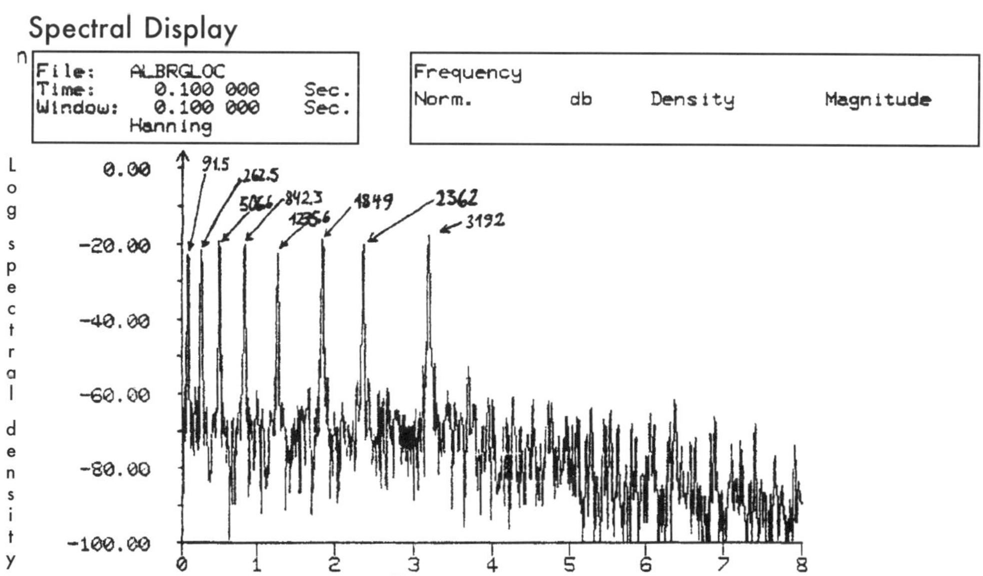

Figure 4b. Spectrum, analogue sample of "ideal xylophone"

The lowest component frequency was set to 100 Hz with the resulting spectrum of {100, 276, 540, 893, 1334, 1863, 2481, 3187} Hz. The components were phase-locked in the digitized sound, but not in the analog sample, yet all had the same amplitude (±0.5 db in the analog sound). The sounds were loaded into a Synclavier II at 50 kHz sampling rate, and into an EMU Emax II at 39.0625 kHz sampling rate so that notes of any length (quite different from a real xylophone) as well as intervals and pieces of music could be played. The samples were used for testing subjects who were asked to identify the size of intervals as well as to describe their cognitive strategy in trying to judge the interval between each pair of stimuli (a⟷b) played in succession. Ten different intervals were presented in random order and in upward and downward directions.

The second stimulus was simply two hammers clashing sampled with the Synclavier at 50 kHz/16 bit. Although the resulting sound is not very musical, a similar sound effect is present in the final movement of the Mahler symphony no. 6.

This sound is particularly suited to our purpose in that the spectral content contains a double resonance (also often encountered in xylophones because of different grain layers) at the "bottom", a phenomenon that is likely to cause pitch ambiguity. Using the hammer sound, eight intervals were once again created and presented in random order in an interval task analogous to that based on the "ideal xylophone", but certainly more difficult since the sound of the hammers lasts basically for only 0.1 second (see Figure 5a) and, in a certain sense, is a sort of short "click".

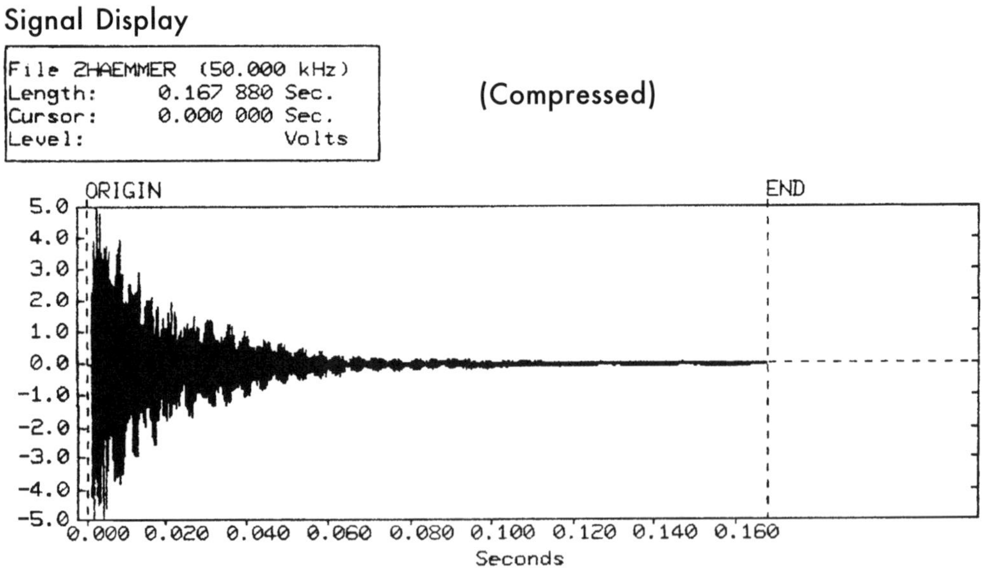

Figure 5a. Two hammers striking, signal display

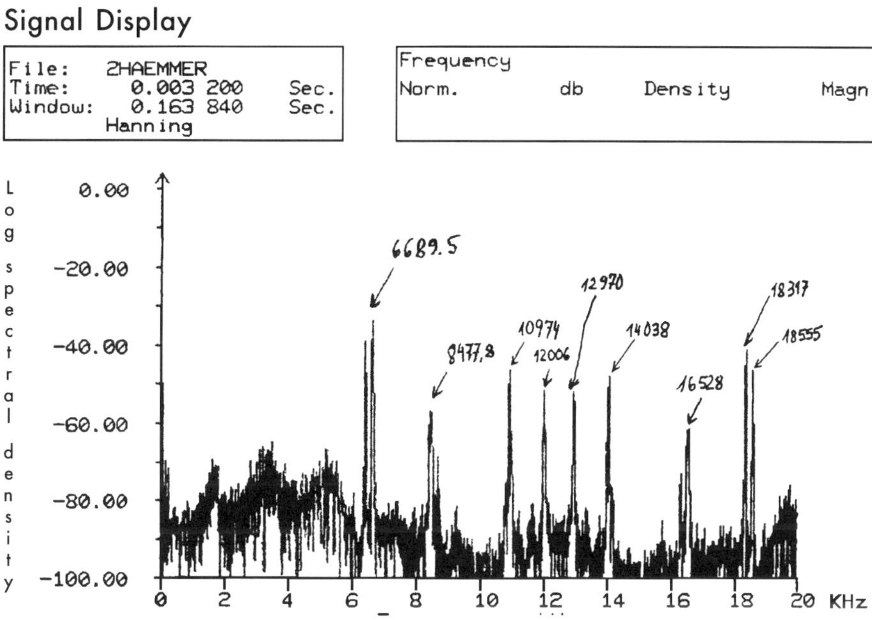

Figure 5b. Two hammers striking, spectral display

A third experiment used the sound of the "ideal xylophone" and only two intervals were presented. However, the conditions in this test were that sounds had been processed by means of (a) flanging, (b) shaping of spectral envelope, and (c) flanging plus filtering of the sounds applied at the same time in order to study the effects of modulation and unusual timbre on pitch.

In addition, using both main stimuli, excerpts of well known melodies (e.g., *Ode to Joy*) were played on the Synclavier II and presented via tape to explore the effect of context and Gestalt recognition.

In the experiments carried out twice in 1991 and 1993, 33 (1991) and 29 (1993) students in a musicology program volunteered as subjects. These subjects had had several years of formal training in music and, prior to admission to the university, had already developed skills such as playing one or more instruments, singing, and reading musical notation. Since the precise amount of training was not relevant to the experiment, this information was not requested of the subjects. The detailed statistical analyses of data from these two studies is discussed elsewhere (Schneider & Beurmann, 1994b). However, the following tables extracted from these analyses illustrate some broad trends:

Table 1

Interval Identification and Recognition Task. Musicology Students in Two Studies (1991 = a; 1993 = b).

Test	Interval	No. Semitones	a/b Median		a/b Variance		a/b SD		a/b Range	
xyl 1	tritone	6	6	5	0.717	1.888	0.847	1.374	5	8
xyl 2	fourth	5	5	5	1.272	1.143	1.128	1.069	7	5
xyl 3	octave	12	7	6	6.371	7.917	2.524	2.814	9	10
xyl 4	M third	4	4	4	2.142	2.527	1.463	1.590	7	9
xyl 5	m third	3	3	3	2.467	0.778	1.57	0.882	10	3
xyl 6	m second	1	1	1	0.172	0.241	0.415	0.491	2	2
xyl 7	M second	2	2	2	4.297	2.851	2.073	1.689	11	6
xyl 8	tritone	6	5	6	2.859	2.091	1.691	1.446	9	6
xyl 9	fifth	7	7	7	5.672	2.180	2.381	1.476	10	7
xyl 10	M third	4	4	4	2.655	3.044	1.629	1.745	9	8
ham 1	fifth	7	5	7	6.933	3.892	2.633	1.973	12	10
ham 2	octave	12	6	7	4.818	9.856	2.195	3.139	10	10
ham 3	M second	2	2	2	2.487	6.172	1.577	2.484	8	7
ham 4	M sixth	9	7	8	8.732	7.852	2.955	2.802	10	10
ham 5	tritone	6	5	5	6.320	7.667	2.514	2.769	10	9
ham 6	M third	4	4	5	5.808	8.247	2.41	2.872	10	10
ham 7	m second	1	1	1	2.735	0.278	1.654	0.528	8	2
ham 8	fourth	5	5	5	12.468	6.744	3.531	2.597	11	10

Table 2

Rank Order of Intervals/Correct Identifications

Sample 1 (1991)				**Sample 2 (1993)**			
Sound	**Interval**	**C.I.***	**Rank No.**	**Sound**	**Interval**	**C.I.***	**Rank No.**
xyl 6	m second	27	1	xyl 6	m second	24	1
ham 3	M second	27	1	ham 7	m second	22	2
ham 7	m second	26	2	ham 3	M second	19	3
xyl 2	fourth	23	3	xyl 2	fourth	19	3
xyl 7	M second	22	4	xyl 5	m third	17	4
xyl 1	tritone	16	5	xyl 7	M second	16	5
xyl 4	M third	15	6	xyl 4	M third	14	6
xyl 5	m third	15	6	xyl 10	M third	13	7
xyl 9	fifth	12	7	xyl 9	fifth	12	8
xyl 10	M third	10	8	ham 1	fifth	11	9
ham 4	M sixth	8	9	xyl 1	tritone	9	10
ham 1	fifth	7	10	xyl 8	tritone	8	11
ham 8	fourth	7	10	ham 8	fourth	8	11
ham 6	M third	7	10	ham 6	M third	7	12
xyl 8	tritone	6	11	ham 4	M sixth	7	12
xyl 3	octave	4	12	ham 2	octave	3	13
ham 5	tritone	3	13	ham 5	tritone	2	14
ham 2	octave	1	14	xyl 3	octave	1	15

* = correct identifications

An analysis of variance of the data was highly significant with respect to interval categories but there were uneven results concerning data of identical categories with respect to the two different sound sources used. It is clear that inharmonic sounds such as those used in the experiments induce pitch ambiguity and therefore make an interval size judgment difficult. The sounds, which have distinct spectra and completely different temporal envelopes, engender uncertainty and force subjects to make distance estimates of the two complex sounds because interval quality has been lost to a great extent. However, simple and popular melodies played with these sound sources were identified by most subjects after listening to one or two phrases. Subjects' responses showed that, when asked about relevant parameters, they were able to identify the melodies through contour and rhythmic pattern recognition, probably stored in long-term memory (Dowling, 1978).

The same strategy, however, does not work well with single intervals when the timbre is completely strange to the listener; even interval and scale patterns that are masked, in this instance by spectral and temporal characteristics of the stimuli used, become difficult to recognize. This interpretation is derived from the data shown in Tables 1 and 2, which clearly indicate that narrow intervals such as the minor and major seconds were identified correctly more of the time than the constitutive musical intervals, of which the octave scored poorly, and the fifth was far from the prominent place it holds in a normal musical context. The loss of interval quality was similar to that found in another experiment in which a fifth was played with the ideal xylophone sound so that the notes of the interval were played in succession, each sound lasting for about 3 seconds with a break of about 2 seconds in between the notes. The signal had been processed by means of a time-axis manipulation (stereo flanging), which added to ambiguity and poor identification (14 correct responses out of 55). The term flanging is used to describe time-axis manipulation of an audio signal by means of a delay line to produce "artificial zeros" in its frequency spectrum; the signal is also shaped by an envelope generator that can vary both the transit time and the delay of the signal. Depending on the amount of flanging applied, both the pitch and timbre of the signal perceived can be changed considerably.

Given this type of inharmonic stimuli, subjects cannot depend on their acquired learning or innate perceptions of interval categories. The ambiguity engendered by the sound sources with respect to pitch and interval causes subjects to attempt distance estimates of pairs of stimuli that are easier to achieve and result in higher scores if these distances d (a,b) are small. In this case, the gap between two successive sounds still indicates closeness of stimuli that otherwise bear little relationship.

As for the strategy of judging interval size, subjects reported two basic approaches, namely (a) making an overall attempt to evaluate the linear distance from sound a to sound b, and (b) trying to analyze the complex sounds and then match partials of one sound to some components of the other. Concerning the first approach, this can be understood as the global estimate known from multidimensional scaling studies, while the second comes close to an additive estimate of differences assigned to several characteristics of sounds that may again be connected to dimensions such as brightness or chroma. According to Torgerson (1961), subjects perceive only a single quantitative relation between stimuli (p. 205) so that stimuli even as complex as these must be finally treated by way of "global distance estimate". This view is corroborated by the behavior of about two-thirds of our subjects, who, indeed, said that they tried to evaluate a single quantitative relation between two successive sounds (xyl a/b; ham a/b) notwithstanding that they had all recognized that the sounds of the ideal xylophone especially contained several if not many spectral components. About one-third of the subjects, however, tried a different strategy and tried rather to single out one component in each sound by which to judge interval size. When asked how many components the xylophone sound might comprise, following close listening to samples played back for 5 seconds each, the vast majority of the 43 subjects believed they were able to distinguish at least three components. In experiments where some 20 subjects had to match a sine wave signal to spectral components, the typical response was three different matches per sample.

This indicates that especially for trained listeners the pitch of these sounds is not one-dimensional even if it is possible to integrate a number of analyzable components into one functional whole (Koffka, 1936), which is then compared to another comparable complex structure (sound a: sound b). (A precise diagram is provided in Schneider & Beurmann, 1994b, p. 31.)

Consequently, the distance estimate here is based on several features rather than on one single attribute, notwithstanding that, in the end, the estimate has to establish the distance of stimuli on a certain dimension, that of pitch. This, however, has long been considered two-componential, or, in some modern approaches, multi-dimensional. If pitch cannot be separated from timbre, as is the case with many complex and especially inharmonic sounds such as those presented here, stimuli tend to evoke a multiplicity of sensations. In particular, those subjects with musical training analytically single out constituents of complex sounds as well as perceive the stimulus as a whole (Terhardt et al., 1982a, 1982b; Parncutt, 1988; Schneider & Beurmann, 1991, 1994a, 1994b).

Thus, in addition to the perception of several pitches, there is the task of assigning an "integration pitch" to the overall configuration of components, transients, modulation effects, etc., which make up the percept. As Carl Stumpf (1983, 1890) argued long ago, analytic listening always involves comparison, evaluation of stimulus features, memory functions, etc., so that apperception can largely be understood in terms of judgment functions. Pitch therefore would have to be regarded as a cognitive concept that is of course based on—although not reducible to—sensation of stimulus features.

Conclusion

The theories and models of hearing presented in this paper discuss pitch mainly as a pattern recognition process in which subjects extract features and the information contained therein from complex stimuli. In the case of inharmonic sounds, spectral components extracted then are often interpreted as approximations of the harmonic series [$f_n = n \times f_i$] as was already discussed in Schouten's (1940) original paper on the residue with respect to perception of bell sounds. Reasoning thus proceeds from harmonic spectra and implies that indeed there is a neural harmonic analyzer, as Keidel et al. (1975) postulated on the basis of neurophysiological discoveries. Moreover, recent experiments have once again indicated that we seem to possess internal octave templates (Demany & Semal, 1988), and clinical studies have shown that pitch perception in humans deteriorates considerably in patients who have undergone a right temporal lobectomy with excision of Heschl's gyri and the surrounding cortex (Zatorre, 1988). A variety of facts and discoveries therefore corroborates the hypotheses related to central pitch and a neural analyzing system that indeed seems to be tuned to harmonic spectra and intervals. This type of pitch processor tends to be increasingly confused in more extreme cases of inharmonic sounds that withstand processes of subharmonic matching or extraction of such components that come close to a harmonic series. For example, ambiguity of a perceived pitch increases if spectral components are densely spaced and have equal relative amplitude.

Pitch perception is of course related to and, in certain respects, dependent on, peripheral spectrum analysis, as has been confirmed by many experiments directed to the so-called critical bandwidth (Zwicker, 1980). Typically, sounds with close peaks in the spectrum caused by, for example, double resonances, are candidates for ambiguity, especially if such twin peaks are located in the low frequency region and are also close enough to each other to produce beats or roughness.

That the time domain is relevant follows not only from effects modulation has on pitch, but also from the simple fact that in inharmonic complexes, periodicity detection will be more difficult than in harmonic sounds. While most listeners easily detect pitch in multi-harmonic sounds and relate it closely to the period of the wave and the fundamental frequency of the harmonic series (Patterson, 1989), with inharmonic sounds there are more factors that are relevant, such as spectral density, internal roughness among components, beats and other modulation phenomena. Thus, with respect to inharmonic sounds, pitch perception has to basically solve five problems:

1. Sufficient resolution of spectral content into distinctive components
2. Detection of periodicity
3. Evaluation of the degree of inharmonicity and of the temporal envelope
4. Integration of 1–3 into one percept
5. Apperception (intentional awareness of percept within a dimensional structure.)

For the detection of pitch by neural networks, several models have been developed (e.g., Sano & Jenkins, 1991; Petroni, Degrassi, & Pasquariello, 1993, 1993) that deal mainly with pitch classes and, in the first place, account for periodic signals with harmonic spectra. Residue pitch here, as in earlier approaches (see earlier section on Models of Pitch Extraction) is treated as pattern recognition of an incomplete signal that is processed by a neural network trained on sounds with harmonic spectra. Pattern recognition with increasing inharmonicity becomes more difficult and, beyond a certain limit, is likely to fail. It can be demonstrated that even the syntactic structure of a completely tonal and harmonic piece cannot be recognized anymore if the texture is realized with the type of inharmonic sound we have generated for our "ideal xylophone". We recorded Sweelinck's famous *Fantasia* (*Opera omnia,* vol. 1, no. 4), which is noted for modal elements, chromaticism, and harmonic structures, into a MIDI sequencer, and then played back the piece in such a way that the timbre shifts gradually from a principal-like organ stop into our xylophone. In a three-part harmonic texture, layering of three inharmonic sounds generates chords of high spectral density that are difficult to analyze and comprehend, even by skilled subjects. Though relations among lowest spectral components of the notes played remain unchanged, shift of spectral energy distribution, and inharmonic sounds produced thereby, cause ambiguity to such an extent that even musically trained subjects no longer can follow the syntax of an otherwise totally tonal context. Even though subjects can assign pitch to sounds of bandpass filtered noise under certain conditions, peripheral auditory analysis and the neural harmonic analyzer referred to above may lose track of signals that by their spectral complexity cannot be sufficiently resolved in the cochlearic filter bank, related to a harmonic series, and processed as a type of residue pitch.

Acknowledgment

For support in the preparations of experiments, the author thanks A. E. Beurmann of the University of Hamburg.

References

Boer, E. de. (1975). On the "Residue" and auditory pitch perception. In W. D. Keidel & W. D. Neff (Eds.), *Handbook of sensory physiology, vol. 5* (pp. 479–583). Heidelberg/New York: Springer.

Boer, E. de. (1977). Pitch theories unified. In E. F. Evans & J. P Wilson (Eds.), *Psychophysics and physiology of hearing* (pp. 323–334). New York: Academic Press.

Bregman, A. S. (1990). *Auditory scene analysis: The perceptual organization of sound.* Cambridge, MA/London: MIT Press.

Coninx, F. (1977). *On the perception of changes in amplitude and frequency of acoustic signals.* Doctoral dissertation, University of Utrecht. (Published in a limited edition.)

Demany, L, & Semal C. (1988). Dichotic fusion of two tones one octave apart: Evidence for internal octave templates. *Journal of the Acoustic Society of America, 83,* 687–695.

Dowling, J. (1978). Scale and contour: Two components of a theory of memory for melodies. *Psychological Review, 85,* 341–354.

Evans, E. F., & Wilson, J. P. (Eds.). *Psychophysics and physiology of hearing.* London/New York: Academic Press.

Gaese, B., & Ostwald, J. (1990). Coding of sinusoidally frequency and amplitude modulated stimuli in the auditory cortex of the rat. In N. Elsner (Ed.), *Brain-perception-cognition: Proceedings of the 18th Göttingen neurobiology conference* (p. 151). Stuttgart/New York: Thieme.

Goldstein, J. (1973). An optimum processor theory for the central formation of pitch of complex tones. *Journal of the Acoustic Society of America, 54,* 1496–1516.

Goldstein, J., & Srulovicz, P. (1977). Auditory-nerve spikes intervals as an adequate basis for aural frequency measurement. In Evans & Wilson (pp. 337–346).

Handel, S. (1989). *Listening: An introduction to the perception of auditory events.* Cambridge, MA/London: M.I.T. Press.

Hesse, H. P. (1972). *Zur Wahrnehmung von Tonhöhe und Klangfarbe als Problem der Hörtheorie.* Köln: A. Volk.

Houtsma, A., & Goldstein, J. (1972). The central origin of the pitch of complex tones: Evidence from musical interval recognition. *Journal of the Acoustic Society of America, 51,* 520–529.

Hudspeth, A. (1985, November). The cellular basis of hearing: The biophysics of hair cells. *Science, 230,* 745–752.

Keidel, W. D. (1992). Das Phänomen des Hörens: Ein interdisziplinärer Diskurs, T.1, 2. *Naturwissenschaften, 79,* 300–310; 347–357.

Keidel, W. D. (Ed.). (1975). *Physiologie des Gehörs. Akustische Informationsverarbeitung.* With contributions by E. David, P. Finkenzeller, S. Kallert, W. D. Keidel, K. H. Plattig, G. Rinsdorf, & M. Spreng. Stuttgart: Thieme.

Keidel, W. D., & Neff, W. D. (Eds.). (1974–1976). *Handbook of sensory physiology, vol. V,* 1–3. Berlin/Heidelberg/New York: Springer.

Keidel, W. D., & Kallert, S. (1979). Physiologie des afferenten akustischen Systems. In J. Berendes, R. Link, & F. Zöllner (Eds.), *Hals-Nasen-Ohren-Heilkunde in Praxis und Klinik,* Bd. 5, 2 (pp. 1–106). Stuttgart: Thieme.

Khanna, S., & Leonard, D. (1982). Basilar membrane tuning in the cat cochlea. *Science, 215,* 305–306.

Khanna, S., Ulfendahl, M., & Flock, A. (1989). Waveforms and spectra of cellular vibrations in the organ of Corti. *Acta Otolaryngologica* (Stockholm). *Suppl. 467,* 189–193.

Koffka, K. (1936). *Principles of Gestalt psychology.* London: Kegan Paul, Trench, Truebner.

Merzenich, M. M., Roth, G. L., Anderson, R. A., Knight, P. L., & Colwell, S. A. (1977). Some basic features of the central auditory nervous system. In Evans & Wilson, pp. 485–495.

Merzenich, M. (1981). Some recent observations on the fundamental organization of the central auditory nervous system. In Y. Katsuki, R. Norgren, & M. Sato (Eds.), *Brain mechanisms of sensation* (pp. 1–19). Chichester/New York: Wiley.

Moore, B. (1982). *An introduction to the psychology of hearing.* 2nd ed. London/New York: Academic Press.

Moore, B. (Ed.). (1986). *Frequency selectivity in hearing.* London/New York; Academic Press.

Nordmark, J. (1970). Time and frequency analysis. In J. Tobias (Ed.), *Foundations of modern auditory theory, vol. 1,* (pp. 55–83). London/New York: Academic Press.

Pantev, C., Hoke, M., Lehnertz, K., Lütkenhöner, B., Anogianakis, G., & Wittkowski, W. (1988). Tonotopic organization of the human auditory cortex revealed by transient auditory evoked magnetic fields. *Electroencephalography and Clinical Neurophysiology, 69,* 160–170.

Parncutt, R. (1988). *Harmony: A psychoacoustical approach.* New York/Heidelberg/Berlin: Springer.

Patterson, R. (1973). The effects of relative phase and number of components on residue pitch. *Journal of the Acoustic Society of America, 53,* 1565–1572.

Patterson, R. (1989). The tone height of multi-harmonic tone. In (n.e.) *The first international conference on music perception and cognition, Kyoto, Japan, October 1989* (pp. 119–124). Kyoto, Japan: University of Kyoto, Faculty of Fine Arts.

Patterson, R., & Wightman, F. (1976). Residue pitch as a function of component spacing. *Journal of the Acoustic Society of America, 59,* 1450–1459.

Petroni, N., Degrassi, F., & Pasquariello, G. (1992). *Detection of pitch in random acoustic signals by neural networks.* (Preprint.) Bari, Italy: University of Bari.

Petroni, N., Degrassi, F., & Pasquariello, G. (1993). Detection of pitch and residue pitch in random acoustic signals. In J. Laaksarno & J. Louhivuoi (Eds.), *Proceedings of the first international conference on cognitive musicology, Jyväskylä, August 1993* (pp. 20–37). Jyväskylä: Department of Music.

Petsche, H. (Ed.). (1989). *Musik – Gehirn – Spiel: Fourth Karajan symposium, Vienna, 1988.* Basel/Boston/Berlin: Birkhäuser.

Pickles, J. (1988). *An introduction to the physiology of hearing.* 2nd ed. London: Academic Press.

Plomp, R. (1976). *Aspects of tone sensation: A psychophysical study.* London: Academic Press.

Plomp, R., & Smoorenburg, G. F. (Eds.). (1970). *Frequency analysis and periodicity detection in hearing.* Leiden: Sijthoff.

Reinecke, H. P. (1964). *Experimentelle Beiträge zur Psychologie des musikalischen Hörens.* Hamburg: Sikorski.

Ritsma, R. (1970). Periodicity detection. In R. Plomp & G. F. Smoorenburg, pp. 250–263.

Romani, G. L., Williamson, S., & Kaufman, L. I. (1982, June). Tonotopic organization of the human auditory cortex. *Science, 216,* 1339–1340.

Sano, H., & Jenkins, B. (1991). A neural network model for pitch perception. In P. Todd & D. G. Loy (Eds.), *Music and connectionism* (pp. 42–53). Cambridge, MA/London: M.I.T. Press.

Schneider, A., & Beurmann, A. (1991). Tonsysteme, Frequenzdistanz, Klangformen und die Bedeutung experimenteller Forschung für die Vergleichende Musikwissenschaft. In C. Floros, H. Marx, & P. Petersen (Eds.), *Hamburger Jahrbuch der Musikwiss, 11* (Laaber 1992) (pp. 179–223). Laaber: Laaber Verlag.

Schneider, A., & Beurmann, A. (1994a). Zur Wahrnehmung von Klängen mit inharmonischen Spektren. In E. T. Hilscher (Ed.), *Festschrift für F. Födermayr* (pp. 45–70). Vienna: Österr. Akad. der Wiss.

Schneider, A., & Beurmann, A. (1994b). Perception of inharmonic sounds: Further experimental findings. *Systematische Musikwiss./Systematic Musicology 2,* Bratislava, 1–31.

Schouten, J. (1940). The perception of pitch. *Philips Technical Review, 5,* 286–294.

Schouten, J. (1970). The residue revisited. In Plomp & Smoorenburg, pp. 41–54.

Shofner, W., & Young, E. (1985). Excitatory/inhibitory response types in the cochlear nucleus: Relationships to discharge patterns and responses to electrical stimulation of the auditory nerve. *Journal of Neurophysiology, 54,* 917–939.

Stumpf, C. (1883/1890). *Tonpsychologie, vols. 1–2.* Leipzig: S. Hirzel.

Terhardt, E. (1972). Zur Tonhöhenwahrnehmung von Klängen. *Acustica, 26,* 173–199.

Terhardt, E., Stoll, G., & Seewann, M. (1982a). Pitch of complex signals according to virtual-pitch theory: Tests, examples, and predictions. *Journal of the Acoustic Society of America, 71,* 671–678.

Terhardt, E., Stoll, M., & Seewann, M. (1982b). Algorithm for extraction of pitch and salience from complex tonal signals. *Journal of the Acoustic Society of America, 71,* 679–688.

Tobias, J. (Ed.). (1970). *Foundations of modern auditory theory, vols.1–2.* London/New York: Academic Press.

Torgerson, W. (1961). Distances and ratios in psychophysical scaling. *Acta Psychologica, 19,* 201–205.

Walliser, K. (1969). Zusammenhänge zwischen dem Schallreiz und der Periodentonhöhe. *Acustica, 21,* 319–328.

Warren, R. (1982). *Auditory perception: A new synthesis.* New York/Oxford: Pergamon Press.

Whitfield, I. (1967). *The auditory pathway.* London: Arnold.

Whitfield, I. (1977). "Auditory space" and the role of the cortex in sound localization. In Evans & Wilson, pp. 475–484.

Wightman, F. (1973). The pattern-transformation model of pitch. *Journal of the Acoustic Society of America, 54,* 407–416.

Zatorre, R. (1984). Musical perception and cerebral function: A critical review. *Music Perception, 2,* 196–221.

Zwicker, E. (1982). *Psychoakustik.* Berlin/Heidelberg/New York: Springer.

RHYTHMIC FACILITATION OF MOVEMENT SEQUENCING: EFFECTS ON SPATIOTEMPORAL CONTROL AND SENSORY MODALITY DEPENDENCE

Michael H. Thaut, Susan H. Brown, Jennifer Benjamin, and J. David Cooke

Aim of Investigation

The observation that complex motor behavior can be stimulated and organized through musical rhythm has been documented across all ages and cultures. Physical activities requiring repeated and coordinated rhythmic movements are often paced by music or chants. Indeed, the universality of the function of music to elicit and structure physical response suggests an intrinsic biological importance of music and rhythm to integrate and organize complex motor activity (Merriam, 1964). Surprisingly, however, our understanding of the physiological mechanisms involved in this phenomenon is very poor, and it is this paucity of scientific knowledge that has contributed to the rather limited acceptance of rhythmic auditory stimulation in, for example, motor rehabilitation. To further elucidate the evidence in our recent research work that rhythmic auditory cues can facilitate gait performance in patients with stroke (Thaut, McIntosh, Prassas & Rice, 1993) and Parkinson's disease (McIntosh, Thaut, Rice & Miller, 1994), we have set up a number of experiments to study underlying mechanisms in interactions between the auditory and the motor systems. Of initial interest were two questions for us:

1. Can auditory rhythm improve the even timing of sequential arm movements during tasks with different spatial requirements when compared to uncued timing? and
2. Is the ability to recall and reproduce temporal stimulus sequences through arm movements enhanced by stimulus presentation in the auditory mode compared to the visual and tactile modality?

Results from these studies were intended to give us a better understanding of how the central nervous system translates rhythmic auditory stimulation into efficient motor control strategies and how peripheral rhythmic input might be utilized in motor rehabilitation.

Methods: Rhythmic Sequencing Study

The effects of rhythmic auditory cueing on the spatiotemporal organization of sequential movements were examined in a forward arm-reaching task with five healthy subjects, ages 19 to 23. Each sequence was comprised of four movements made to different target locations oriented vertically in front of the subjects. Each sequence consisted of five targets (distance between adjacent targets = 8 cm) requiring alternating flexion and extension movements about the elbow (Figure 1).

Elbow movement was recorded using electrogoniometers at a sampling rate of 100 Hz. Extension/flexion reversal points were used to determine contact point on the target marker. Two tasks were examined: (a) alternating (right arm followed by left arm) and (b) simultaneous (movements of both arms) (Figure 2).

In each task, subjects were instructed to touch target markers (3 cm in diameter) in a given order at a regular rate of 2 Hz. Subjects were given several minutes to visually examine the target sequence and memorize it, so learning would not play a role in their performance. Subjects first performed each task without auditory cueing. In this condition,

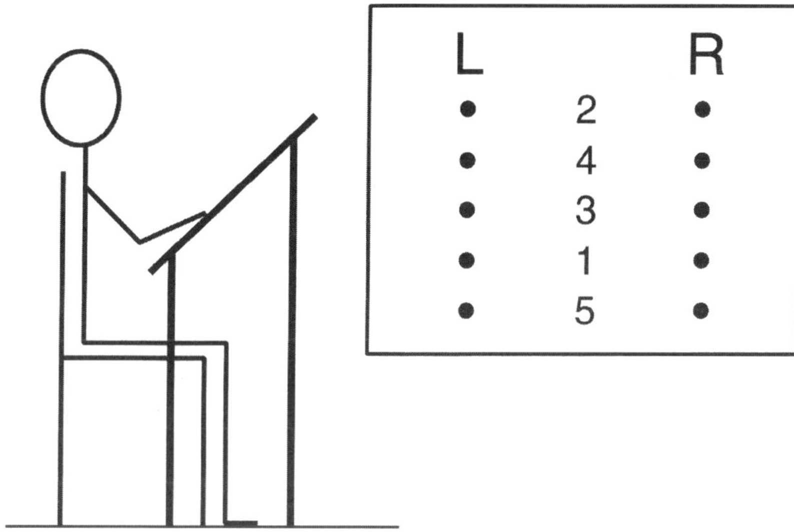

Figure 1. Experimental setup: Tilt table with target surface laid out in a sample sequence.

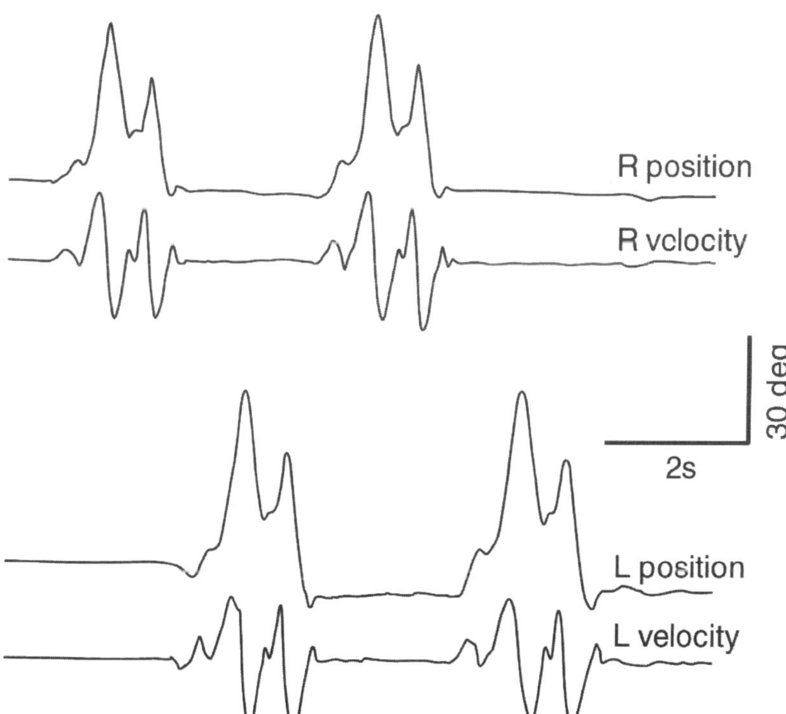

Figure 2. Goniometer traces for position and velocity of elbow flexion-extension movements during a target tracking task with alternating arm movements (upper traces = right arm; lower traces = left arm).

subjects tapped out the desired movement frequency with their finger before starting the movement sequence. In the second condition, subjects moved in time to a rhythmic auditory cue delivered as a 2 Hz metronome beat imbedded in an instrumental musical background.

Results: Rhythmic Sequencing Study

Without auditory cueing, subjects were unable to produce sequential movements with even timing. In contrast, rhythmic auditory cueing led to a significant ($p < .05$) decrease in variability of movement duration, particularly for alternating movements in which variability, as expressed by coefficients of variation, decreased between 30 to 60 percent (Figure 3).

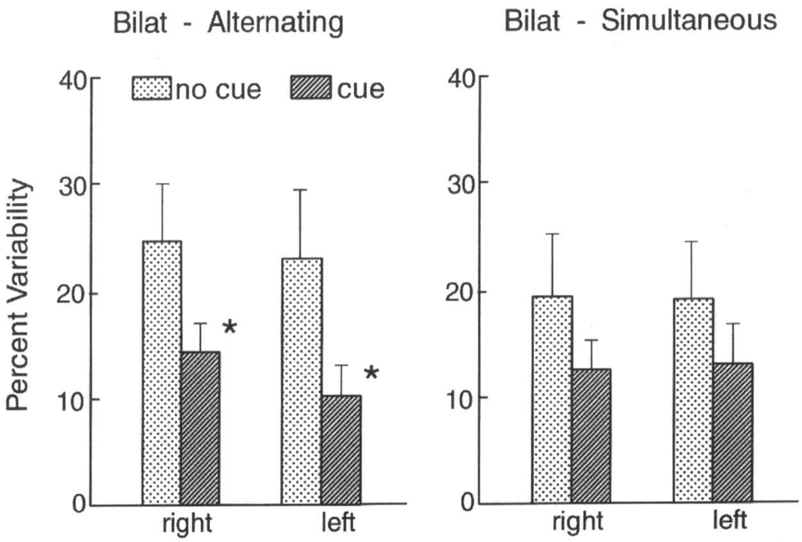

Figure 3. Graphic display of coefficients of variability for alternating and simultaneous right and left arm movements with rhythmic cueing (cue) and without cueing (no cue).

Thus, movement durations remained relatively constant despite a threefold increase in intertarget distance. In addition, auditory cueing in the alternating task led to a significant reduction in variability in the time required to switch movements from one arm to the other. The data suggest that, in the presence of a rhythmic auditory cue, arm movement velocity was appropriately scaled so as to produce evenly timed movement sequences whereas without rhythmic pacemaker movement durations were driven by the spatial requirements of the intertarget distance, that is, durations increased with target distance (Figure 4).

Methods: Sensory Modality Study

Temporal beat patterns were delivered to three groups of college age subjects (n = 6 per group) in the visual, auditory, and tactile sensory modality, respectively. Subjects were

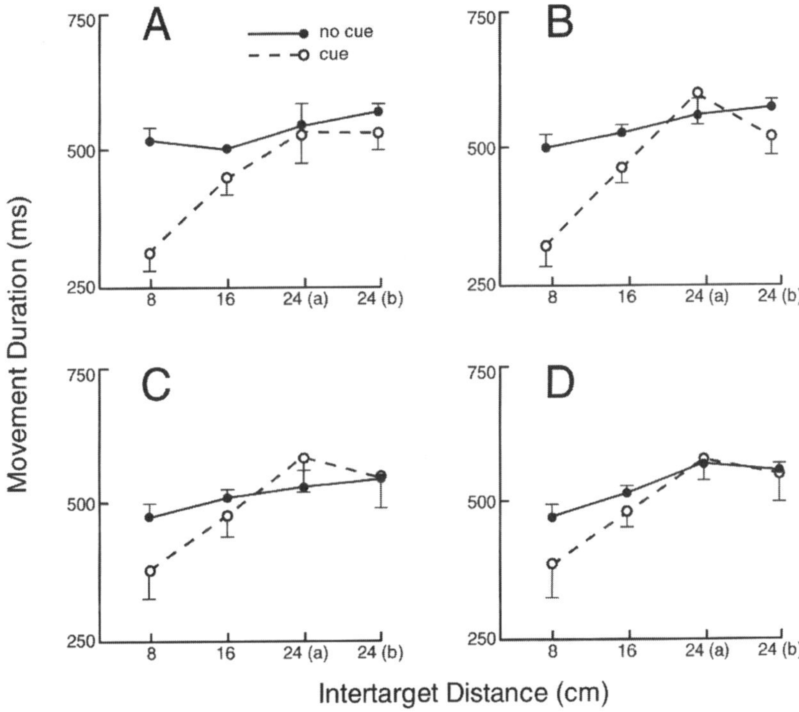

Figure 4. Movement durations (y-axis) plotted as a function of target distance (x-axis) for 4 representative subjects. All 4 plots show a linear dependency of movement durations on target distance without cueing and a change of durations to even timing regardless of target distance with cueing.

asked to tap out the sequences with the ulnar side of the hand unto a padded target plate, using a flexion-extension movement about the elbow. The target plate was located on an adjustable tilt table surface right in front of the subjects, so subjects did not need to visually guide their movements. The auditory beats were presented as 1000 Hz tone bursts via headphones; the visual cues were presented as red LED 75 cm away in a perpendicular plane to the subject's eyes; and the tactile stimulus was delivered via a rotator cuff attached to the nonmoving forearm. In each sensory modality the stimulus had a plateau time of 50 msec. The timing sequences ranged from 3 to 11 stimuli and consisted of random beat intervals of 250, 500, 750 and 1000 msecs. Each pattern was presented three times. Subjects were asked to observe each timing pattern, and then tap it back as accurately as possible. There were no time constraints on the subject's response time. All experiments were conducted in a darkened room to enhance visual perception of the LED and provide environmental consistency across sensory modalities.

Results: Sensory Modality Study

Interstimulus interval (ISI) recall was considered accurate when the subject stayed within +/- 20% of the intended duration. Auditory cueing resulted in a significantly greater number of accurate ISI reproductions as compared to tactile (short patterns: $p < .03$; long patterns: $p < .0001$) or visual cueing (short: $p < .002$; long: $p < .0001$) In analyzing percent accuracy of interval duration (1/relative error), auditory cueing resulted in greater overall accuracy in reproducing intended interval durations as compared to tactile (short: $p < .001$; long: $p < .001$) or visual (short: $p < .0006$; long: $p < .03$) (Figure 5). Representative traces of movement responses for each sensory modality are shown in figure 6.

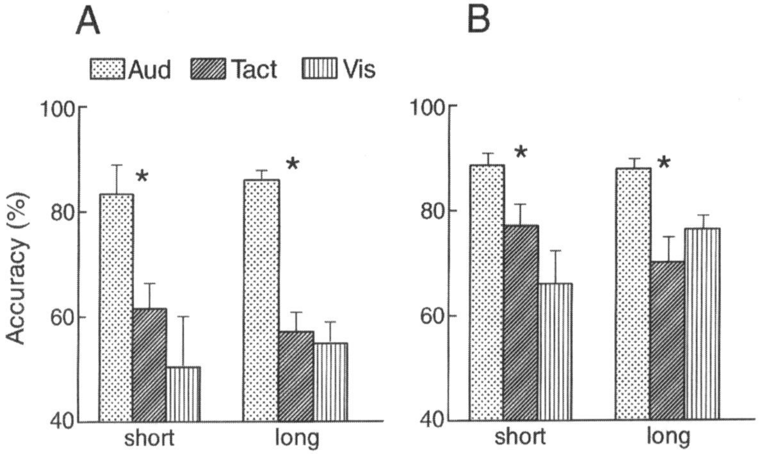

Figure 5. Accuracy of interstimulus interval reproductions (A) and percent accuracy of interval durations (1/relative error) (B) for auditory, tactile and visual stimulus presentations.

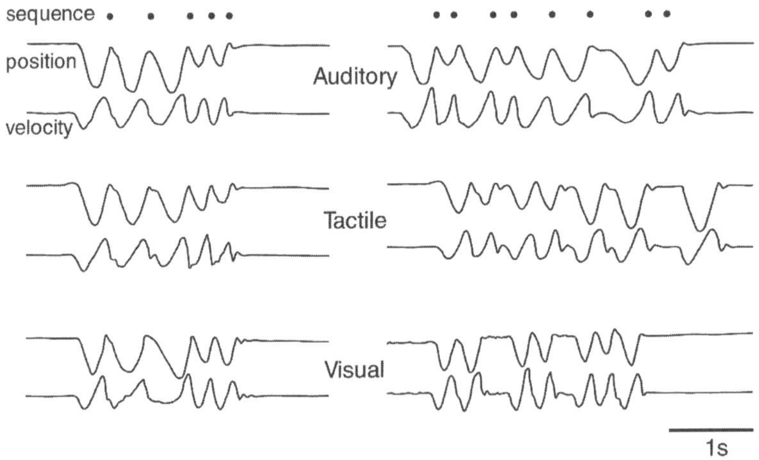

Figure 6. Representative position and velocity profiles of one subject's elbow flexion-extension movements during recall of a short (left side) and long (right side) stimulus sequence. The dots above the curves represent the stimuli, the distance between the stimuli represent the time intervals between the stimuli. Reversal points of the movement profiles indicate target contact. Clearly visible is the close tap to stimulus interval consistency in the auditory modality whereas tapping in the tactile and visual modality are characterized by irregular stimulus intervals and missing stimuli in the tapping sequence.

Conclusions

Without rhythmic cueing movement durations within a sequence varied systematically with changes in intertarget distance. Internal clock output to maintain even movement durations was unable to override the spatial constraints of the movement task. The presence of a rhythmic pacing signal as external clock source facilitated the ability to adequately scale movement kinematics so as to maintain even movement durations in the face of changing spatial demands.

In tasks in which timing information was conveyed through different sensory modalities, the ability to reproduce temporally varying stimulus patterns into movement patterns was greatest when the pattern was delivered in the auditory modality. Regardless of pattern length or complexity, the auditory system was more effective in the transfer of timing information into correctly timed motor sequences.

Both studies shed new light on the efficiency of rhythmic auditory cueing in facilitating the spatiotemporal organization of complex, sequential movements. In the first study, whereas spatial task constraints confounded internal rhythmic timing mechanisms, auditory rhythm as an external clock structure produced stable movement durations during varying spatial tasks demands. In the second study, temporal pattern recall was enhanced in the auditory modality.

It is well known that the auditory system is a fast acting system with brief peripheral delay at the transduction level in response to external stimulation (Abeles, Prut, Bergman, Vaadia, & Aertsen, 1993). Since acoustical stimuli evolve continually along a time axis and cannot be 'frozen' in time or space without losing essential characteristics of the information, the auditory system must analyze temporal information quite rapidly. Indeed, comparisons between neural and behavioral response times to auditory and visual stimulation have shown a small but consistent advantage for the auditory modality (Chapman, Spidalieri, & Lamarre, 1986). At the present, we do not know where rhythmic acoustical patterns are translated into rhythmic motor patterns in the brain. However, the results of the two studies we report here underline the importance and efficiency of auditory rhythm to act as external clock source and temporal control template for programming and execution of complex movement sequences.

References

Abeles, M., Prut, Y., Bergman, H., Vaadia, E., & Aertsen, A. (1993). Integration, synchronicity, and periodicity. In A. Aertsen (Ed.), *Brain theory* (pp. 149–181). New York: Elsevier.

Chapman, C. E., Spidalieri, G., & Lamarre, Y. (1986). Activity of dentate neurons during arm movements triggered by visual, auditory, and somesthetic stimuli in the monkey. *Journal of Neurophysiology, 55*, 203–226.

McIntosh, G. C., Thaut, M. H., Rice, R. R., & Miller, R. A. (in press). Stride frequency modulation in Parkinsonian gait using rhythmic auditory stimulation. *Annals of Neurology.*

Merriam, A. P. (1964). The anthropology of music. Evanston IL: Northwestern University Press.

Thaut, M. H., McIntosh, G. C., Prassas, S. G., & Rice, R. R. (1993). Effect of rhythmic auditory cueing on temporal stride parameters and EMG patterns in hemiparetic gait of stroke patients. *Journal of Neurologic Rehabilitation, 7*, 9–16.

II.

MUSIC, SPECIFIC POPULATIONS, AND THERAPY

A CALL FOR RESEARCH ON THE EFFECTS OF POPULAR MUSIC ON ADOLESCENT BEHAVIOR

Joe Stuessy

Music affects behavior. It is wonderful that in the past few decades, the body of research has grown steadily and has strongly confirmed what people since Damon and Plato intuitively understood, namely, that music affects human behavior.

As the evidence continues to mount, however, we are confronted with a good news/ bad news situation. For if music can have positive effects, then we must also admit that it can have negative effects. Although I would prefer not to be the bearer of bad tidings, I am afraid that appears to be my role. Since the mid 1980s, I have been involved in a national debate about the relationship between certain types of popular music and adolescent behavior. In that debate, it has been my position that music can be one of the factors influencing negative behavior. One of the most frustrating things about this debate, no matter what position one takes, is that there is little or no valid research on the topic. And that is why I am here to talk to you today.

The Need for Research

An entire generation of youth is growing up today surrounded by styles of music that explicitly encourage violence. Young people absorb the music in large quantities for many hours per day. Critical observers, including psychiatrists whose specialty is adolescents, law enforcement personnel, music educators, and attorneys, have speculated that there is a direct causal relationship between the musical environment and violent behavior. Parents have also speculated that the music may have more subtle effects, such as attitudinal changes regarding authority, sex, and drugs.

In light of the number of subjects potentially affected (millions of teens and preteens), and their well-publicized actions (including murders, suicides, rapes, etc.), there is a shocking paucity of objective research in this area. Although some studies have clearly established a correlative relationship between aberrant behavior and musical preference, few, if any, have probed the causal aspect of this phenomenon. As a result, we must rely on anecdotal evidence for our conclusions. I will now describe three incidents in which music appears to have been involved and then conclude with my plea for an active research agenda in this area.

Case One

For legal reasons, I shall avoid using real names in the following case studies. The first case involves a young man ("Robert") who had fallen under the spell of a powerful and charismatic friend who was fascinated with Satanism. Robert was not a strong personality and came from what it often called a dysfunctional family. When I was growing up, we referred to people like Robert as "leeches" because, lacking their own individual strength, they latched on to a peer whom they perceived as popular and attractive. They became inseparable from the hero figure, usually adapting their own persona to reflect that of their idol. Thus, the leech would modify hair styles, clothing styles, and even ways of walking and talking; in addition, he would also modify attitudes, philosophies, and musical preferences. That is what happened with Robert.

Robert's hero was an attractive and popular student in the school. Unbeknownst to all but his closest associates, the hero was also a Satanist. [It is not clear whether he was a serious Satanist, or merely posed as a Satanist in order to enhance his anticultural image with his more impressionable associates, including Robert.] A small group of four boys, including the leader and Robert, began reading Satanic propaganda, practicing Satanic rituals, and listening to a certain style of heavy metal rock music often called black metal. Such music has lyrics that praise Lord Satan, denigrate traditional religions, and are generally rather dark and morose in tone. The music is often described by normal listeners as sounding angry.

Robert's group gradually moved from reading and talking about Satanism to actually performing animal sacrifices. For some time, they had agreed that the real thrill would be a human sacrifice. On a given evening, the group's leader informed Robert and another friend that it was time to take the big step. The victim was to be the fourth member of the group, a boy who was considered the weakest member. All four boys loaded themselves into a vehicle and headed for a remote rural area. (Later testimony indicated that some alcohol and drugs were consumed.) On the way to the site, they repetitively played a song by their favorite rock group that spoke of bleeding brains and violence.

When they reached their destination, they proceeded to sacrifice a cat. Then three of the boys turned on the fourth member and beat him to death with baseball bats. They threw the body down a nearby well.

No one would claim that the music made these young men commit murder. However, one can speculate that the music was one of the factors in their behavior. Listening over and over to such music for a period of months or years may have had the effect of reinforcing certain attitudes. And the repetitive listening on the way to the sacrificial site may have had the effect of enhancing their psychological state for the big adventure.

Case Two

Frank and his friend also came from a dysfunctional family. They were heavily into drugs and alcohol and listened repetitively to a style of heavy metal rock that often dealt with suicide as a solution to life's problems. On a certain evening, both boys were in Frank's room getting stoned and listening repetitively to a favorite song about suicide. Later testimony revealed that there was a subaudible track mixed into the recording that repeated the words, "Get a gun; shoot, shoot."

At a certain point in the evening, the boys decided to take a gun and go to a nearby park and shoot themselves. They did so, but miraculously, Frank lived. He had blown most of his face off, but somehow survived. He later testified that while listening to the music, he and his friend had felt an irresistible urge to shoot themselves. Frank stated in very clear terms that he felt the music had affected their actions.

Frank eventually died from his wounds. Again, we are left with troubling questions. As always, other factors were involved (drugs, alcohol, dysfunctional family, easily accessible weapons, etc.). But among those factors was the music telling them to do exactly what they did. In spite of all the other factors, could it have been the music that literally triggered their immediate behavior?

Case Three

The third case involves a style of music known as "gangsta rap." This style often has lyrics that preach violence against women, police, and Caucasians (especially white cops). Warren was almost obsessed with gangsta rap music. When he was arrested for murder at the age of 19, he had some 900 tapes in his possession. Friends testified that he listened constantly to the music. They further said that he was actually a rather mild mannered young man, until he put on his headphones. Suddenly, his demeanor would change and he became "bad", changing his posture, his walk, his attitude.

But our story must go much further back. Warren's mother simply did not want to be bothered with raising a child and his father was not a part of the household. At a very young age, Warren was turned over to his grandmother, who had racist tendencies. In court testimony, she said that she thoroughly distrusted white people and felt that the world would be a better place if there were no white people in it. When an attorney asked her if she had communicated that attitude to Warren, her response was, "You damn right I did!"

By the age of 9 Warren was dealing drugs off the back of his bicycle. He also began stealing cars. Between the ages of 9 and 19, Warren had been arrested for over 300 car thefts. He simply stole a car, was arrested, turned loose, and, needing a new set of wheels, stole another car! Not surprisingly, Warren became associated with a gang, which led to frequent violent encounters with the police. He grew to hate cops—especially white cops.

On the night in question, Warren was speeding down a rural highway in a stolen car. On the cassette player in the car, Warren was playing one of his favorite rap albums. The album contained a song that described an incident in which a young black man is pulled over by a white officer; the young man shoots the officer. Ironically, Warren looked into his rear view mirror and saw a state trooper behind him with his red lights flashing.

Warren pulled over and saw the white state trooper walking up to the stolen car. As Warren later testified, "the cop was grinnin' so I knew he was going to jack me around." Warren was listening to the music; he saw the cop approaching; everything began to flood together in his mind—Grandma, the gangs, the drugs, the numerous arrests, the white cops, and all those years of gangsta rap.

Now the cop was at his window. "Fuck the police; I ain't gonna take this shit!" He fired the gun. The officer—a husband and father of two children—was dead. Only a year earlier, he had been decorated for saving an entire family in a burning house.

Was the music a factor in Warren's behavior? I think so. I believe it acted in two ways. First, over the years, the messages in the music reinforced Warren's distrust and hatred for police—especially white police officers. Second, at a moment of maximum tension, the music playing at the time acted as a triggering device for Warren's actual behavior.

If you doubt that the music was a factor in Warren's behavior, try a slightly different scenario. Keep all the other factors the same (Grandma, the drugs, the gangs, etc.). But change the music so that Warren had listened to years of the Carpenters. And, as he was pulled over that night, the music playing on the cassette was Barry Manilow. With only those changes, would Warren have shot the officer? Of course, I do not know for sure and neither do you. But I would suggest that just by changing the music, Warren would have been **less likely** to have used his gun. If that is true, it is impossible to deny that the music was a factor in his behavior.

Implications of Correlational and Anecdotal Studies

Some will argue, of course, that it is not so much the music as the lyrics that are the real operative factors. But studies have shown that we absorb and retain text more readily when it is attached to music. How many of you learned the alphabet by singing it?

Others will argue that I am confusing the chicken with the egg. Indeed, studies have shown that dysfunctional adolescents have a strong preference for music that contains negative lyric themes and certain musical characteristics. So does the person's attitude lead to certain musical preferences, or do musical preferences lead to certain attitudes? I cannot answer that question, but I can suggest that if one has a given attitude, repetitive listening to certain music can reinforce that attitude.

We must acknowledge, of course, that many other factors play powerful roles in any given behavior. In the three cases cited earlier, there were the factors of drugs, alcohol, dysfunctional families, peer influences, and the like. Indeed, anecdotal studies suggest that aberrant behavior is caused by the accumulation of a matrix of such factors (including music), but that music may act as a "triggering mechanism" for a specific behavior.

The Challenge to Researchers

Last week, someone in our local newspaper asked why it seems that the current generation of youth is so terribly violent. I submit that it hardly takes a rocket scientist to figure that out. From an early age, children are surrounded by violent television shows, violent video games, violent movies, and violent music. Can anyone then wonder why they behave so violently?

I am thrilled to learn of all the research that has been described at this conference. I am only a musician, not a researcher and must rely on people like you to prove my theories right or wrong. Each of you is dealing with some subset of the big question: How and why does music affect us? I would urge you to consider the immense implications of research into the more specific question of how popular music affects adolescent behavior. With what seems to be an entire generation involved in a virtual epidemic of violence and sexual promiscuity, it seems only reasonable to heed the observations of those who are closest to the action. Because of our belief that music affects behavior, we must consider the possibility that certain styles of popular music may be one of the powerful players in this epidemic. And if the music is one of the influential factors, we need to know it and we need to know how that influence operates.

The required research is complex. At the very least, we must seek answers to the following multifaceted questions:

1. What particular physiological, affective, and behavioral responses are elicited in teen and preteen listeners by certain popular musical styles?
2. Are there discernible relationships among specific musical elements and specific responses?
3. What relationships exist between various physiological and behavioral responses?

Within each of these basic questions lies a myriad of subquestions. The challenge is a daunting one. But the importance for society, now and in the future, is massive. We must begin.

SKINHEADS AND VIOLENCE: BLAME IT ON OI!-MUSIC?

Renate Müller

Introduction

Not with hatred shall we persecute those who hate—we want justice, we do not want revenge. To begin with this main idea of Simon Wiesenthal's 1992 book *Recht, nicht Rache, Erinnerungen (Justice, Not Revenge)* does not mean that the incomprehensible injuries of victims of xenophobic violence are trivialized. It does mean, however, that certain questions must be addressed: What are the social conditions that lead to hostility and violence against foreigners? Can skinhead violence be attributed to their hate-filled songs? and What can be done about xenophobic violence, which is primarily a crime committed by young people?

My position, which will be argued from theoretical and empirical perspectives, is vulnerable for the following reasons: It is apologistic because I am attempting to understand indefensible behavior; and it may be seen as politically naive because I regard skinheads as members of a youth culture.

The opposing view would hold that barbarians do not have any culture (Treptow, 1993).

My empirically-based arguments derive from:

1. Results of a biographical long-term study (Heitmeyer, Buhse, Liebe-Freund, Möller, Müller, Ritz, Siller, & Vossen, 1992);

2. Results from analyses of reports and court records on violent xenophobic delinquents, and of escalating incidences of violence against foreigners like those in Rostock in 1992 (Willems, Würtz, & Eckert, 1993);

3. Results of journalistic inquiry and a survey on skinheads (Farin & Seidel-Pielen, 1993);

4. Street workers' reports on projects of so-called "accepting youth work" (Heim, Krafeld, Lutzebäck, Schaar, Storm, & Welp, 1992; Krafeld, Möller, & Müller, 1993);

5. Secret service reports (Skinheads n.d.; Skinheads, 1992; Skinheads, 1993);

6. Examination of the lyrics of skinhead songs, based on 53 taped songs from six different skin bands, and the lyrics of nearly 100 more songs from 16 skin bands, most of which were submitted to me by the secret service.

Statement of Problem

This paper will focus on those persons and groups who approve or even commit crime and violent acts against foreigners and who stand up for xenophobic violence, such as that found in songs. We do not know how many of the 18 millions of young persons in Germany between the ages of 13 and 29 are in this subpopulation (Zinnecker & Fischer, 1992, p. 21). Most young persons (82%) seem to disapprove of skinheads (p. 218).

Acts of violence against foreigners have increased since 1991. Two hundred and fifty acts of violence between 1987 and 1990 were followed by nearly 10 times as many in 1991. This came to nearly 2500, 76% of which, however, did not include assaults against persons. In 1992, more than 6,300 cases were registered, which is nearly three times as many as in 1991 (Willems et al., 1993, pp. 7–10). No further increase was observed in 1993 (Leyendecker, 1993, p. 70).

According to analyses of delinquency reports and court records, 90% of acts of violence against foreigners emerge out of group processes. In addition, 25% of the offenders are politically motivated with ties to rightist groups (these are the older offenders over 25); 10% are criminals (brawlers), former juvenile delinquents, and also over 25 years of age; 60% are members of youth cultures (e.g., skinhead cultures), or they are at least fellow-travelers in similar recreational groups (Willems et al., 1993, pp. 76–81).

The last mentioned group constitutes offenders who commit violence against foreigners. What kind of young people are drawn toward hostility and violence against foreigners? Why do young people searching for identity seek membership in violence-oriented and xenophobic youth cultures?

Theoretical Approach

Self-Socialization and Identity Building

The theoretical construct of the argument is based on symbolic interaction and the social use of symbol systems that include language, clothing, and music. Becoming a member of the skinhead culture is conceptualized as a process of self-socialization (Müller, 1995). The use of Nazi symbols as well as oi!-music and violent behavior is viewed as an important part of identity building. The underlying theory includes the concept of the individual choice of socializing environments and cultural codes that ascribe social meaning to aesthetic objects. Modern societies, which are not homogenous but culturally diverse, offer options of membership in different subcultures and corresponding life-styles. There are plenty of musical cultures that define themselves by musical style. Thus, cultural identity and ways in which that identity is manifested become a matter of individual choice. Individuals socialize themselves by their choice of membership in cultures, and their efforts to become familiar with the chosen symbol systems. Youth cultures can be viewed as centers of self-socialization.

Everybody is his or her own identity builder and style setter. Symbols available in the culture are selected to dress up in front of others and to fulfill others' expectations. Symbols become estranged from their traditional meanings; new meanings are affixed to them and they become part of new symbol systems used in new contexts. Symbols are also used to evoke traditional meaning for example, when skinheads used working clothes, boots, and bald heads to refer to their proletarian origin. This point will be discussed later.

Skinhead Culture: The Social Use of Symbols

The view that skinhead culture is related to youth and youthful protests rather than a political movement can be supported by skinheads' own utterances in interviews, song lyrics, and statements made in court. A contrasting position holds that skinhead power is a new national-socialistic, Fascist, rightist political movement rather than a youth culture (Bähr, 1993; Butterwegge, 1993).

My research has uncovered many songs whose theme is social problems like drug use and homelessness. Therefore, one might as well say that skinhead culture in many respects is the ideal authentic and autonomous youth culture, as youth theorists would have it: emanating from the underground, not manipulated by mass media, maladjusted, critical, shocking, and creative.

The Clothing. The skinhead outfit often is called martial, which, according to the secret service, is a distinguishing characteristic of skinheads (Skinheads, n.d., p. 3; Skinheads, 1992, p. 2). This is not entirely accurate, although skinheads often wear bomber jackets, battle clothes, and parachutist boots. The skinhead outfit is also proletarian, consisting of bald heads, working clothes, boots, and suspenders, all of which symbolize a proletarian culture. Bald heads are a symbol of former oppressions. Laborers who had protested against oppressive measures were punished by having their heads shaved, thus robbing them of their dignity and identity. The new meaning of this symbol of oppression is "proud to be a proletarian". In fact, short hair is practical during fights, and skinheads love fighting. In addition, bald heads mean a demarcation against longhaired intellectuals like hippies (Farin & Seidel-Pielen, 1993, pp. 23–24).

Contrary to popular opinion, Doc Martens boots are orthopedic shoes with air-cushioned soles, well known among orthopedists as "Dr. Maertens", and produced in Munich. A British businessman and boots manufacturer bought the license in the early 60s and called the steel-core security shoes "Dr. Martens" because he misspelled "Maertens". Doc Martens are also found in the closets of Madonna and U2 (Dolak, 1993, p. 32). They are also very popular outside of MTV.

The Community. The first skinheads appeared in the early 70s in London as protesters against the loss of their turf in London's traditional laborers' quarters, thus expressing a sense of feeling alienated in their own country. They shared this feeling and a music genre called ska with London's West Indian immigrants (Farin & Seidel-Pielen, 1993, pp. 23–37). According to Clarke (1979), skinhead culture means the symbolic recovery of community in an environment of collapsing traditional, territorial and social structures. One feels as though he is in a big family. Companionship and solidarity are depicted by members as the most important features of skinhead culture (Farin & Seidel-Pielen, 1993, pp. 6–14). This constitutes a sense of collective solidarity against oppression by those who want to order you about (Clarke, 1979, p. 171).

Nazi Symbols. The use of Nazi symbols by many young people is not necessarily an indicator of a political attitude; on the contrary, it is a way to shock. Nazi symbols rank highest among taboos in German society. Therefore, there is nothing better to serve as a means to shock.

One way to use symbols socially within youth cultures is the following: a meta-communicative utterance of demarcations, on the one hand, and of solidarity on the other. Thus symbols are used to define social relations rather than to communicate content. The message is not "Look at us, we are Nazis," but "Look at us, we don't belong to you. We are breaking your taboos, and we enjoy your anger about it. We are hated, but now you finally have good reason to hate us. We gave it to you because you hate us anyhow."

Violence as a Symbol. Males in lower class cultures are body-oriented. Body orientation is expressed in usually violent defense of territories. Although we may not like this, the idea did not originate with skinheads (Farin & Seidel-Pielen, 1993, pp. 37–38; Clarke, 1979).

Within restrictive social environments such as lower class milieus, the strategy is not one of argument, but of violence. Those who were physically abused as children mistake violent behavior for a normal way of human communication and, even, of personal attention.

The experience of violence means an experience of risk: Violence invites risk to oneself and others of injury and even death. Those who commit violent acts risk punishment and discrimination. Violence is daring. The conscious seeking for extreme experiences that test the body's limits, such as surfing on cars, subway trains, and elevators, or the use of drugs, or horror movies, or violence against foreigners can be seen as objections of youth against oppression of their cultural identity by the educational system. When a person does not see any way that his identity will be accepted, violence becomes a means to validate this identity.

Oi!-Music. Oi! stands for joy. Joy, in this case, means to drink and dance until you fall down. "Strength thru Oi!" was a record title that was a takeoff on "Strength through Joy" (Kraft durch Freude"), a leisure time organization in Nazi Germany that offered the opportunity of a holiday to women and children. Oi!-oi!-oi! is the skinheads' cry. They have changed the German vowel "eu" to "oi" in their songs, band names, and fanzines, for example, Doitschland, Noie Werte, Froinde, Kraft durch Froide.

Music, oi!-music, that is, seems to be the social glue in skinhead culture. Oi!-music can be viewed as a central means of expression within the skinhead culture (Farin & Seidel-Pielen, 1993, p. 192).

Oi!-music developed in London at the end of the 60s (Farin & Seidel-Pielen, 1993, pp. 23–37). Skinheads joined with Black immigrants from the West Indies to use West Indian rock music known as ska. They selected ska because of its pulsing liveliness and its great difference from the music of the mods and hippies, groups to which the skinheads did not want to belong.

Ska developed into Reggae, which meant that it slowed down and started to express political ideas of Black immigrants. Therefore, because of the change in structure, plus nationalistic influences in Great Britain at the time, part of the skinhead culture separated from the West Indians both musically and politically. Two bands, "Screwdriver" and "No Remorse", the idols of today's German skin bands, founded "White Skinpower", which musically merged punk and ska and politically turned out to be white racism. Skinhead culture and oi!-music reached the continent at the end of the 70s. In Germany as well as in Great Britain, the skin scene divided into right and left groups:

1. The leftist groups, including s.h.a.r.p. skins, which means "skinheads against racial prejudice", and red skins gathered around bands that attracted punks as well as skins such as "Sham 69" and "4Skins".

2. The right-wing groups, also called "Fascho-Skins" by the German secret service, or "Party-Skins", which means they contact right-wing organizations. These groups are believed to be politicized oi! skins, with leanings toward racism.

3. The largest group of skinheads is derived, according to the secret service, from the so-called oi! skins. Their primary goal is oi!, joy, and they are not interested in political agitation (Skinheads, n.d., pp. 3–4; Skinheads, 1992, pp. 3–4). However, they do have problems with foreigners that are articulated in skinhead songs, which are often hate filled.

When skinheads meet in concert, they all sing along and dance a kind of "jump'n dance", which is the same as the punks' dance. This is called "Pogue" or "Pogo", wherein people jump against each other. Outsiders such as subculturally uneducated adults look upon this as an aggressive fighting dance. According to the body-oriented ethic of male lower class cultures, however, Pogo might be seen as an expression of solidarity in body contact as well.

Skinheads express their problems with foreigners through their songs, which are furiously screamed and driven rather than sung. An example of this genre is "Asylantek" sung by the skinhead band "Blut und Ehre". The message is: There are too many asylum seekers; a flood of asylum seekers is threatening our country; it is a lie that they are persecuted; the government is supporting asylum seekers instead of the German homeless.

Oi!-music is a means of expressing skinheads' tabooed ideas about foreigners, the German nation, and violence, but it is also a vehicle for expressing the skinhead concept of community. An example of this is "Deutsche Skinheads", a song about the skinhead community sung by the skinhead band "Werwolf vereint". The feeling of being hated is also a frequent subject of skinhead songs and is connected with self hatred. A more detailed discussion of this point will be presented later in the paper.

The musical style of oi!-music is very near to punk, on the one hand, and to heavy metal, on the other. Yet, oi!-music is usually produced on a very low professional level. Skin bands have one or two electric guitars, an electric bass, and drums; a synthesizer is seldom used. The structure of the songs is very simple: Introduction, verse, chorus, and, maybe, a guitar solo. Rhymes are often awkward, and verses rather than choruses are often repeated. The poor professional level is due partly to the fact that the records are mostly self-produced and often copied. Many "bootlegs" exist, the quality of which is even worse than the originals. The low professional level of their music production gives listeners of skin bands the feeling that their lives are on a par with those of their idols (Farin & Seidel-Pielen, 1993, p. 61).

One of the two most popular skinhead bands is the group "Störkraft", whose name means "jamming power, interferential power, or, trouble-making power". The chorus of the song "Kraft für Doitschland" says: "We are the power, the power, the power, the power for Germany, the power that cleans up Germany. We are the power, the power, the power, the power for Germany. Be proud of your country" (Translated by the author).

Oi!-music integrates the elements of skinhead culture and seems to be the most important means of expression. Perhaps this is the reason why oi!-music is blamed for acts of violence against foreigners committed by skinheads.

There are many such unsupported claims like the following: Musical elements such as loudness, speed, distortion, lyrics, and rhythm in oi!-music call forth strong emotions like aggression and hatred that are immediately transposed into acts of violence (de la Motte-Haber, in Ley, 1993, p. 32; Bähr, 1993, p. 12; Skinheads, 1993, p. 10). Effects caused by the music are compared to those of drugs that promote violence (Funk-Hennigs, 1994, p. 19). The patterns of behavior among skinheads are said to be strongly influenced by skin bands (Skinheads, 1993, p. 1). These assertions that claim there is a linear relationship from the song to the act of violence are made without:

1. Considering the variety of attitudes and patterns of opinions within the skinhead scene that is reflected in the diversity of skinhead songs; and

2. Taking into account the meaning of skinhead culture in terms of their members' cultural identities.

The so-called "stimulation hypothesis" is implied in the claim that music arouses acts of violence. Media research, however, does not confirm this theory in empirical studies (Kunczik, 1993, p. 100). Thus, the application of the "stimulation hypothesis" to musical impact on skinhead violence is not clear. In addition, research to date has not produced a high correlation between certain musical elements and the arousal of aggressive emotions, or, even more significant, aggressive behavior (Behne, 1993, 1994).

In the debate about violence, it is conceded, however, that there are some extreme personal and social conditions such as severe neglect or demoralization that, although not yet sufficiently investigated, may, under the influence of media violence, arouse acts of violence (Kunczik, 1993, pp. 103–106). Likewise, there may exist conditions under which music becomes a medium that arouses violence.

From studies of delinquency reports and court records, it is known that, in some cases, oi!-music was present immediately before acts of violence against foreigners were committed (Willems et al., 1993, pp. 86–87). Oi!-music is mentioned in tandem with several other conditions that seem to lead to a propensity toward violent acts. These conditions include:

1. Dysfunction or, at least, problems within the family unit;
2. Poor school records; and
3. The alchemy among oi!-music, alcohol, personal negative experiences with, as well as rumors about foreigners (Willems et al., 1993, pp. 108–109).

These research results concerning xenophobic crime offenders correlate with the view that music is a part, although not the main part, of a process of self-socialization toward violence against foreigners.

If we are taking into consideration the musical impact of xenophobic violence (and especially the effects of rightist lyrics) we should refer to the research of Brown and Schulze (1990, p. 89): "...When we ask 'What does this text mean?' we must also ask 'for whom?'" Who are skinheads? Why do they seek identity through the use of something as highly tabooed as Nazi symbols, racist and nationalistic lyrics, violence, and a kind of music, oi!-music that expresses all of these elements in one medium?

Skinheads' Self-Socialization

The answers to these questions may be partially determined by the following assertions: Skinheads have negative self images and they feel like foreigners in their own country. Skinheads' problems are denied.

Negative Self Image. Skinheads develop negative self images because during their socialization they are not accepted as individuals in their family or in school (Heitmeyer, et al., 1992, p. 357). Skinheads are also not accepted as members of an autonomous youth group. They chose membership in skinhead culture because they found acceptance there, a chance to be, perhaps for the first time in their lives. It does not matter that the attention they draw from outside the skinhead culture is negative and is either hatred or fright. By terrifying others, their identity is validated and, at the same time, their sense of community is affirmed. The following are examples of lyrics from their songs:

1. "Ugly and Mean" by the skinhead band "Bomber":

   I am the personification of evil

'I am bad' is written on my face
Children run away, parents are terrified
I am the reincarnation of evil
I am ugly, mean, bad, and brutal
For others I am a torture. (Translated by the author)

2. "The Dirty Pig Next Door" by skinhead band "Kahlkopf":

I introduce myself
I announce myself
I am the dirty pig next door. (Translated by the author)

An LP cut by the most popular German skinhead band "Störkraft" is called "Dreckig, kahl und hundsgemein", which means "dirty, shorn, and low-down". It is clear that the hatred expressed in skinhead songs is partly the hatred they feel for themselves.

"Foreigners in Their Own Country". Skinheads feel disadvantaged, outcast, and threatened by foreigners, and so they feel themselves aliens in their own country. According to Willems et al. (1993), the following characteristics are shared by all those committing acts of violence against foreigners: a feeling of deprivation and discrimination, and a sense of fear and hostility against foreigners. (p. 137, p. 140)

Young people who lack orientation, have low esteem, and feel a sense of powerlessness, perceive foreigners as threatening. They fear foreigners as rivals in several contexts: their home ground and neighborhoods, workplaces, perks, and government handouts. Last but not least, they fear foreigners as sexual competitors (Fischer, 1992, pp. 146–147; Willems et al., 1993, pp. 104–105). Many of these skinheads also experienced violence at the hands of foreigners (Heitmeyer et al., 1992, pp. 360–361).

Denial. In fact, young people who fear foreigners are themselves discriminated against because nobody takes their problems and fears seriously. For this reason and also because nobody communicates with them, their readiness to act violent escalates to brutality.

For example, the secret service looks upon skinheads' grievances against foreigners as specious. While in Great Britain, skinheads' protests against social injustices were taken seriously, the perception in Germany is that skinheads are protesting against imaginary problems (Skinheads, n,.d., p. 2; Skinheads, 1992, p. 1).

Therefore, to the skinheads, becoming a member of a xenophobic youth culture is perceived as a step that immediately brings with it a feeling of belonging, acceptance, and having found kindred spirits. This imparts a missionary touch to skinheads, the feeling that they are the only ones to save the German nation. Unfortunately, this sentiment is often validated by other segments of the German population that have been badly neglected by the government and politicians. This was the case in Rostock-Lichtenhagen, where the source of tensions between local residents and foreigners was the fact that the "Asylbewerberheim" (asylum) was unbearably overcrowded. This provides an explanation, though not an excuse, for the reliance skinheads could place on local residents' acceptance of, and applause for their acts of violence (Willems et al., 1993, pp. 118–128).

Practical Consequences and Preventive Measures

In order to solve the problem of xenophobic violence committed by youth in German society, two issues must be addressed: The problems caused by the German youth, and the problems they themselves have. This has been neglected far too long. Why has nobody talked to skinheads? Why has nobody listened to skinheads? It seems obvious that the taboos skinheads break are so powerful that rational argument is not possible. Therefore, skinheads are stereotyped and stigmatized as Nazis, and their problems are swept under the carpet. The first positive step, therefore, is to reflect upon the taboos.

Taboos

Taboos such as the following must be discussed and discarded: (a) You must not have problems with foreigners; (b) You may not use Nazi symbols; and (c) You must not be drawn to mob experiences like mass rallies or meetings.

Problems with Foreigners. When Rostock residents aired their grievances about foreigners through letters to the editor of the German newspaper *Die Zeit*, this was interpreted as "Shame on Germany" (Sommer, 1992, p. 1). Those who rail against people who fear foreigners and call them racist do not themselves experience problems with foreigners; for intellectuals, foreigners are not a problem. Thus, the real problems are never aired and remain taboos. Consequently, arguments become irrational, emotional, and unfair. A more effective approach would be to take seriously the problems skinheads are experiencing with foreigners.

Denial of these problems seems to result in escalation of brutality according to the following pattern of thinking: If the problems we experience are denied, we are going to solve them on our own. This seemed to be also the attitude of the above mentioned residents in Rostock-Lichtenhagen whose problems have been badly neglected by the government and the politicians (Willems et al., 1993, pp. 118–128). Denial results in the fact that legitimate sorrows and problems can only be articulated within right wing groups, that people who articulate these problems are stigmatized as fascists (p. 146) and that they only experience support by right wing groups.

On the other hand, according to reports on projects of "accepting youth work", listening to skinheads and accepting their personalities and problems—without sharing their views and attitudes—seems to be a means of de-escalation. This point will be argued in more detail in the section about "accepting youth work".

The Use of Nazi Symbols. In Germany, it is illegal to use Nazi symbols. There are legal regulations that are so complicated and unreal that the real Neo-Nazis amuse themselves often by tricking courts and the judiciary in general (*Der Spiegel*, 1992, pp. 41–50).

A more effective method would be to change the status of these Nazi symbols from taboos to new contexts and meanings, through playful and ironical handling of these symbols and the exposure to ridicule of their representatives (e.g., Hitler). On the other hand, taboos surround the representatives of Nazi symbols with an aura. This, in fact, was the goal of Goebbels' propaganda, a strategy that distanced Nazis from criticism and from discovery of the inherent ridiculousness of their tenets. To make fun of these highly charged tabooed symbols would strip them and their representatives of any aura.

Examples include Chaplin's Hitler-movie, Hartfield's collages, and the German movie "Schtonk!" about the fake Hitler diary. Beyond that, I agree with Wiesenthal, who argues that we should encourage the discovery of the ridiculousness of Neo-Nazis as well as that of Hitler and Himmler by showing movies of their speeches (Wiesenthal, 1992, pp. 424–425). Instead these movies are tabooed in Germany because it is assumed that they glorify fascism. Recently (February 1994), an exhibition of Hitler portraits initiated by historians was attacked as glorification and became such a scandalous issue that it could not be shown in Germany any longer. The same happened to a movie called "Beruf: Neonazi" ("Profession: Neonazi"), which mainly contained information about Bela Ewald Althans, a young Neo-Nazi, and which was only broadcast by one TV station. The aura that isolates Nazi representatives from criticism still remains, and we are a long way from playing with Nazi symbols.

Fascination by the Masses. We need to talk about the fascination masses can develop for ideologies and their symbols; in order to do this, we must first admit that this fascination exists. It might be useful to point out that the iconography and choreography of Hitler's leadership behavior and the response of the exultant masses exhibit amazing parallels to the self stylizing and limelight seeking of rock stars and the concomitant ritualistic behavior of their fans at concerts.

We need to be aware that these mass rituals and the fascination that surrounds them, which we know from speeches of Hitler and Goebbels are also part of demonstrations and concerts against xenophobia and their oceans of candle lights. Skinhead songs, too, refer to the fascination of and by the masses, for example, in the song "Volk steh auf" by the skinhead band "Triebtäter". This song fascinates by starting with a famous Goebbels speech arousing exultant shouts of the masses accompanied by skinhead music. It is the breaking of a taboo to admit the fascination generated by this song.

Youth Work Program

Youth who commit acts of violence against foreigners or who are prone to do so need options for alternative ways to build their identities. They need communication and acceptance in order to develop positive self concepts, and their problems must not be ignored. We need to give them something to be responsible for, something that has cultural meaning for them, for example, meeting places and musical instruments that are a means to express their cultural identity. In this way, they may gain a sense of control over their environment.

These ideas are successfully realized in projects where skinheads and right wing youth are accepted by social workers who are street workers (Heim et al., 1992; Krafeld et al., 1993). The main principle behind *Jugendarbeit* (youth work program) is to accept young people who engage in violence against foreigners. This means to accept them as personalities and to listen to them without sharing their attitudes and—what is very important—without trying to change their attitudes, too. This is not a concept of integration or assimilation of skinheads into youth work groups where skinheads do not ever experience acceptance either by other young people or by social workers. *Jugendarbeit* is a new type of social work, especially developed for the skinhead problem. It is based on concepts of symbolic interaction: to listen to a person and to take a person's problems seriously allows a person the possibility to change negative self-images to more positive ones. As we know from reports on *Jugendarbeit*, skinheads feel accepted for the first time in their lives by others outside their group: "We have been coming here for years! Nobody ever spent any time with us! And nobody ever talked to us! We appreciate you treating us differently!" (Heim et al.,

1992, p. 20) Skinheads do not want to be changed by social workers, and street workers do not want to change them. But what happens are changes in the following direction: for the first time in their lives, they look upon themselves differently, from the point of view of a person who accepts them without sharing their ideas or being shocked. They start to communicate their ideas to people who are different from themselves. They start to reflect upon themselves because their ideas look different when they are articulated in front of people who do not share these ideas but do accept their personalities. From this point of view, some of them start to change their attitudes. *Jugendarbeit* gives them something that they might lose but do not want to lose: rooms in which to meet, rooms they must take care of, and people who accept them.

Jugendarbeit does not solve the problems skinheads are facing in their social environments, but it seems to be a promising way of overcoming the present silence towards skinheads. Thus it becomes a paradigm for interaction with skinheads in other social contexts such as school.

Youth Culture in the Education System

Prevention measures are desperately needed in the educational system. As it stands, children and youth do not have the opportunity to develop and assert their cultural identity in the present system. Current curricula do not recognize youth culture as a subject in school; it is not only not present, but is even discouraged. Music lessons, especially, present to German children works from other cultures, for example, a Mozart symphony, an Israeli dance, or a Beatles song, as more valuable pieces than those from the students' repertoires. In other cultures, such as that of the United States, the same problem prevails when youth music, whether it be rap, heavy metal, or rock, is ignored. The dominance of works from classical collections in our educational systems to the exclusion of youth culture and more popular and native genres does not invite tolerance for foreign cultures. How can children learn to tolerate foreign cultures if their own culture is denied? A more useful approach would be to encourage and include creative and cooperative exchanges with youth cultures and their musical expressions that include punk, heavy metal, hiphop, and oi! and to place these in the educational system. As a member of the state curriculum committee for music education in Germany as well as a music educator in the primary and secondary systems, I have worked toward this end. In order to relate to the body orientation of youth cultures, I have developed especially a concept of rock dance (Müller, 1992, 1993).

Summary

Oi!-music is part of skinhead culture that defines itself and is defined by society as a phenomenon in opposition to the mainstream and dominant culture. Skinheads are socialized by experiences of being not accepted—neither as individuals nor as members of an autonomous youth culture. They feel disadvantaged and cast out. Skinheads are discriminated insofar as the problems they have with foreigners are socially denied and ignored. Within the above theoretical framework, and according to empirical results, it is rather the case that the social deprivation of cultural identity to skinheads is more to blame for violence against foreigners than oi!-music as part of skinhead culture. From this perspective, the following are some practical consequences and preventive measures: Children and adolescents need acceptance to gain positive self-concepts. Cultural identity cannot be developed if a youth culture is not only not present but even discriminated against in educational institutions.

References

Bähr, J. (1993). Devotionalien aus Gewalt, Blut und Knochen. Rechtsrock bildet die Basis für ein faschistoides Denken der Jugend. *Neue Musikzeitung, 1*, 12–13.

Behne, K.-E. (1993). Wirkungen von Musik. *Musik und Unterricht, 4*(18), 4–9.

Behne, K.-E. (in press). Wirkungen von Musik. In S. Helms, R. Schneider, & R. Weber (Eds.), Kompendium der Musikpädagogik. Kassel: Bosse.

Brown, J. D., & Schulze, L. (1990). The effects of race, gender, and fandom on audience interpretations of Madonna's music videos. *Journal of Communication, 40*, 88–102.

Butterwegge, C. (1993). Zur modischen Fehldeutung des Rechtsextremismus/Rassismus als Jugendrevolte und soziale Protestbewegung. *deutsche jugend, 41*, 483–487.

Clarke, J. (1979). Die Skinheads und die magische Rückgewinnung der Gemeinschaft. In J. Clarke, P. Cohen, P. Corrigan, J. Garber, S. Hall, D. Hebdige, T. Jefferson, R. McCron, A. McRobbie, G. Murdock, H. Parker, & B. Roberts (Eds.), *Jugendkultur als Widerstand* (pp. 171–175). Frankfurt am Main: Syndikat.

Dolak, G. (1993). Dynastien, Aussenseiter, Newcomer: Familien Maertens und Funck. Auf Luftpolstersohlen in den Mode-Olmp. *Süddeutsche Zeitung, 88*(17), 32.

Farin, K., & Seidel-Pielen, E. (1993). *Skinheads.* München: C. H. Beck.

Fischer, A., & Zinnecker, J. (1992). Einleitendes zur Jugendstudie. Jugend '92. In Jugendwerk der Deutschen Shell (Ed.), vol. 1, *Lebenslagen, Orientierungen und Entwicklungsperpektiven im vereinigten Deutschland* (pp. 9–22). Opladen: Leske & Budrich.

Fischer, C. (1992). Skinpower Germany: Mein Leben ist aufregender. *Jugend, 1*, 141–155.

Funk-Hennigs, E. (1994). Zur Musikszene der Skinheads: Ein jugendkulturelles und/oder ein rechtsextremistisches Phänomen unserer Gesellschaft? In H. Gembris, R.-D. Kraemer, & G. Maas (Eds.). *Musikpädagogische Forschungsberichte 1993* (pp. 11–39). Augsburg: Dr. Bernd Wissner.

Heim, G., Krafeld, F. J., Lutzebäck, E., Schaar, G., Storm, C., & Welp, W. (Eds.). (1992). *Akzeptierende Jugendarbeit mit rechten Jugendcliquen.* Bremen: Steintor.

Heitmeyer, W., Buhse, H., Liebe-Freund, J., Moller, K., Müller, J., Ritz, H., Siller, G., & Vossen, J. (1992). *Die Bielefelder Rechtsextremismus-Studie: Erste Langzeituntersuchung zur politischen Sozialisation männlicher Jugendlicher.* Weinheim und München: Juventa.

Krafeld, F. J., Möller, K., & Müller, A. (1993). *Jugendarbeit in rechten Szenen: Ansätze – Erfahrungen – Perspektiven.* Bremen: Ed. Temmen.

Kunczik, M. (1993). Gewalt im Fernsehen: Stand der Wirkungsforschung und neue Befunde. *Media Perspektiven, 3*, 98–107.

Landesamt für Verfassungsschutz Baden-Württemberg (Ed.). (1992), *Skinheads.* Stuttgart.

Landesamt für Verfassungsschutz Baden-Württemberg (Ed.) (1993). *Skinheads. Musik – Bands – Magazine, 1993.* Stuttgart.

Ley, R. (1993). Der Rock von rechts: Gefahr Oi-Musik—Bundesprüfstelle muss immer häufiger eingreifen. *Hamburger Abendblatt, 233*, 6, 10, 32.

Leyendecker, H. (1993). Fremdenhass: "Direkt platt schlagen". *Der Spiegel, 52*, 61–72.

Müller, R. (1992). *Rock- und Poptanz mit Kindern und Jugendlichen: Rocktanzspiele, Choreographien, Tanzprojekte.* Regensburg: Bosse.

Müller, R. (1993). *Rock- und Poptanz im Musikunterricht der Grundschule und der Sekundarstufe I.* Freie und Hansestadt Hamburg, *Behörde für Schule, Jugend und Berufsbildung (Ed.).* Hamburg: Amt für Schule.

Müller, R. (in press). Selbstsozialisation: Eine Theorie lebenslangen musikalischen Lernens. In K.-E Behne, G. Kleinen, & H. de la Motte-Haber, *Musikpsychologie, Jahrbuch der Deutschen Gesellschaft für Musikpsychologie, 11.* Wilhelmshaven: Florian Noetzel.

Niedersächsisches Innenministerium (Ed.). (n.d.). Skinheads. *Fakten und Hintergründe.* Hannover.

Sommer, T. (1992). Das Schandmal des Fremdenhasses. Scham genügt nicht: Die Ausländer brauchen unseren Schutz. *Die Zeit, 42*, 11. Oktober, 1

"Das Kreuz mit den Haken". (1992). *Der Spiegel, 52*, 41–50.

Treptow, R. (1993). Jugendkultur im Umbruch? Fragen an die Jugendkulturkritik. *Kulturpolitische Mitteilungen, 60,* 20–21.

Wiesenthal, S. (1992). *Recht, nicht Rache. Erinnerungen.* 2[d] ed. Frankfurt am Main/Berlin: Ullstein.

Willems, H., Würtz, S., & Eckert, R. (1993). *Fremdenfeindliche Gewalt. Eine Analyse von Täterstrukturen und Eskalationsprozessen.*Bundesministerium für Frauen und Jugend und von der Deutschen Forschungsgemeinschaft (Eds.). Bonn: Bundesministerium für Frauen und Jugend.

Zinnecker, J., & Fischer, A. (1993). Jugendstudie '92. Die wichtigsten Ergebnisse im Überblick. *Jugend '92, 1,* 213–227.

MUSIC THERAPY IN EARLY REHABILITATION OF PATIENTS WITH ACUTE MYOCARDIAL INFARCTION

Joseph Escher, Eric Dayer, and Leo Anthenien

Introduction and Purpose

Myocardial infarctus patients belong to a special group within an internal medicine department (Langosch, 1989). They are suddenly torn from everyday life and separated from their family, friends, and colleagues. During the first days of their stay in the intensive care unit—mostly in a fully conscious state—they are confronted with a total loss of independence. Contrary to subjective perceptions of their own capabilities, they are for awhile immobilized with absolute bedrest and are thus dependent on help from others for everyday matters such as personal hygiene. Because of the infarction, the polarities of "autonomy vs. dependence", "above vs. below", "active vs. passive" are suddenly modified, often as a first-time experience. Most of these patients live with a feeling of immanent death and, thereby, suffer pain and fear. Their central organ—the heart—has failed; it is "hurt", "heart broken" (Condrau & Gassmann, 1989). The symbolic meaning of this vital organ comes to the front of a person's awareness in such a dramatic moment of life (Nager, 1993), and the emotional reactions are manifold. They depend on the patient's personality, life history, affective life situation, treatment conditions, etc. The most serious consequences of this sudden intrusion of illness include a shaken personality with major identity crises and a strong narcissistic component. The life threat caused by acute myocardial infarction, as well as the unfamiliar surroundings of the intensive care unit, undoubtedly lead to an enormous psychophysical stress (Hannich, Wendt, & Lawin, 1983; Bernhard, & Schäfer, 1984; Klapp, 1985; Hannich, 1987).

In "life-event" studies, researchers have attempted to classify the biopsychosocial meaning of life crisis (Holmes & Rahe, 1967; Irwin, Daniels, Bloom, Smith, & Weiner, 1987; Irwin, Patterson, Smith, Cadwell, Brown, Gillin, & Grant, 1990; Overmier, 1988). However, it is important not to attribute all of these crisis problems to one cause. Susceptibility to stress reactions varies individually, because complex-multifactorial influences are involved that depend on stress-related influences, or protective factors such as personal defense mechanisms, coping behavior and the like (Kropiunigg, 1990).

Since Ader (1981) coined the term "psychoneuroimmunology", some stress studies have included the evaluation of immunological parameters in order to prove biopsychosocial associations (Ader, Felten, & Cohen, 1991). Data come from various surveys, or reports of natural stress situations (e.g., painful loss events, acute illness), or experimental stress induction (Jemmott & Locke, 1984; Klosterhalfen & Klosterhalfen, 1989; Reichlin, 1993; Hodel, 1993). When the immune system is depressed, extreme psychosocial strain can lead to an increased incidence of infections. An example of this kind of stress would be the loss of a partner (Bartrop, Luckhurst, Lazarus, Kiloh, & Penny, 1977; Schleifer, Keller, Camerino, Thornton, & Stein, 1983; Kiecolt-Glaser, Fisher, Ogrocki, Stout, Speicher, & Glaser, 1987). Immunology is also gaining in importance in studies of psychiatric disease (Kaschka & Aschauer, 1990).

Where neuroimmunological disorders and their effects are concerned, music therapy may play a significant role in maintaining optimal rehabilitation conditions in acute disease situations. In various studies during the past years, it was shown that music had a positive influence on the subjective feelings and psychophysiology of a person (Spintge & Droh, 1992; Escher, Höhmann, Anthenien, Dayer, Bosshard, & Gaillard, 1993). Concerning the modification of immunological parameters, Maranto (1991) as well as Nolan (1991) suggested that music had an effect of stimulating the immune system of cancer patients who had undergone a bone marrow transplant procedure.

By using music therapy in early infarction rehabilitation, we aimed at reducing the immediate effects of major stress and at building up through a patient-music therapist relationship the ability to work on and attack the disease. At the same time, patients received on admission a booster injection of tetanus toxoid and of pneumococcal antigen. Over a period of 3 weeks, we analyzed the antibody response to thymo-dependent and independent antigens in those patients treated with music, as well as those who were not, so that we could look for the prolonged influence of stress on the humoral immune response.

Method

Description of Subjects

We randomly assigned to two groups 20 patients with enzymatic and electrocardiograph modifications compatible with a definite diagnosis of myocardial infarction. Thus 10 patients had music therapy treatment, while the other group served as controls. The age of the 20 patients ranged from 52 to 70 years and the sample consisted of 17 men and 3 women. We excluded from the study all patients over 70 years of age.

Experimental Setting

During the first day of hospitalization in the intensive care unit, we measured the patients' antibodies in relation to tetanus and pneumococcal antigens in the serum. At the same time, we fortified the patients with 0.5 ml Te-Anatoxal®(Berna) and Pneumovax-23®(MSD). Fourteen and 21 days later, we drew blood again to test for antibody titers to tetanus and pneumococcal antigens. Anxiolysis and sedation were standardized to avoid confounding variables. Every patient received 1.5mg of bromazepam three times a day. The treatment of the myocardial infarction followed international guidelines. When ventricular failure was absent and there was no evidence of another contraindication, we normally used a beta-antagonist treatment.

Patients in the first group had music therapy interventions during their entire stay in the hospital. This took place according to the patient's convalescence schedule, which consisted of three approximately 1-week segments, three music therapy treatments per segment, with a total of about nine music therapy sessions. It is impossible to be more precise about the general music therapy treatment interventions because they were applied according to the individual needs of the patients. At the end of their hospitalization, all patients in both groups were questioned concerning the various implications of the infarction event. Those patients who had had music therapy were not interviewed by the music therapist but by a person not involved in music therapy who questioned both groups of patients.

Monitoring of Immune Parameters

In order to follow the humoral antibody response of the patients, we examined the rise of the antipneumococcal and antitetanus antibodies over the 3 weeks following

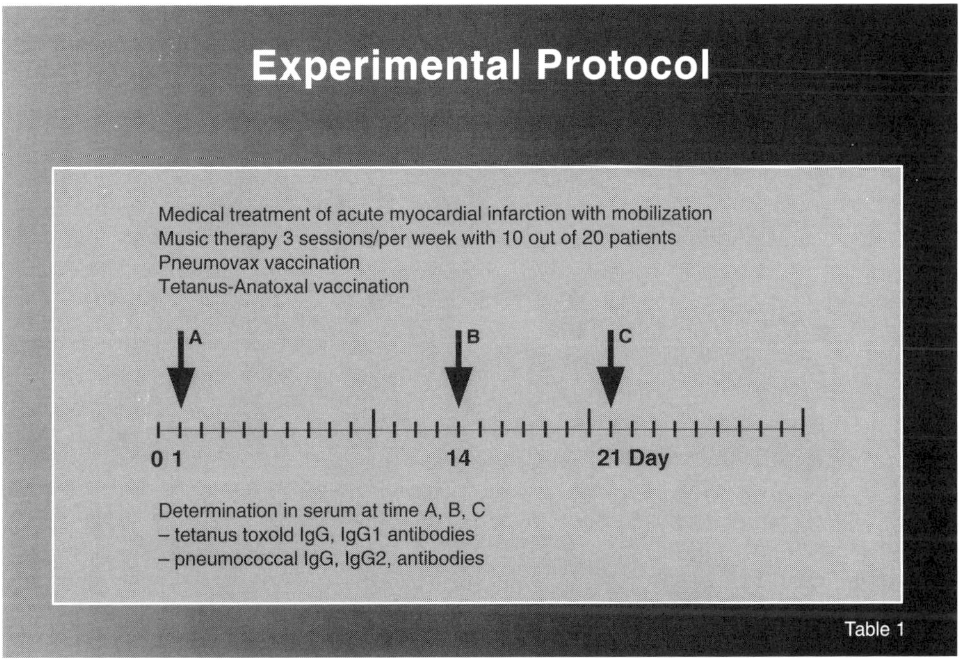

Table 1

admission to the hospital. We injected subcutaneously 0.5 ml Te-Anatoxal®(Berna) and Pneumovax-23®(MSD) on the first day of hospitalization. Antibody titers were compared with the prebooster vaccination titers.

Antibody determination. Antipneumococcal and tetanus antibodies in the serum were detected by an enzyme-immunoassay (Binding Site, Birmingham, England, lot 552) according to manufacturer specifications.

Statistical analysis. We used *t*-tests and the Wilcoxon nonparametric test to compare the two groups of patients (Statistica, Statsoft, Tulsa, Arizona, USA).

Music Therapy Treatment: Phase I

Patient situation:	Absolute bedrest, sedatives, drowsiness.
Focus of therapy:	Rest and relief from strain in order to keep the activity of the heart as low as possible.
Music therapy:	Trophotropic pieces selected from patient choices.

Here the functional side of music comes into play, that is, the music therapist chooses trophotropic pieces from among the patient's personal choices. The selected music contain rhythms without strong accentuation, flowing legato melodies, with distinctive consonances and little dynamic change (Decker-Voigt, 1991, pp. 71–75). Musical selections included second movements of classical works, popular German and French music in slower tempi, as well as sounds of nature combined with flute melodies. This kind of music has a soothing effect on mind and body, provided it does not arouse excitatory memories. During this phase the patient is passive, although he may feel the need to talk about the infarction event. The music therapist's attitude towards the patient is characterized by the effort to convey an ambiance of protection and security.

Music Therapy Treatment: Phase II

Patient situation:	Bed rest; the patient now feels the need to do something on his own again. He feels his strength coming back.
Focus of therapy:	Relationship established between the systole and the diastole of the heart and social behaviors of "giving – taking", "activity – passivity".
Music therapy:	Music connected with patient's life story and interests.

Functional music is now replaced by associative music. More and more music that is connected with the life-story of the patient, or is of special interest to him, is now heard. The main topics often include work, one's profession, or everyday life stresses. The symbolic meaning of the physiological functional principle of the heart—systole and diastole—with its continuous change of "giving – taking", of "activity – pause" is discussed during psychotherapy. This encourages associations between the physiology of the heart disease, the event of the infarctus, on the one hand, and an opportunity to analyze this pathology in terms of the patient's personal life structure, on the other.

Music Therapy Treatment: Phase III

Patient situation:	Return to independence. Patient can walk around and perform some physical tasks. Feeling of personal power returns.
Focus of therapy:	Balancing out sympathicus and vagus influx, that is, between the "driving" and "breaking" forces.
Music therapy:	Free choice by patient. No restrictions.

The course of the session is largely determined by the patient. There are no further restrictions as far as music is concerned. The period of rehabilitation after the hospital stay becomes the main topic. The patient becomes aware of the fact that life situations during the following weeks and months will still be strongly affected by the infarction, for example, coping with the future, the family situation, professional problems, circle of friends, restrictions in goal-planning, determining the rehabilitation program and its length, and, finally, reentering the work force. In a sense, music therapy once again, follows physiological development, and the music therapist tries to regulate and harmonize in a symbolic way the polarity between "driving" and "breaking" forces. Attempts to translate this into action by means of a musical improvisation usually fail because of the patient's self-imposed pressure to do well and fear of failure.

Concluding Questionnaire

Before leaving the hospital, the patient was asked to respond to the following questions during a final interview:

1. "Do you recall an incident of special importance that occurred in the time preceding the infarction? If yes, which incident?" (This question is asked to establish the relationship of an event with the infarction.)

2. "Do you see a connection between this or another incident and your infarction? If yes, how?" (This would establish a causal-correlation relationship.)

3. "Looking back now, after the infarction, what would you change in your present life-style?"

4. "How, in your opinion, will the disease influence your future life-style?"

5. "Can you mention anything specific that, due to the infarction, will cause you to change your life-style?"

6. "Did you have any stressful experiences during your stay in hospital? If yes, what were they?"

7. "Did you, on the other hand, have any experiences that brought you relief? If yes, what were they?"

For questions 3–5, the interviewer offered accordingly a few alternatives in relation to descriptors such as "familiar", "professional", "handling leisure time", "handling health", and, if appropriate, "sex life".

Results

Humoral Antibody Response through Music Therapy

The antibody response to both pneumococcal and tetanus antigens peaked at day 14 with an average tenfold increase, There was a wide variation in the percentage of increase of the antibody titers in all groups (range: 1.78–3243).

The titers of the thymo-dependent IgG and IgG1 antitetanus antibodies showed no significant differences when the group treated with music therapy was compared with the control group (see Figure 1).

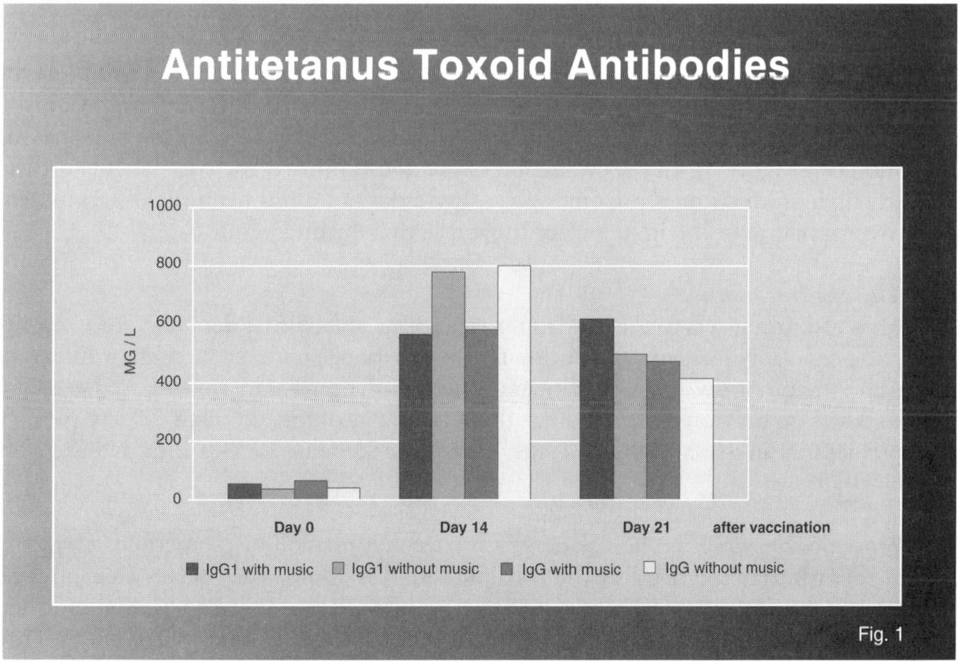

Fig. 1

Although there was a difference in the mean of the titers of the thymo-independent IgG2, but not in the total IgG, antipneumococcal antibodies (see Figure 2), a *t*-test showed it was not significant due to the dispersion of the values.

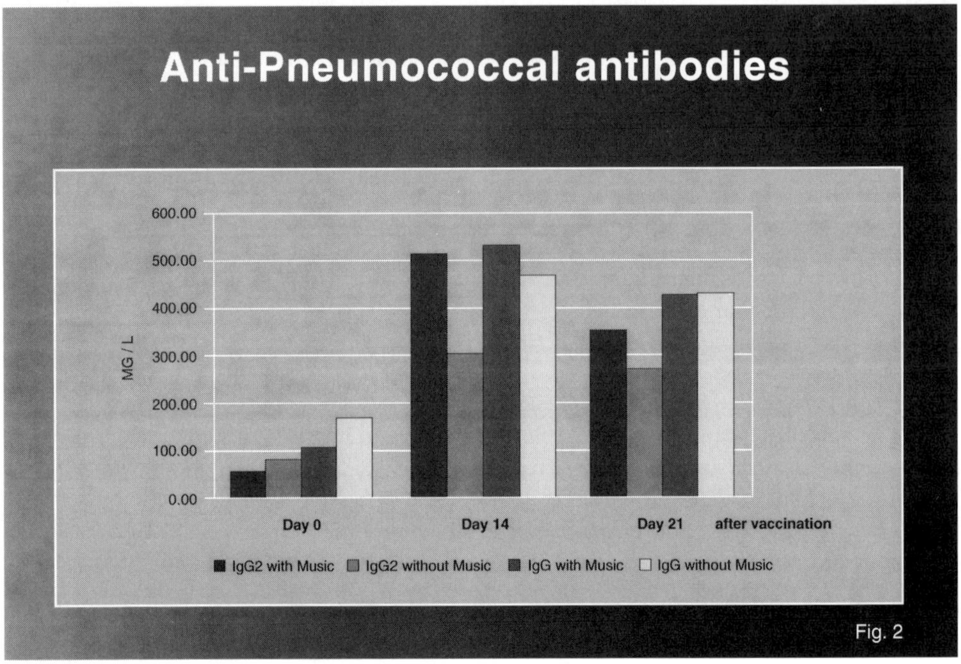

A slightly significant higher production of the IgG2 antipneumococcal antibodies by patients in the music therapy group was observed only after using a nonparametric Wilcoxon test comparing the medians of the two groups of patients at day 14 after the pneumovax-vaccination (see Figure 3). In the evaluation of the questionnaire, the two patients with an extremely high production of pneumococcus-IgG2 did not differ from the others in their subjective estimation of the influence of the music therapy intervention.

Music Therapy Intervention

How a person reacts to the sudden invasion of an acute illness depends, among other things, on personality makeup. According to our experience with music therapy interventions over a period of 4 years with patients suffering myocardial infarction, we have concluded—based on previous studies—that there are two groups: the high anxiety patients and those who are in denial (Beutel, 1988; Kächele & Steffens, 1988; Heim, 1989; Köhle & Gaus, 1990).

High anxiety patients. These patients are extremely meticulous, sometimes almost *too* exact in following instructions in the rehabilitation program. They sense their physical weakness and speak about it. They feel unsure of themselves and are anxious about their heart, asking questions about the cause of the infarction. Many respond well to music. They

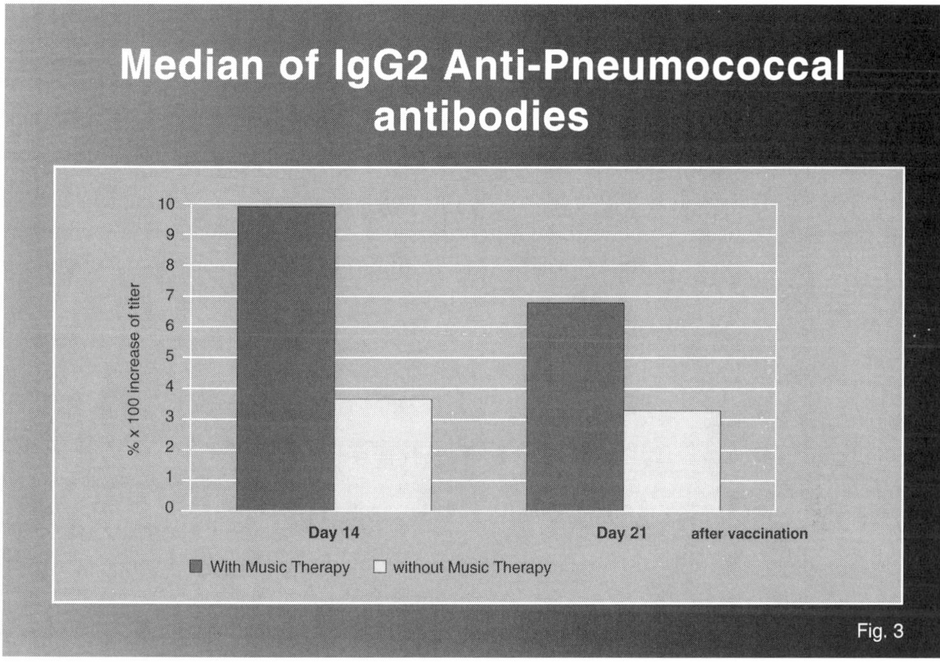

are mostly unable, or find it difficult to talk about emotions, but allow themselves to be touched by music to the depth of their soul. These men and women are mostly conscientious and sensitive. They tend to subvert deeply personal matters due to their intrapsychological pressure to do well (Type A-Behavior, Friedman & Rosenman, 1974). Under the influence of the shock of the infarction, they become aware of this dynamic and, in the effort to recover, again put into action the self-imposed pressure to do well, for example, by resolving to plan a healthier future. In their anxiety regarding their heart problem these patients are now able—contrary to their hitherto existing everyday habits—to allow themselves regressive needs, such as proximity, passivity, being cared for and sheltered, and letting loose. This offers a valuable starting point for music therapy. The music therapist's caring attitude and the response to music legitimizes these needs and is at the same time nourishment for the emotionally "hungry" heart.

Patients in Denial. These patients deny the seriousness of their heart disease and the emotions that arise from the illness. They are unable to perceive fear or any real degree of affliction. They usually are not very involved in the rehabilitation program and very soon lose any concern they may have had about the infarction. They respond to music in a rather superficial way and attend the music therapy sessions only because they were suggested or ordered by the doctor. Therapy with these patients can be tedious. Nevertheless, at some time in the intervention a degree of response is noted, or the patient shows some kind of acknowledgment of the disease and even manifests some grief about it. If a therapist eventually succeeds in engaging the patient in a discussion about professional and family matters, or the patient's interest in music is discussed, therapy can be of some value. This happens in spite of a certain superficial response and in face of the actual crisis.

With both groups, it was worthwhile beginning with music therapy in the intensive care unit. During this phase, the patient's and his relatives' distress is strongest. The immanence of mortal danger is still clearly perceptible. This deep distress opens up an opportunity—especially for those in denial—to make use of a psychotherapeutic exchange. During the entire period of the study, it proved to be difficult for nearly all patients to talk about intimate "matters of heart" such as love, loneliness, and, yearning. These topics, which are possibly decisive in the emergence of myocardial infarction, can however be touched by music. Here especially we see the special benefit of music therapy with myocardial infarction patients during the acute phase of their disease.

Coping of patients after an acute myocardial infarction with and without music therapy

	with MT	without MT
Recognizing the necessity of change in the arrangement of the present way of life after the infarction event (Question 3)	90%	40%
Influence of the infarction event in arranging the future way of life (Question 4)	80%	60%
Already planned changes in the arrangement of the future way of life after the infarction event (Question 5)	70%	40%

Table 2

Questionnaire

The answers of the first group of patients to the questions concerning important "life-events" before the infarction and hospital treatment did not differ from those of the second group.

However there is a highly significant difference between the two groups concerning answers about a change between past and future attitudes towards the disease. Responses to the questionnaire of patients treated with music therapy were more positive than those of the control-group:

To questions 1 and 2: Five out of 10 patients recalled an important event prior to the infarction.

There was no difference between groups in number of positive responses.

To question 3: Still under the scare of the infarction, nine out of 10 patients in the therapy group made life-style changes, whereas only four out of 10 patients in the control-group did likewise. In all cases, the change involved a certain cardiovascular risk behavior, above all, reduction of stress ("more calmness", "more leisure time" etc.)

To question 4: Eight out of 10 patients in the therapy group saw immediately how the illness impacted plans for their future life, whereas only six out of 10 in the control-group were able to do so.

To question 5: In the music therapy group, 7 out of 10 patients directly envisioned changes in their life-style after the infarction, whereas only 4 out of 10 in the control-group could do this.

To questions 6 and 7: In both groups, only 2 out of 10 patients noted stressful events during their hospital stay while 15 (eight of them from the music therapy group) of the total number of patients mentioned relief-providing events. This response referred to treatment in general; only two patients mentioned music therapy specifically.

Discussion

It has been established that an acute heart infarction, with the associated mandatory treatment in an intensive care unit, implies an important biopsychosocial stress for a patient. Relevant research reports that immunological measures indicate biological stress reactions. Music, that is to say music therapy, is claimed by its practitioners to produce a positive influence on the subjective experience of stress and that, through psychoneuroimmunology, these effects are measurable. Beginning with this hypothesis, we wanted to investigate how music therapy treatment during the intensive treatment after infarction, could modify the humoral immune response to recall antigens, such as tetanus toxoid and pneumococcal antigen injected on the first day of hospital admission.

Our hypothesis was only partly confirmed. In our study, we were able to show an increased IgG2-antibody production against the pneumococcal antigen in the group of patients who were treated with music therapy early after the infarction. The other antibodies measured at the same time periods—the IgG-pneumococcal antibodies as well as the IgG and IgG1-tetanus antibodies—however, showed no statistical differences between the music therapy group and the controls.

The significance of the results must be regarded with caution because of dispersion of the values (see Figure 4) and the alpha level ($p = 0.05$).

Moreover, we had expected an increased titer of the thymus-dependent antitetanus antibodies, which should have been directly influenced by the music therapy, supposedly diminishing stress. On the contrary, we measured increased thymus-independent, antipneumococcal antibodies in the music therapy group of patients. The meaning of such a finding remains unexplained. There were several limitations to our study:

1. Our expectations were extrapolated from animal response to stress and may not be transposable to humans.

2. The sample may simply have been inadequate.

3. The dispersion of the titers suggests confounding variables that would have to be controlled in order to allow a true evaluation of the effect of the music therapy intervention.

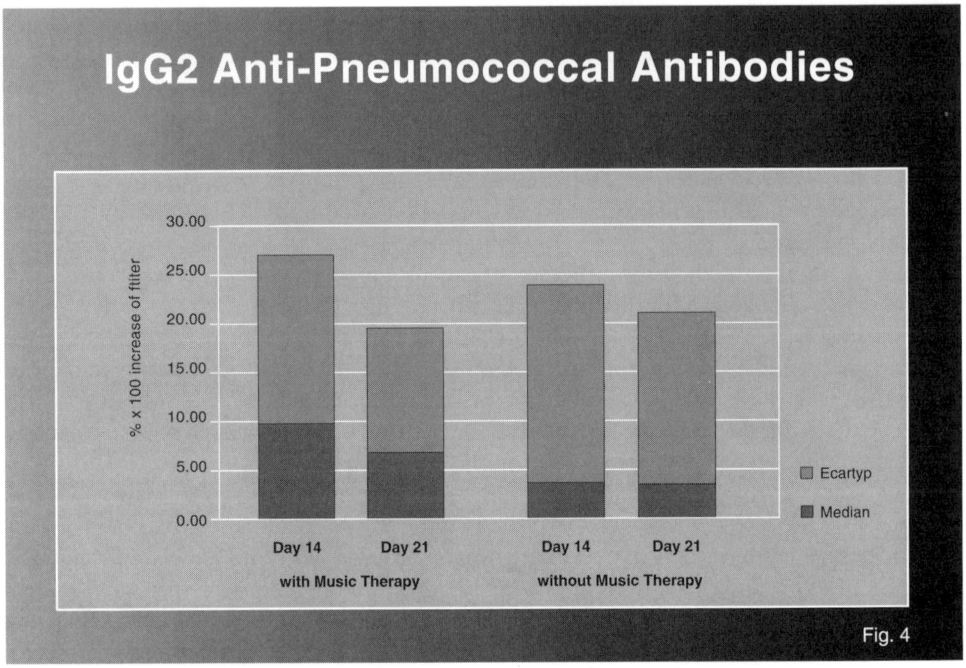

Fig. 4

The wide variety of personalities, the multiple variables influencing the patient after the myocardial infarction (nursing team, physiotherapist, doctor, private surroundings, etc.) are surely factors that, as a whole, can modify in the last analysis the balance of the psychological effect on the humoral immune response. Music therapy can only be seen as one of many factors that could have a positive influence on the immune system.

Even though a highly significant positive difference in the humoral response is lacking between the two groups, there is no doubt that music therapy influences in a positive way—in the sense of reducing stress—patients' well being. In our opinion, a future study with a larger sample of more standardized groups of infarctus patients could show the influence of music therapy on biological parameters, in particular on immunocompetency.

The questionnaire completed at the end of the treatment contained only a few statements concerning life-events relevant to the infarction. However, life events need to be explored by means of a more specific questionnaire containing several items.

Four-fifths of all the patients treated with music therapy gave positive responses—with regard to the realities of their disease—to the three questions regarding exchanges in their present and future life-styles. Barely half of the patients in the control group did likewise. We see this as a clear indication, that a patient treated with psychotherapy usually gets down to the bottom of the problem, looking at life, as it has been up to the present and as it can be in the future. Obviously, psychotherapy—in this case, music therapy—supports introspection, enabling the patient to reflect more on personal life-style. Emphasis rests on cognitive decisions to change things; in our study, however, we found no equivalent on the affective level. Answers to questions concerning negative or positive experiences during hospital treatment showed no difference in the two groups. These results correspond with the reports from other studies: The patient with myocardial infarction values above all the stay in the intensive unit (Klapp, 1985). It is Köhle and Gaus (1990) who primarily report the healing influence of psychotherapeutic intervention as far as reducing mortality. In our music therapy treatment, the two music therapists are, in the context of liaisons, fully integrated in the medical team. This is of special value. We know of the fears and somatic complications that can turn up when a patient is moved from the intensive care unit to the ward ("moving-arrhythmia"). From this aspect, it is of great value when the music therapist can continue to be with the patient, making constant care possible—something that is neglected in the usual somatic treatment setting.

Thus, it was our personal impression that music therapy, in the sense of an adjunctive psychotherapy, is suitable for patients with an acute myocardial infarction, helping to reduce stress,, and improving acknowledgment and acceptance of the disease. Although—in a strictly scientific sense—the statistical results of this music therapy study turned out to be insignificant, we believe—based on empirical judgment—that we have introduced a psychotherapeutic element in the acute treatment of infarction patients in the intensive care unit, an ambiance that is usually characterized by machines and drugs. This unusual cooperation of an intensive care medical doctor with a psychotherapist is a modest attempt to follow the postulate of critical medicine (Nager, 1986; Spoka, 1987; Rechenberger & Werthmann, 1988). We must be conservative in the scientific interpretation of the results. An excessive interpretation of benefits obtained up to now through numerous psychoneuroimmunological research studies should not be overstated. An experienced immunologist warns: "To date, we have very little knowledge of the relationship among psyche, the immune system and disease" (Grob, 1990, p. 106).

Nevertheless the connection between music therapy and psychoneuroimmunology remains a fascinating branch of research.

References

Ader, R., Felten, D. L., & Cohen, N. (Eds.). (1991). *Psychoneuroimmunology.* New York: Academic Press.

Bartrop, R. W., Luckhurst, E., Lazarus, L., Kiloh, L. G., & Penny, R. (1977). Depressed lymphocyte function after bereavement. *Lancet, 1*, 834–836.

Bernhard, P., & Schäfer, J. H. (1984). Seelische Belastungen internistischer Patienten aus der Intensivbehandlung und ihre Auswirkung auf die Interaktion mit dem Behandlungsteam. In U. Tewes (Ed.), *Angewandte Medizinpsychologie* (pp. 200–208). Fachbuchhandlung für Psychologie. Frankfurt am Main: Verlagabteilung.

Condrau, G., & Gassmann, M. (1989). *Das verletzte Herz.* Zürich: Kreuz-Verlag.

Decker-Voigt, H. H. (1991). Aus der Seele gespielt. Eine Einführung in die Musiktherapie. München: Goldmann Verlag.

Escher, J., Höhmann, U., Anthenien, L., Dayer, E., Bosshard, C., & Gaillard, R. C. (1993). Musik bei der Gastroskopie. *Schweizerische Medizinische Wochenschrift, 123,* 1354–1358.

Friedman, M., & Rosenman, R. H. (1974). *Type A behavior and your heart.* New York: Knopf.

Grob, P. J. (1990). Immunsystem und Psyche. *Psychosomatische Medizin, Schweiz, 18,* 98–107.

Hannich, H. J., Wendt, M., & Lawin, P. (Eds.). (1983). *Psychosomatik der Intensivmedizin. Symposium in Münster.* New York, Stuttgart: Georg Thieme Verlag.

Hannich, H. J. (1987). *Medizinische Psychologie in der Intensivbehandlung. Untersuchungen zur psychologischen Situation.* New York: Springer-Verlag.

Heim, E. (1989). *Krankheit als Krise und Chance. Warum wir krank werden, was wir daraus lernen für uns und im Umgang mit anderen.* München: Moderne Verlagsgesellschaft.

Hodel, L. (1993). *Psyche und Immunität. Eine ausgewählte Literaturstudie der Psychoneuroimmunologie bei gesunden Personen.* Unpublished doctoral dissertation, University of Zürich, Faculty of Medicine.

Holmes, T. H., & Rahe, R. H. (1967). The social readjustment rating scale. *Journal of Psychosomatic Research, 11,* 213–218.

Irwin, M., Daniels, M., Bloom, E. T., Smith, T. L., & Weiner, H. (1987). Life events, depressive symptoms and immune function. *American Journal of Psychiatry, 103,* 437–441.

Irwin, M., Patterson, T., Smith, T. L., Caldwell, C., Brown, S. A., Gillin, J. C., & Grant, I. (1990). Reduction of immune function in life stress and depression. *Biological Psychiatry, 27,* 22–30.

Jemmot, J. B., & Locke, S. E. (1984). Psychosocial factors, immunologic mediation and human susceptibility to infectious diseases: How much do we know? *Pychological Bulletin, 95,* 78–108.

Kächele, H., & Steffens, W. (1988). Bewältigung und Abwehr. Beiträge zur Psychologie und Psychotherapie schwerer körperlicher Krankheiten. Berlin: Springer-Verlag.

Kaschka, W. P., & Aschauer, H. N. (Eds.). (1990). *Psychoimmunologie.* Stuttgart: Georg Thieme Verlag.

Kiecolt-Glaser, L. K., Fisher, L. D., Ogrocki, P., Stout, J. C., Speicher, C. E., & Glaser, R. (1987). Marital quality, marital disruption and immune function. *Psychosomatic Medicine, 49,* 13–34.

Klapp, B. F. (1985). *Psychosoziale Intensivmedizin. Untersuchungen zum Spannungsfeld von medizinischer Technologie und Heilkunde.* Berlin: Springer-Verlag.

Klosterhalfen, W., & Klosterhalfen S. (1989). Psychologische Faktoren, Immunität und Krankheit. In H. Speidel & B. Strauss, (Eds.), *Zukunftsaufgaben der psychosomatischen Medizin* (pp. 135–156). Berlin: Springer Verlag,

Köhle, K., & Gaus, E. (1990). Psychotherapie und Herzinfarktpatienten während der stationären und poststationären Behandlungsphase. In T. von Uexküllx (Ed.), *Psychosomatische Medizin* (pp. 691–714). München: Urban & Schwarzenberg,

Kropiunigg, U. (1990). *Psyche und Immunsystem. Psychoneurologische Untersuchungen.* Vienna: Springer Verlag,

Lange-Schmidt, I. (1989). *Körperantwort. Die Leib-Seele-Beziehung und das Herz. Zum ganzheitlichen Verständnis psychosomatischer Erkrankungen. Kassel:* Prolog Verlag.

Langosch, W. (1989). *Psychosomatik der koronaren Herzkrankheiten. Edition Medizin, VCH (Psychologie in der Medizin).* Basel: Weinheim.

Maranto, C. D., & Scartelli, J. (1991). Music in the treatment of immune-related disorders. In R. Spintge & R. Droh (Eds.), *MusicMedicine* (pp. 142–153). St. Louis: MMB Music.

Nager, F. (1986). Medizintechnik aus ärztlicher Sicht. In F. Gutzwiller & G. Kocher (Eds.), Probleme mit der apparativen *Medizin zu teuer, unkoordiniert, unmenschlich?* (pp. 29–40). Schriftenreihe der SGGP, Band 10. Horgen.

Nager, F. (1993). *Das Herz als Symbol.* Basel: Editiones Roche.

Nolan. P. (1991). Bone-marrow-transplantation. In R. Spintge, & R., Droh (Eds.), *MusicMedicine* (pp. 209–212). St. Louis: MMB Music.

Overmier, B. J. (1988). Psychological Determinants of When Stressors Stress. In D. Hellhammer, I. Florin, & H. Weiner (Eds.), *Neurobiological Approaches to Human Disease* (pp. 236–259). Toronto: Hans Huber.

Rechenberger, H. G., & Werthmann, H. V. (Eds.). (1988). *Psychotherapie und Innere Medizin. Grundlagen und Anwendungen.* München: Verlag J. Pfeiffer.

Reichlin, S. (1993). Neuroendocrine-immune interactions. *New England Journal of Medicine, 329*(17), 1246–1253.

Scartelli, J. (1991). Music therapy and psychoneuroimmunology. In R. Spintge, & R., Droh (Eds.), *Music Medicine* (pp. 137–141). St. Louis: MMB Music.

Schleifer, S. J., Keller, S. E., Camerino, M., Thornton, J. C., & Stein, M. (1983). Suppression of lymphocyte stimulation following bereavement. *JAMA, 250.* 374–377.

Spintge, R. & Droh, R. (Eds.). (1992). *MusikMedizin. Physiologische Grundlagen und praktische Anwendungen.* Stuttgart: Gustav Fischer Verlag.

Sroka, K. (1987). *Herzkrank. Ein menschliches Konzept der Herzkrankheit. Alternativen zur Schulmedizin.* Hamburg: n.p.

Tsao, C. C., Gordon, T. F., Maranto, C. D., Lerman, C., & Murasko, D. (1991). The effects of music and biological imagery on immune response (S-IgA). In C. D. Maranto (Ed.), *Applications of Music in Medicine* (pp. 85–121). Washington, DC: National Association for Music Therapy.

THE OMNICHORD: AN INSTRUMENT FOR REHABILITATION

Arthur Harvey

The use of musical instruments for therapeutic and rehabilitative purposes is commonplace worldwide. One instrument that has proven to be exceptionally versatile and adaptable for any situation, from special education to geriatric programs, is the Omnichord, made by the Suzuki Corporation and available in several models. It is the immediacy of its music making capability and diversity in producing those elements that qualify it as a musical instrument and place it in the category of serious resources for the development of therapeutic and rehabilitative music programs. In the last decade, I have introduced the Omnichord in therapeutic music training workshops around the world and have had positive feedback from people in a variety of environments and cultures.

For a musical instrument to be considered a vehicle for use in rehabilitation, it must make *music*, the act of creating *sounds*, organized rhythmically, melodically, harmonically, and in patterns. The Omnichord is an electronic sound generated instrument that utilizes modern technology to extend, expand, and combine the capabilities of the traditional autoharp, a rhythm machine, and a keyboard into one portable, lightweight "superinstrument". The instrument can be powered by either batteries, or AC or DC current, and many be additionally amplified, patched into a MIDI setup, or used with headphones.

With a strong conviction that music making ought to involve creative processes as well as facilitate creative responses, one can use the Omnichord to play it in many ways and produce a wide variety of musical sounds. In recent years, using the Omnichord with many individuals, both handicapped and nonhandicapped, I have had the Omnichord'S sound source, the strum plate, played with everything from fingers and hands to elbows, chin, nose, shoulder, knuckles, and even toes. In recent months, I have used the Omnichord in a wide variety of situations with positive responses:

1. In a therapeutic music program with severely and profoundly retarded adults at Waimano Hospital and Training School (Pearl City, Hawaii).
2. In an early childhood Toddler Program.
3. In a special education program for autistic children in an Intermediate School.
4. With an elderly individual who is visually impaired.
5. In an upper elementary class of learning disabled students.

I began a new program of therapeutic music with multihandicapped individuals begun at Waialae Baptist Church, Hawaii, where I served as Minister of Music for the last 3½ years. This population included blind/CP, deaf/blind, autistic/blind, orthopedically handicapped/retarded, and OH/blind/retarded individuals. In each of the above situations, the Omnichord has proven to be the one instrument that *all* individuals can interact with and be actively involved in the process of music making.

The Omnichord offers 10 choices of tone quality, rhythm patterns with a wide spectrum of tempi, and every major, minor, diminished, augmented, minor 7th (dominant 7th) and major 7th chord. The advanced models also have a chord memory capability that allows the player to preprogram 80 chords in progression for playback with either a large hand button or a foot adapter.

The versatility of the Omnichord can be illustrated in the many situations in which it has been used in recent years. A sample of some of the other programs in which the Omnichord has been a source of music making and therapeutic music experiences includes:

1. In my monthly Singing Seniors program for Sing-Along times.
2. In an oncology unit.
3. In an Alzheimer's unit.
4. In nursing homes.
5. In two state hospitals for chronically ill and elderly patients.
6. In Very Special Arts Festivals for group singing.
7. In a class of trainable retarded children.
8. In a preschool choir program.
9. In a Christmas caroling program at homes and in hospitals.
10. In a rehabilitation program with brain-damaged individuals.

There are many therapeutic benefits that can be associated with the use of the Omnichord that include (a) motor development, (b) perceptual development, (c) social development, (d) language development, and even (e) cognitive or precognitive development. The playing of the Omnichord can provide alternative communication opportunities as well as expressive possibilities for many disabled individuals with limits in their communicative/expressive skills. I have seen increases in range of motion, muscle strength, digital dexterity, attention, eye tracking, auditory perception, eye-hand-motor skills, emotional release, memory, alertness, and focused and appropriate behavior, through the use of the Omnichord. I have used it for language development in special education classes for song writing, diction, and articulation practice.

In recent weeks, we have seen major developmental steps in several of the participants in our therapeutic Omnichord program due to the adaptability of the instrument as well as the immediate musical feedback available with limited skills. One client responded so well to the use of the Omnichord that she initiated behavior for the first time during our sessions. Her parents realized that their disabled daughter had potential greater than they had previously thought and have already enrolled her in additional programs. Another client has increased the use of the left hand, one that had limited muscle strength, through alternating strumming patterns from left to right hand while playing familiar songs.

The ease of learning the Omnichord and the immediacy of its music making capabilities have made it an excellent instrument for training staff with limited or no previous musical training. At Waimano Hospital and Training School, I was hired to develop a therapeutic music program for the clients and provide training for all the staff. As a result, I created songbooks during each of three successive summers that included requested songs the staff used with severely and profoundly retarded adults. These books contained play, folk, Hawaiian, seasonal and patriotic, and popular songs. They were written in such a way as to minimize musical notation, while providing a means for a musical performance on the Omnichord. In addition to the clients, the staff have also benefited from more musical experiences. There was a noticeable attitudinal improvement in both staff and clients and a decrease in personnel change for the first few years after the beginning of the therapeutic music program.

Because we know that music can produce both significant and potentially rehabilitative psychological and physiological changes in individuals, it is necessary to have a means of making music that is accessible, transportable, adaptable, and authentic musically. I have found the Omnichord to be an instrument that is uniquely qualified to meet these requirements.

RHYTHMIC AUDITORY STIMULATION AS AN ENTRAINMENT AND THERAPY TECHNIQUE: EFFECTS ON GAIT OF STROKE AND PARKINSON'S PATIENTS

G. C. McIntosh, Michael H. Thaut, and R. R. Rice

Introduction

Beginning in 1988, we incorporated music therapy into our neurologic rehabilitation program. This was initially done with the aim to increase enjoyment and participation in therapy activities through the stimulating effects of music. Quite early on, however, the physical therapists and occupational therapists working with our patients noted and reported observations suggestive of motor facilitation. Some patients were observed performing motor activities to musical accompaniment that, prior to the inclusion of music, were not within their capabilities. In order to evaluate these observations of motor facilitation, we first studied the effect of rhythmic cueing on stride parameters and electromyography (EMG) patterns in the gait of normal individuals (Thaut, McIntosh, Prassas, & Rice, 1992). We found improvement in stride parameters, especially stride symmetry, and EMG patterns, especially the consistency of muscle contraction within the stride cycle (Thaut et al., 1992). These studies suggested that auditory rhythm served as a peripheral timing signal that improved stride rhythmicity and positively affected muscle activity by producing more focused motor unit recruitment patterns. Based on these observations in normal individuals, we decided to explore "rhythmic auditory stimulation" (RAS), the term we have coined for this technique, as a potential facilitative measure in a neurologic rehabilitation setting.

In the 3 years since this study of gait in normal individuals, we have conducted three further studies to determine the potential entrainment effects and rehabilitation therapy effects of RAS. The first study investigated RAS gait entrainment in a group of stable patients who had suffered a post cerebrovascular accident (CVA) within a period of 1 month to 2 years (Thaut, McIntosh, Prassas, & Rice, 1993). We then initiated a study, not yet completed, of RAS as a gait training technique with stroke patients during their initial rehabilitation. Our most recent study has investigated the effects of RAS in gait training for patients with Parkinson's disease (PD).

RAS Gait Entrainment Post CVA

Method

This initial rehabilitation study was done with 10 subjects who had a prior CVA involving a cerebral hemisphere. Five of the subjects had either thrombotic or hemorrhagic events affecting the right cerebral hemisphere, and five had events affecting the left cerebral hemisphere, typically in a middle cerebral artery distribution. Various characteristics of these subjects including type and localization of the CVA and major neurologic deficits are outlined in Table 1.

The subjects were evaluated while walking for 6 meters at free speed along our laboratory walkway to determine their baseline walking ability. Measurements were taken and an analysis made of gastrocnemius surface EMG and temporal stride parameters by way of computerized foot switches. In addition, selected biomechanical variables were monitored by way of video analysis. The second walk in this entrainment study was done with the

Table 1. *Description of Subjects*

PATIENT CODE ID	SEX	AGE	POST STROKE (Months)	CVA TYPE	NEUROLOGIC DEFICITS
10	M	64	3	Right hemispheric infarction with hemorrhagic conversion	Mild left hemiparesis and left sensory inattention, diabetic neuropathy with bilateral footdrop
2	F	49	9	Left intercerebral hemorrhage. Arteriovenous malformation	Right hemiparesis with essentially plegic right upper extremity, fluent aphasia
3	M	87	24	Right intracranial hemorrhage	Right hemiparesis and nonfluent aphasia. Right homonymous hemianopsia.
4	M	74	5	Left thalamic hemorrhage	Left hemiparesis and mild left sided sensory deficits
5	M	71	11	Right thalamic hemorrhage	Left hemiparesis involving upper extremity much more than lower extremity, moderate left sided sensory inattention
6	M	65	2	Right lacunar infarct. Left internal capsule	Mild left hemiparesis with intact sensation and perception
7	F	80	2	Left parietal ischemic stroke	Right hemiparesis, fluent aphasia, sensory inattention, visual field defect on the right, alexia with agraphia
8	M	70	4	Right intracranial hemorrhage	Mild left hemiparesis and no sensory deficits
9	M	67	2	Intercerebral hemorrhage. Left internal capsule	Right hemiparesis with dysarthria and no sensory deficits
10	M	77	4	Left middle cerebral artery distribution infarction	Mild right hemiparesis with mild sensory inattention, intact language function

subjects having matched RAS cadence to the free speed gait cadence to determine if immediate entrainment effects occurred without interference from practice. Instrumental Renaissance Dance style music in 2/4 meter with an embedded metronome beat (50 millisecond square wave at 500 Hz) to enhance the tempo was used for RAS. Tempo was varied to match each subject's gait cadence. The music was recorded on a synthesizer and replayed using a sequencer as a variable tempo driver.

Results

In this stroke entrainment study, a clear pattern of auditory to motor synchronization emerged for most subjects. The subjects significantly improved their stride symmetry and weight bearing time on their paretic side ($p < 0.05$). Stride variability also decreased to a significant degree ($p < 0.05$). The stride parameter findings from the RAS entrainment study in stroke patients are diagramed in Table 2 using the mean percentage change from the nonrhythm condition as the measure of relative improvement.

Table 2. *Mean Percentage Change (MPC) from Nonrhythm Condition for Temporal Stride Parameters (n = 10)*

STRIDE PARAMETERS	MPC Trial 1	MPC Trial 2	MPC Trial 3	Total MPC
Increase in weightbearing (Stance) time on the affected side	2.0	3.3	6.0	3.8*
Decrease in stride variation	15.9	27.1	32.5	25.2*
Increase in stride symmetry	7.5	21.9	34.8	21.4*

*Significant at $p < .05$

Subjects also showed a more balanced muscular activation pattern on EMG between the paretic and nonparetic limbs. A decrease in integrated amplitude variability of EMG on the paretic side was also noted. These EMG changes were significant ($p < 0.05$), and are outlined in Table 3 using the mean percentage change for the nonrhythm condition as the measure of relative improvement.

Table 3. *Mean Percentage Change (MPC) from Nonrhythm Condition for Gastrocnemius EMG Parameters (n = 10)*

EMG PARAMETERS	MPC Trial 1	MPC Trial 2	MPC Trial 3	Total MPC
Increase in Amplitude (µV/msec)				
Affected Side	4.8	11.4	16.3	10.8*
Nonaffected Side	-7.7	-8.3	-9.6	-8.5 (ns)
Decrease in Amplitude (µV/msec)	14.9	15.1	19.5	16.5*
Decrease in Amplitude (µV/msec) during Swing Phase	2.9	11.8	16.6	10.4*

*Significant at $p < .05$ ns = nonsignificant

RAS In Stroke Rehabilitation Gait Therapy

Method

In the stroke rehabilitation study, we have so far analyzed the potential therapeutic effect of RAS in gait training with four patients in the experimental group compared to four matched patients in the control group. The subjects were brought into the study when they were able to walk for 5 meters with hand-held assistance, usually a few weeks into their stroke rehabilitation program. Each subject was pretested using EMG, temporal stride analysis, and video analysis of selected biomechanical variables. The experimental group was trained for 6 weeks daily using RAS as the main gait training technique incorporated into a conventional stroke rehabilitation program. The control group, on the other hand, received daily conventional gait training with no RAS. Both groups were trained by qualified physical therapists familiar with gait rehabilitation post CVA.

Both groups were matched by age, Barthel index score, gender, and site of lesion. After the 6 weeks of rehabilitation therapy, the subjects were posttested measuring the same parameters and using exactly the same techniques for which they had been pretested. No music was used during either pretesting or posttesting measurements. For the RAS therapy group we prepared 10 instrumental pieces from various musical styles including country and western, classical, big band, dance, and American folk with enhanced beat function using a synthesizer and sequencer. Study subjects in the RAS group selected their preferred musical style. All music was digitally recorded and played back by way of synthesizer with a sequencer serving as a variable tempo driver so the tempo could be adjusted to the subject's preferred stride. Therefore, as stride velocity increased during the rehabilitation period the tempo could be adjusted appropriately.

Results

In the stroke rehabilitation study (which is still underway), current data analysis with eight subjects shows considerable gains after 6 weeks of RAS therapy over conventional physical therapy in both velocity and stride length (Figure 1).

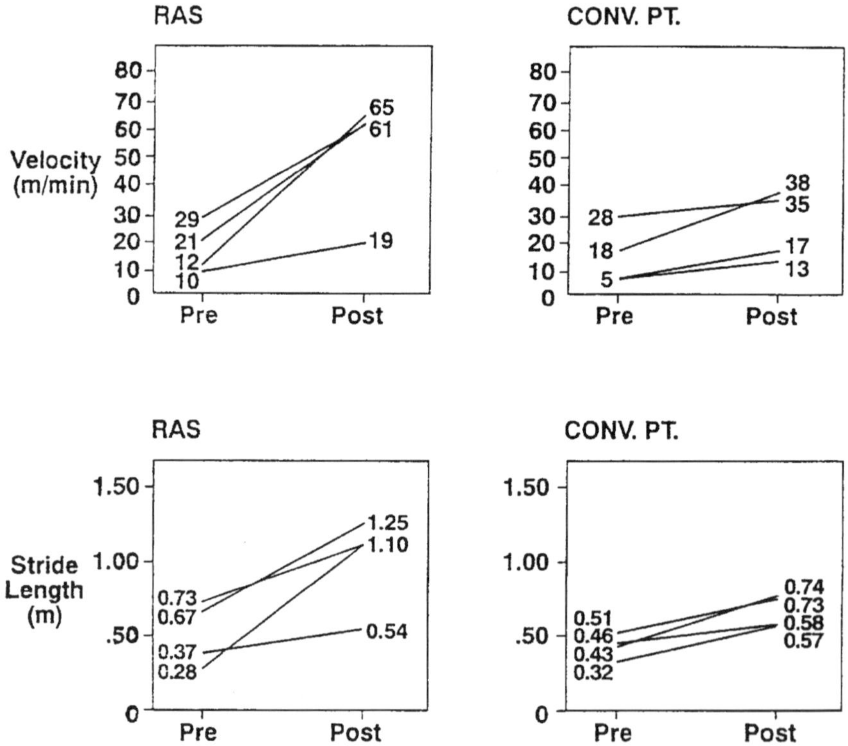

Figure 1. The graphs above show the changes in gait velocity pre- and post-rehab program for those patients treated with RAS and conventional physical therapy. The graphs below show the changes in stride length pre and post-rehabilitation for RAS and conventional physical therapy.

Minimal changes were noted in cadence. Improvement in EMG variability was also seen to a greater degree in the RAS group. An example is shown in Figure 2.

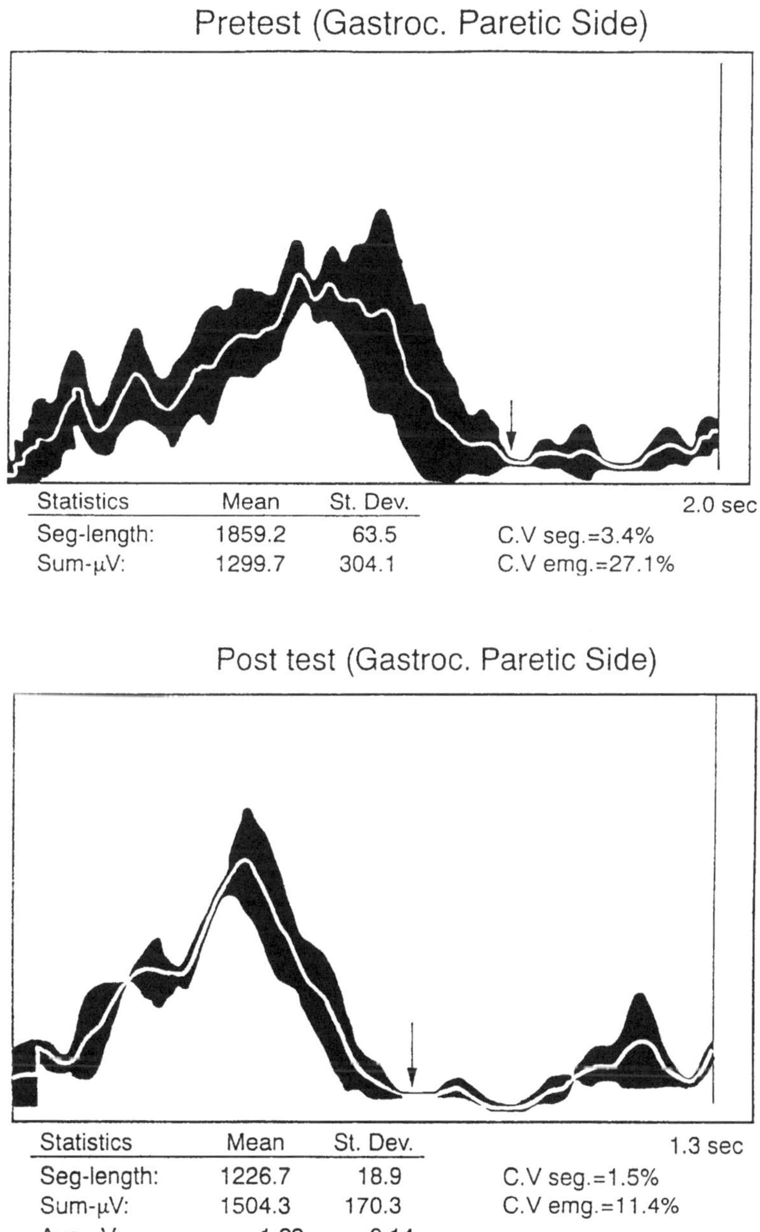

Figure 2. Reduction in variation of the EMG pattern in the gastrocnemius muscle on the paretic side from the pre-test (above) to post-test (below).

RAS Gait Entrainment in Patients With Parkinson's Disease

Method

An entrainment study with six PD patients has been completed. In this study the subjects walked four times for 6 meters. Initially, the subjects were asked to walk at maximal speed without rhythmic cueing. They were then evaluated using RAS matched to that same maximum speed. The third trial was conducted with RAS at 10% increased tempo over the maximum speed gait tempo. Finally, the subjects were studied without RAS to determine if there was any short term carryover effect. Only temporal stride parameters were recorded. The subjects in this study had varied duration and severity of disease, and all were medicated with dopaminergic medications. All measurements were made 60–90 minutes after a dosage of medication. The same musical styles and digital audio technology available in the stroke rehabilitation study were used in the PD study.

Results

In the entrainment study with PD subjects, four of the six subjects improved their walking speed with RAS demonstrating close phase coupling of their stepping patterns with the external pacemaker. One subject walked faster but consistently stepped ahead of the beat. The subject with the most severe motor impairments was not able to speed up gait cadence with RAS. The improvements noted in gait velocity and stride length were both significant at $p < 0.05$ and are outlined in Table 4.

Table 4. *Mean Values (x) of Stride Parameters of PD Patients*

n = 6	Baseline	RAS (10% faster)	Carryover
Velocity (meters/min)	34.2	42.3	42.7
	Baseline vs. RAS: $p < 0.05$		
Cadence	91	100	98.5
	Baseline vs. RAS: $p < 0.05$		
Stride Length (cm)	74	88	83
	Baseline vs. RAS: $p < 0.05$		
Symmetry	0.82	0.88	0.88

Discussion

Grillner and Wallen (1985) have described locomotion as depending on two factors. The first essential factor for locomotion based on their theory is rhythmic neural activity of a central pattern generator that provides the oscillatory network requisite for rhythmic locomotor output. The second essential factor is that of sensory input necessary for timing and shaping the locomotor pattern. A central pattern generator is a network of neurons, usually interneurons, that when activated is capable of producing automatic patterned movements. In the studies from our laboratory over the past 3 years (described above), we have sought to determine if peripheral rhythmic auditory stimulation can function as an external oscillator whose signal periodicity can entrain temporal parameters of gait and underlying neuromuscular activity by way of influences over the purported central pattern generator for gait (Figure 3).

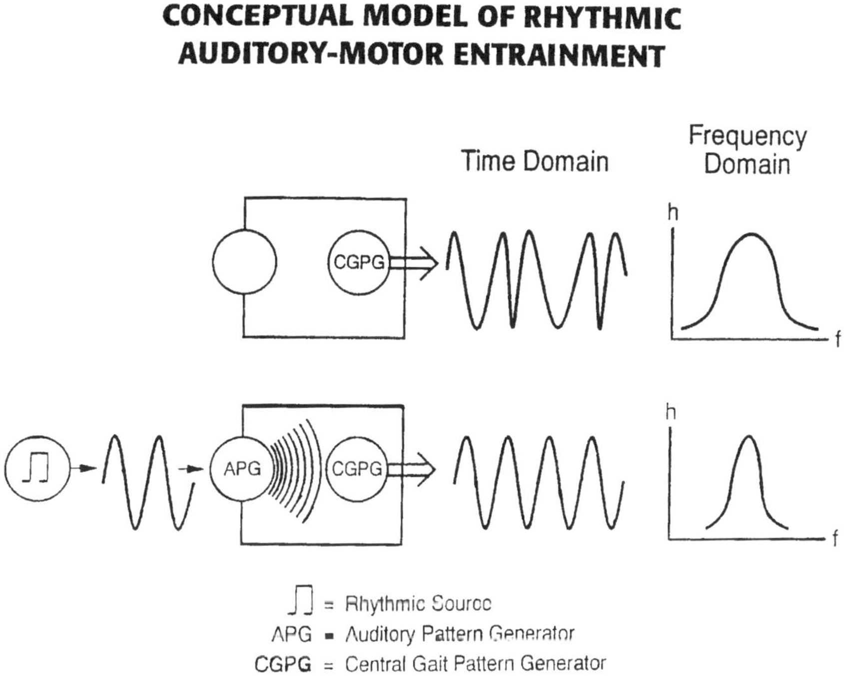

Figure 3. The conceptual model for rhythmic auditory motor entrainment indicates a central pattern generator that operates in a time domain and a frequency domain (above). When rhythmic source, which has a set signal periodicity, affects the auditory pattern generator, then this has a direct effect on the central pattern gait generator to produce a greater rhythmicity and less variation in the frequency domain (below).

Specifically we have been interested in studying these potential entrainment effects as neuromuscular rehabilitation techniques to retrain motor control in individuals with neurologic damage to their motor systems, in our studies more specifically stroke and PD.

We have demonstrated a strong facilitatory effect of RAS on gait performance in both stroke subjects and in PD subjects. The amount of facilitatory effect noted in both groups is somewhat surprising because the gait deficits in stroke and PD have very different kinesiologic features and are brought about by differing neuropathologies. The mechanism of this facilitatory effect remains elusive to us, although we have developed some theoretical ideas based somewhat on the work of others.

Rossignol and Melvill-Jones (1976) have described the potential priming effect of sound on the motor system. This study used the H-reflex to monitor audio-spinal influences in man and recognize the possibility of rhythmic movement synchronized to sound. It is our opinion, based on the studies we have performed to date, that rhythmic auditory cues are able to access central pattern generators for gait in the nervous system and augment motor control by using timing as a coordinating unit in the generation of complex movement sequences. Our observations are in line with those previously described by Rossignol and Melvill-Jones (1976), but use entrainment and therapy paradigms. In addition, the synchronization effect observed in our studies supports the notion that there is an anticipatory structure of RAS that may facilitate motor control on a motor program level. The efficiency within the musical performance context to build and execute complex motor programs using rhythmic clock structures as coordinative constraints has been previously described by Shaffer (1981). By utilizing musical rhythm in therapy, we may actually be accessing motor programming strategies of an anticipatory nature similar to the ones used by skillful performers in music.

At the present time, we have ongoing studies in normal elderly populations, further studies with PD patients, and analysis of the effect of this technique in children with cerebral palsy. We are also analyzing in greater detail some of the temporal relationships of specific stride parameters to changes in tempo in hopes of developing a better understanding of the neurophysiologic mechanisms behind our observations of auditory motor facilitation in man.

References

Thaut, M. H., McIntosh, G. C., Prassas, S. G., & Rice, R. R. (1992). Effect of rhythmic cueing on temporal stride parameters and EMG patterns in normal gait. *Journal of Neurologic Rehabilitation, 6,* 185–190.

Thaut, M. H., McIntosh, G. C., Prassas, S. G., & Rice, R. R. (1993). Effect of rhythmic cueing on temporal stride parameters and EMG patterns in hemiparetic gait of stroke patients. *Journal of Neurologic Rehabilitation, 7,* 9–16.

Griller, S., & Wallen, P. (1985). Central pattern generators for locomotion with special reference to vertebrates. *Annual Reviews in Neuroscience, 8,* 233–261.

Rossignol, S., & Melvill-Jones, G. (1976). Audio-spinal influences in man studied by the H-reflex and its possible role in rhythmic movements synchronized to sound. *Electroencephalography and Clinical Neurophysiology, 41,* 83–92.

Shaffer, L. H. (1981). Performances of Chopin, Bach, Bartok: Studies in motor programming. *Cognitive Psychology, 13,* 326–376.

THE NATURE OF THE TUNE AND TEXT IN THE PRODUCTION OF SONGS IN ALZHEIMER'S TYPE DEMENTIA

Julene K. Johnson and Hanna K. Ulatowska

Abstract

The present case study was a 2-year, longitudinal investigation of the production of familiar songs by one subject with dementia of the Alzheimer's type (DAT). In the context of song production, characteristics of the breakdown of language (i.e., text) and music (i.e., tune) were explored. In addition, a cognitive and language profile was compiled for comparison. Results of this longitudinal case study revealed that the tune and text of familiar songs showed differential breakdown during the progression of Alzheimer's dementia. When the subject progressed into moderate stages of the disease, systematic errors in the song texts at the level of words were observed. A large proportion of the initial text errors were semantically and phonologically related to the original text. Components of the tune remained relatively preserved at this time, and the integrity of the song was maintained by text insertions. An eventual disintegration of the tune, however, occurred as the subject became severely demented. During this time, the tune became monotonic, and rhythmic organization was lost. Text errors continued to occur and were less related to the original text. The subject, however, continued to attempt to produce songs.

Introduction

Recently there has been a growing interest in the heterogeneous nature of cognitive impairments in persons with dementia of the Alzheimer's type (DAT). Because cognitive impairment is a primary disturbance in DAT, an understanding of the multidimensionality of cognition is a priority. Most research thus far has concentrated on deficits of memory (Brandt, Spencer, McSorley, & Folstein, 1988; Nebes, 1989). However, recent research on other aspects of cognition, such as language and communication, attention, and visuospatial skills has uncovered problems in other aspects of cognition (Salmon, Heindel, & Butters, 1991). Investigations addressing the unique patterns of cognitive preservations and deficits will contribute to a better understanding of the complex nature of this neurological disorder. The cognitive neuropsychological approach to the study of DAT supports detailed case studies and longitudinal followings in the attempt to isolate functionally relevant cognitive subsystems (Schwartz, 1990; Shallice, 1990).

Music Cognition in DAT

One area of cognition that has received little attention in the Alzheimer's literature is music cognition. The study of music processing provides a unique way to investigate another aspect of cognitive functioning in DAT. A few studies have addressed the use of music in the care of persons with DAT in terms of sensory stimulation (Dietsche & Pollman, 1982; Norberg, Melin, & Asplund, 1986) and music therapy (Claire & Bernstein, 1990; Lipe, 1991; Olderog-Millard & Smith, 1989; Pricket & Moore, 1991). These studies report that music activities have a positive effect on various behaviors (i.e., attention, communication, and group participation). Other authors using dichotic listening tasks have concluded that central auditory functioning is impaired in DAT (Grimes, Grady, Foster, Sunderland, & Patronas, 1985; Mohr, Cox, Williams, Chase, & Fedio, 1990).

A preservation of music functioning in DAT has recently been documented in several case studies. Three cases report a preservation of music production (Crystal, Grober, & Masur, 1989; Beatty, Zavadil, Bailly, Rixen, Lavadil, Franham, & Fisher, 1988; Polk & Kertesz, 1993). The subjects were able to perform, from memory, previously learned piano compositions. The subject described by Beatty et al. (1988) could play and identify scales and sight-read a brief, unfamiliar piano piece but had difficulty in identifying time and key signatures, distinguishing among music styles (e.g., waltz and march), and labeling familiar tunes. Crystal et al. (1989) also reported an inability to provide titles for familiar classical works. The important finding in these studies, however, is that some aspects of music knowledge remain intact despite impairments in other areas of cognition. It is difficult to explain these patterns of music cognition without a detailed understanding of how music functioning relates to other cognitive functioning. In addition, the generalizability of preserved music abilities in persons *without* music training must also be addressed.

Polk and Kertesz (1993) documented a second case in which the subject presented with primarily right posterior cortical atrophy, spatial agraphia, and a visuopractic deficit. This subject had impairments in melodic and rhythmic organization that were compared to a preservation of language functions. The concurrent evaluation of music and language in DAT has only been conducted by Polk and Kertesz. Although minimal literature is available concerning music cognition in DAT, there are many reports concerning language functioning in DAT. Numerous disruptions in language functioning have been documented (Bayles & Kaszniak, 1987; Kempler, 1991; Ulatowska & Chapman, 1991). Although the associations of music and language have not been extensively investigated in DAT, a moderate body of literature examining the patterns of music and language deficits in focal brain damage is available.

Music and Language in Brain Damage

Aspects of language and music functioning have been simultaneously evaluated in other neurologically impaired subjects, such as in those who have suffered a stroke or undergone a temporal lobectomy (see Zatorre, 1984; Marin, 1982 for reviews). These associations between language and music functioning of brain-damaged persons have been considered for several centuries. The literature describes numerous patterns of preservations and deficits of both language and music abilities. As early as 1745, Dalin noted a preserved singing ability in an aphasic (Benton & Joynt, 1960). Others also reported preserved music abilities in subjects with concurrent aphasic disorders (Morgan & Tilluckdharry, 1982; Assal, 1973; Geschwind, Quadfasel, & Segarra, 1968; Luria, Tsvetkova, & Futer, 1965); in other cases, a breakdown of music abilities has occurred (Brain, 1941; Jellinek, 1956). The disorder of music functioning, termed *amusia,* has been documented in persons with and without aphasia (Marin, 1982; Zatorre, 1984). Although the literature points to no clear conclusions about the relationship between music and language functioning in these cases, most studies have not systematically investigated this association.

In addition to studying music and language as systems, aspects of music (i.e., tune) and language (i.e., text) can be studied in the context of songs. Although many studies address song production in brain damaged populations, few cases document specific aspects of the tune or the text. Yamadori, Osumi, Masuhara, and Okubo (1977) evaluated the singing abilities of Broca's aphasics and found that 6 of the 24 subjects had some impairment of singing. The subjects who had difficulty singing were only able to hum the tune, producing no song text. They also reported that three additional subjects produced a few paraphasic errors in the text while singing, while the others produced songs of good quality. This study, however, did not provide any explanation for this finding. Morgan and Tilluckdharry (1982) also reported a preservation of singing in two subjects with severe Broca's aphasia. Early cases by several authors (Jackson, 1871; Kast, 1885; Knoblauch, 1890; Mann, 1898; Jossmann, 1927) acknowledge impairments of singing, but these cases lack detailed documentation. Farat (described in Knoblauch, 1890) classified two types of aphasics who could sing: those who could sing with text and those who could sing the melody without text. Other studies mention singing abilities in articles addressing aphasia but do not give a detailed account (Smith, 1969; Heilman, Tucker, & Valenstein, 1976; Geschwind, Quadfasel, & Segarra, 1968; Gott, 1973). Thus, the studies concerning the analysis of song production in neurologically impaired individuals have not been comprehensive.

Singing and speech abilities have also been assessed following intracarotid injection of sodium amytal, which induces a transient loss of function in the ipsilateral cerebral hemisphere. Gordon and Bogen (1974) and Borchgrevink (1980) described the effects of this procedure on singing and speech production. Although the accounts of singing were not described in detail, Borchgrevink (1980) noted that following left carotid injection, the rhythmic elements of singing familiar songs were impaired, while the ability to produce melodies was preserved. Singing was less disturbed than speech. Conversely, following right intracarotid injection, language remained relatively intact; rhythmic aspects in singing were preserved, while the melody was described as being "monotonic". Changes, if any, in the song text, however, were not documented during this procedure. Thus, the melodic and rhythmic elements, in addition to speech and music functions, were found to be differentially affected in sodium amytal experiments.

Background on The Use of Songs

The context of a song provides a setting in which language and music are associated in time. Texts of songs are composed of connected language in the form of song lyrics and can consist of a variety of language forms. For instance, song lyrics are sometimes narrative in form, and others consist of repetitions of phrases. The production of songs, unlike other forms of music, is a dynamic event that requires an interaction of a text with rhythmic and melodic motion of the tune. A moderate repertoire of songs is commonly known by the average American, especially older Americans. Most persons have experienced singing to some degree during their lives. Singing can be done without formal music training and is common during several social events, such as Christmas, school, and religious ceremonics. Songs, therefore, are ecologically salient. The study of song texts in DAT will provide a contrast to documentation of numerous impairments of language in DAT (Bayles & Kaszniak, 1987; Ulatowska & Chapman, 1991; Kempler, 1991)

Purpose of Study

The present case study is a 2-year, longitudinal investigation of the production of familiar songs in one subject with DAT, specifically one with no formal music training. In the context of song production, characteristics of the breakdown of text (language) and tune (music) can be explored. The following questions were examined: (a) Do cognitive functions mediating music cognition remain intact through the progression of DAT? (b) What is the longitudinal nature of the tune and text in the production of familiar songs in DAT? (c) Are the text and tune differentially affected in the breakdown of song production?

Method

Subject

D.N. was followed for 2 years, beginning shortly after the diagnosis of probable DAT by a local Alzheimer's Research Center in December 1989. She is a 76-year-old, right-handed female who was diagnosed with probable DAT (according to NINCDS-ADRDA criteria; McKhamm, Drachman, Folstein, Katzman, Price, & Stadlan, 1988), following a neurological examination consisting of computed tomography, MRI, EEG, spinal tap, and blood tests. She had no previous history of neurological abnormalities. She earned a bachelor's degree in education and worked as a teacher and an office clerk. It is important to note that she had no formal music training, although she participated in church music activities throughout her life. Her father was an amateur vocalist, and her husband plays several instruments for a hobby. In addition, she and her husband regularly attended community music concerts, even into the course of the disease. A premorbid sample of her singing ability from 1969 was also available that revealed average competence in singing.

She was selected as a candidate for a case study after observation of selective disruptions and preservations of cognitive functioning. It was noticed that the subject had impairments in language and cognition, yet was able to sing familiar songs. This case study, however, was not selected on the basis of unusual or particularly unique patterns; but instead, it is hoped that she represents a typical case. When relatively little is known about an area, an in-depth case study approach can be more informative than group studies. Furthermore, the heterogeneity documented in the progression of DAT has been used to argue for case study research (Schwartz, 1990). In group studies, subject variation is not adequately addressed. Therefore, the decision to conduct an in-depth case study supported the goal to provide detailed, longitudinal documentation of multiple areas of cognition.

In addition to documenting specific aspects of music functioning, a profile of language and cognitive abilities was also compiled. The overall battery consisted of a music assessment, focusing on song production, and a battery of standardized language and cognitive assessments. The examiner met with the subject on a weekly basis at her residence for a duration of 2 years.

Basic Music Assessment

The assessment of music abilities included evaluations of basic music skills and the production of familiar songs. Because music cognition involves various levels of representation, it is important to assess the intactness of a basic level of music functioning in addition to the more complex music behavior of song production.

Basic music abilities were assessed via tasks requiring rhythmic and melodic reproduction and song title completion. The tasks were adapted from the amusia assessment battery of Wertheim and Botez (1959). To assess short-term memory for rhythmic phrases, the subject was asked to reproduce (by finger tapping) rhythmic patterns (up to five beats in length) modeled by the experimenter. The subject was also asked to vocally reproduce short melodic phrases (up to five pitches in length) modeled by the examiner. Melodic reproduction was utilized to assess short-term memory for unfamiliar melodic phrases.

A song title completion task was used to assess recall of song titles. The association of language and music in songs occurs at different levels and in different contexts. For instance, language and music can be associated in the following ways: verbal descriptions about music, verbal categorization of types of music (e.g., "folk songs" or "patriotic music"), the text (or lyrics) of songs, and the singing of songs on nonsense syllables. The elicitation of song titles is an additional way to assess language associated with songs. We commonly refer to songs by their titles. In this context, the possible relationship between the ability to produce song titles and the ability to produce the complete song can be addressed. Both Beatty et al. (1988) and Crystal et al. (1989) reported an impaired ability to generate song titles in two cases with DAT. A repertoire of well-known song titles from the 1930s to 1950s was selected. From this list, the examiner verbally cued the first few words of each song titles and asked the subject to complete the phrase. For instance, titles included, "Let Me Call <u>You Sweetheart</u>" and "For He's a <u>Jolly Good Fellow</u>", and the subject was asked to complete the verbal cue with the underlined portion of the title.

Song Production Evaluation

The evaluation of music components was also done in the context of singing familiar songs. A repertoire of familiar songs was initially established, using 50 songs with well-known titles (from the 1930s through 1950s). The subject was asked to check those titles that were familiar to her. "Familiar songs" were defined as being those songs that the subject checked and could recall at least part of the text or tune. Songs indicated by the subject as familiar included primarily folk songs and hymns. Using songsheets of these familiar songs and no accompaniment, the subject sang a variety of these familiar songs during the 2-year period of study. To control for practice effects, some songs were presented each week, and others were presented at less frequent intervals. Throughout the study, it was noted that songs presented more frequently did not differ in quality from those presented less often. Sessions were audio recorded and later transcribed.

Time periods (Time 1–4) refer to intervals of 4 months. Time 1 (10/91–12/91) begins 4 months prior to the time when changes in singing abilities occurred. Seventy-five versions of songs sung by the subject during the four time periods were selected from the transcriptions as being most representative of her singing ability. From these 75 songs, a collection of 10 songs per time period (or 40% of the total songs) was randomly selected for further analysis. The 10 songs included versions of "Amazing Grace", "Rock of Ages", and "Jesus Loves Me". During each time period, three samples of "Amazing Grace" and "Rock of Ages" were selected, and four samples of "Jesus Loves Me" were selected. Selection of the same songs over time provided comparisons within and between songs.

Qualitative analysis of songs. Analysis of the songs included overall qualitative ratings of the tune and text and additional analyses of the tune and text. Selection of the variables operationally defining the tune and text were selected based on empirical research regarding features of a tune and text. The importance of pitch and rhythmic elements in contributing to a meaningful melodic sequence has been addressed by many authors (Monahan &

Carterette, 1985; Handel, 1989; Dowling, 1973). Dowling and Harwood (1986) discuss evidence for the importance of pitch elements in the memory for melodic features. Sloboda & Parker (1985) provide analyses of both melody and rhythm in their study of vocal reproductions of unfamiliar melodies. An additional variable of "musical interpretation" provided a category that addressed expressive variation in the tunes. Music interpretation is difficult to define and can be quantified in the correct use of phrasing and dynamics. Based on the findings of these researchers, the following variables were selected for rating the tune: pitch accuracy (proximity of recalled pitches to original pitches), rhythmic accuracy (similarity of recalled rhythmic patterns to original rhythmic structure), and appropriateness of musical interpretation (musically correct expressive variation of the tune).

In the present study, overall qualitative ratings of song texts were also made. Song texts, like ordinary discourse, have structural organization. In the case of familiar songs, the text is prescribed more distinctly than in discourse of conversation. Song texts are usually recalled verbatim, much like the recitation of a previously memorized text (e.g., poems or prayers). Therefore, the production of a "good" song text relies on exact reproduction. There are no studies that rate the quality of song texts, but there are examples of rating systems that are applied to assess other types of discourse (Ulatowska, Allard, & Donnell, 1988; Ulatowska, North, & Macaluso-Haynes, 1981). The quality of articulation of the song text is another dimension that can be assessed. The rating of articulatory agility is one domain used in the *Boston diagnostic aphasia examination* (Goodglass & Kaplan, 1983). Based on the previous studies of rating quality of texts, the variables selected to assess the quality of the song text included word accuracy and articulation.

It was important that longitudinal aspects of changes in song production were recorded. Therefore, overall ratings of the quality of song production were made during each time period. A 5-point Lickert scale (see Figure 1) was utilized to rate the variables for the tune and text. Evaluations of the tune and the text were made separately on the scale. Each of the variables was rated on the 5-point scale with 5 being of good quality (as in an average singer) and 1 being of poor quality. A mean for each of the tune and text variables was calculated separately. Two raters with at least a bachelor's degree in music judged the overall quality of the tune and text according to the specified variables.

Song text analysis. In addition, further analyses of the text were undertaken after the observation of differential breakdown of the tune and text. The total number of text errors per song was determined. Then a mean percentage of text errors per time period was calculated. Also, the text errors were categorized according to the type of error they represented. The categorization scheme for classification of the text errors was adapted from Goodglass and Kaplan (1983), Hodges, Salmon, and Butters (1991), and Li and Williams (1991). Hodges et al. (1991) found that the profile of naming errors on the *Boston Naming Test* distinguished subjects with DAT and Huntington's disease. In the present study, the types of errors were considered over time to determine if the nature of the errors changed.

Language and Cognitive Assessment

The Boston naming test (Kaplan, Goodglass, & Weintraub, 1983) and the *Boston diagnostic aphasia examination* (Goodglass & Kaplan, 1983) were utilized in the assessment of language function. A communicative questionnaire (Ulatowska et al., 1988) filled out by the subject's spouse assessed aspects of functional communication. Samples of discourse

Quality

1 _____ 2 _____ 3 _____ 4 _____ 5 _____

poor quality good quality

A. Aspects of TUNE

_____ Pitch Accuracy
- a. Tonal accuracy
- b. Pitch contour
- c. Key relations

_____ Rhythmic Accuracy
- a. Overall tempo
- b. Accuracy of beats

_____ Stylistic Interpretation
- a. Dynamic range
- b. Phrasing

B. Aspects of TEXT

_____ Word Accuracy
- a. Semantic paraphasias
- b. Phonemic paraphasias
- c. Added words
- d. Neologisms
- e. Unrelated words
- f. Unintelligible utterances

_____ Articulation of Text

Figure 1. Rating scale used for qualitative evaluation of tune and text

(e.g., during reminiscence about a song topic or in the retelling of memorable experiences) were also transcribed to determine if similar errors were seen in other examples of discourse. Language was evaluated every 6–8 months using the standardized assessments.

The severity of dementia was determined every 4 months according to the *Global deterioration rating scale* (Reisberg, Ferris, DeLeon, & Crook, 1983). Other neuropsychological tests included the *Mini mental status examination* (MMSE; Folstein, Folstein, & McHugh, 1975) and various subtests (discrimination, visual memory, and visual sequence) from the *Test of visual-perceptual skills* (Gardner, 1982). Combinations of cognitive tests were administered every 6–8 months.

Results

Language and Cognitive Profile

Assessments of language and cognitive functions showed considerable deterioration throughout the study. Longitudinal results of the standardized tests are outlined in Tables 1 and 2. Time periods (Time 1–4) refer to intervals of 4 months, beginning 4 months before changes in song production occurred (9/90). On initial evaluation (2/90), D.N. was assessed to be in the moderate stages of DAT (GDS rating of 4).

Table 1. *Summary of Standardized Language Measures*

BOSTON DIAGNOSTIC APHASIA EXAMINATION subtests	Time 1	Time 2	Time 3	Time 4
1. Auditory Comprehension				
a. Word discrimination	60	60	*	*
b. Body-part identification	100	55		
c. Commands	50	0		
d. Complex ideational	40	30		
2. Naming				
a. Responsive	40	35	*	*
b. Confrontative	60	45		
c. Animal naming	60	30		
3. Repetition				
a. Words	70	70	*	*
b. High-probability	70	30		
c. Low-probability	50	40		
4. Automatic Speech				
a. Automatic sequences	50	30	*	*
b. Reciting	*	40		
5. Reading Comprehension				
a. Symbol discrimination	25	*	*	*
b. Word recognition	80	*		
c. Oral spelling	70	50		
d. Word-picture matching	40	*		
e. Reading sentences	40	50		
BOSTON NAMING TEST	10/30	4/30	*	*

Note: * Indicates that test was not given during the time period due to the lack of understanding of the instructions.

Table 2. *Summary of Standardized Cognitive Tests*

	Time 1	Time 2	Time 3	Time 4
Global Dementia Rating	4	4	5	6
Mini-Mental Status Exam	*	4/30	*	*
Test of Visual-Perceptual Skills				
a. discrimination	8/16	*	*	*
b. Visual memory	1/16	*	*	*
c. Visual sequence	0/16	*	*	*

Note: * Indicates that test was not given during the time period due to the lack of understanding of the instructions.

Initial evaluation of language revealed a confrontation naming deficit that was confirmed with a score of 10/30 on the revised *Boston naming test.* She performed below normal limits on the majority of the selected subtests of the *Boston diagnostic aphasia examination* (auditory comprehension, naming, repetition, automatic speech, and reading comprehension subtests). On the communicative questionnaire, her spouse reported that on most days she had word-finding difficulties and conversed in poorly formed sentences. Twenty-five percent of the time, she used neologisms and spoke in a monotone voice during conversation. At this time, she rarely confused the meaning of words. The clinical course of language deterioration during Times 1 and 2 can be seen in the progressive decline in most of the standardized language and cognitive scores. During Times 1 and 2, increases in the use of neologisms, the use of poorly formed sentences, and confusion of words with different meanings (e.g., "house" for "garage") were reported on the communicative questionnaire.

During Times 3 and 4, however, standardized language and cognitive tests were inappropriate to administer. The subject was unable to understand the instructions of the standardized language and cognitive assessments. At this time, she was assessed to be in the severe stages of dementia (GDS ratings of 5–6 and scores of 0/16 on three subtests of the *Test of visual-perceptual skills*). Deterioration of her language during Times 3 and 4 was evident in conversational discourse that was characterized by empty content, difficulties in word retrieval, and frequent circumlocutions. Syntactic structure and pragmatics of conversation remained preserved. The significant point is that in the moderate stages of the disease, her language and cognitive functioning were particularly impaired. With progression into the severe stages, language and cognitive impairments worsened.

Basic Music Abilities Profile

Tasks used to assess basic music abilities were utilized to support the findings with songs. The overall finding is that rhythmic and melodic reproduction through Time 3 were performed with an accuracy at or above 70%. These tasks were not performed during Time 4. The subject completed the titles of familiar songs with between 78% and 81% accuracy through Time 3. A considerable decrease (13% accuracy) in the ability to complete the titles occurred during Time 4. These results of basic music skills supported the findings in song production. Both basic music abilities and the ability to produce songs remained relatively intact until Time 4.

Song Production

Overall qualitative ratings of both the text and tune, found in Figure 20, revealed that during Time 1, all aspects of singing were normal. The subject easily sang from song sheets with minimal errors in the tune and text. Her repertoire included approximately 40 songs. She sang with appropriate stylistic interpretation and with correct tempi, relatively good pitch, and rhythmic accuracy, although she had some difficulty with lower pitched notes because of the raspy quality of her voice Despite considerable deficits in language and cognition during Time 1, D.N. retained the ability to produce familiar songs.

It was not until Time 2 that qualitative changes in the songs began to occur. As can be seen in Figure 2, overall qualitative ratings of the text declined first, followed by later declines in the quality of the tune. Because of the differential changes in the tune and text, further analyses of the text were conducted to determine the nature of these changes. An-

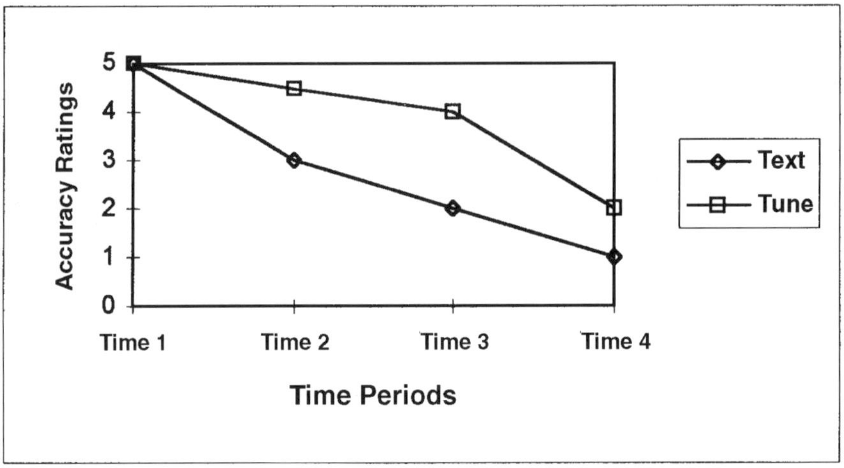

Figure 2. Overall qualitative ratings of tune and text

other observation was that the repertoire of songs sung diminished with time. By Time 4, the subject's repertoire diminished from about 40 songs to about 10 songs.

Song Text Errors

Accuracy of the song texts during the singing of familiar songs was further evaluated. Figure 3 represents the gradual increase in the mean number of text errors per song. The total number of text errors per song was tabulated and then averaged for each time period. Prior to Time 2, no alterations in the song texts were observed. However, beginning in Time 2, errors in the song texts began to occur. Word substitutions were made that most often fit into the overall music structure. In other words, the word substitutions produced were similar in length and syllabic structure to the original text and also coincided well with the tune. See Appendix A for an example of the singing of "Amazing Grace" in which the subject inserted a text that fits the overall music structure. The occurrence of the text errors was infrequent at first and then increased gradually through Time 4. Errors did not occur at the same locations in the text with repeated singing attempts either within or between sessions, although this may be an area for further investigation. Furthermore, errors seemed to be relatively evenly distributed over the duration of the songs.

Substitutions of text phrases were also observed (e.g., "the hope of my house is gone" for "that saved a wretch like me" of "Amazing Grace"), although occurring less frequently than simple word substitutions. In addition, perseverations of paraphasic errors (such as "mesik, music, shusik, sek" for "music") were also found in song texts. These types of errors also occurred in her conversational speech as well as in the reading of nonmusic texts.

Text errors were categorized during all time periods according to the type of error they represented. The following text errors were recorded: semantic and phonologic paraphasias, unrelated words, neologisms, unintelligible utterances, and added words. Table 3 outlines the categories of text errors during each time period. As can be seen, the nature of the text errors changes over time.

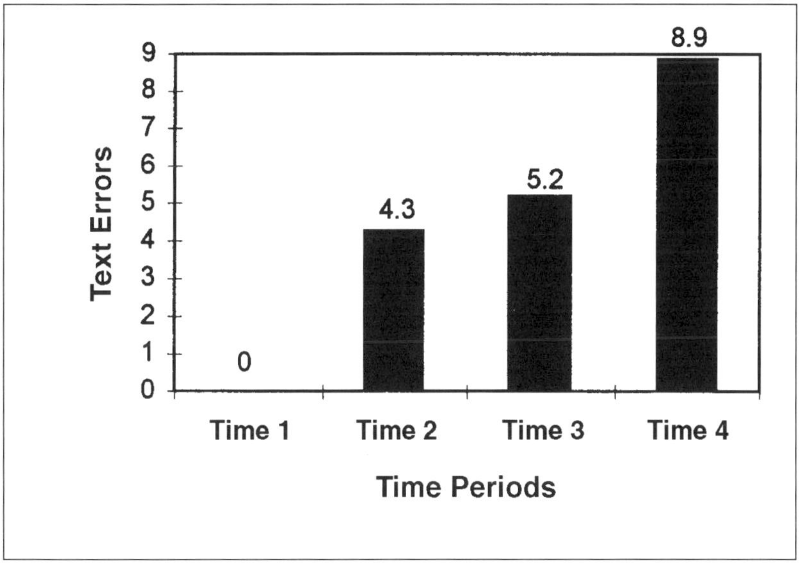

Figure 3. Mean number of text errors per song according to time periods

Table 2. *Number and Category of Text Errors*

ERROR TYPE	Time 1	Time 2	Time 3	Time 4
Semantic Paraphasias	0	12	3	12
Phonemic Paraphasias	0	10	6	11
Added Words	0	7	11	11
Unrelated Words	0	7	15	23
Neologisms	0	0	4	8
Uninterpretable	0	2	4	10
TOTALS	0	38	43	75

During Time 2, the majority of errors are paraphasic errors that are semantically and phonemically related to the original text. For example, "waved" was inserted for "saved", "sound" for "song", "match" for "wretch", and "founs" for "sound". There are minimal occurrences of unrelated words or unintelligent utterances at this time. Increases, however, in the occurrences of unintelligent utterances, added words, and unrelated words can be observed in Times 3 and 4. Thus, the text insertions became less similar to the original text with the progression of dementia.

Another observation was that during Time 3, the amount of time spent humming also increased. This could explain why the total number of text errors did not increase substantially between Times 2 and 3. The occurrence of humming took place most often at ends of phrases. The subject, however, inserted words and continued with a text when possible, even if it was incorrect, and resorted to humming when the original text seemed inaccessible. The propensity to apply a song text, when possible, was evident. Included in later renditions of the songs were more frequent attempts to sing the songs. These repetitions of the songs occurred when errors in the songs were noticed by the subject. She made frequent comments regarding the text errors. For example, while singing the first phrase of "Rock of Ages" she sang, "Rock of ages, clark for me" and then stated, "That's almost the words, I guess." The word "clark" is a paraphasic error for the word "cleft". After several attempts to sing "My Country Tis of Thee", she stated, "I just can't hold on to it". These kinds of statements occurred more frequently during Time 2 and decreased gradually. While repeating a phrase, she most often retained the correct tune.

When comparing the language used in song texts with general language functioning, it can be noted that impairments in general language functioning are seen at an earlier date and with greater intensity. It is not until Time 2 that changes in song texts even occur. At this time, the subject had considerable impairments in language functioning. Therefore, deterioration of language was not initially seen in song texts, although it was observed in other aspects of language functioning. It was not until later in the progression of DAT that a disruption of the song texts occurred.

Tune. As can be seen in the overall qualitative ratings of the tune and text in Figure 2, initially the tune and the text were rated as being of good quality. It was not until Time 3 that significant changes in the tune began to occur. Minimal changes in the melodic, rhythmic, and stylistic aspects of the songs were evident during Times 1 and 2. A decrease in quality of the tune was seen in Time 3 and was characterized by a flattening of the melodic contour, thus becoming more monotonic. The overall rhythmic organization remained relatively intact until around Time 4. During this time, the overall tempo slowed and beat relations within the song were not maintained. These changes in the tune are reflected in the overall qualitative ratings of the tune. It is important to note that the subject continued to attempt to sing the songs, although the integrity of the song was compromised.

Discussion

Results of this longitudinal case study of a subject with DAT reveal that the text and tune during song production show differential breakdown during the course of DAT. In the case of song production, aspects of text production are initially more affected than the music aspects. The most distinctive disintegration is manifested at the level of words. These initial changes in the text occurred without affecting the overall music structure. The types of word substitutions made in the songs are noteworthy. Systematic errors relating more closely to the original text of songs occurred earlier in the progression of dementia. For example, phonologically similar and semantically related paraphasias were the most common text errors (comprising over 50% of the text errors) that occurred during Time 2. Increases in the number of unrelated words, added words, neologisms, unintelligible utterances were observed during Times 3 and 4. As the disease progressed, the text errors related less to the original text. Therefore, a change in the profile of text errors with disease progression was evident.

Several researchers have investigated the types of verbal errors made by subjects with DAT on naming and memory tasks. These naming errors are hypothesized to be semantically-based, thus, reflecting the disruption of the semantic system in DAT (Hodges, Salmon, & Butters, 1991; Lowenstein, D'Elia, Guterman, Eisdorfer, Wilkie, LaRue, Mintzer, & Duara, 1991). In addition, Hodges et al. (1991) also documented longitudinal changes in the error profile during naming performance over a 3-year period. The systematic progression of text errors in song texts could possibly reflect the disruption of the semantic system; however, further research should explore this possibility.

This pattern of the text and tune breakdown has not been documented in any other neurological disorders. As was discussed earlier, several authors have documented an inability to produce a song text while the tune is preserved in aphasics (Yamadori et al., 1977; Morgan & Tilluckdharry, 1982; Geschwind et al., 1968). However, to our knowledge, no other study documents insertions of text errors into a song text. This is not to say, however, that this does not exist. Whether or not this pattern occurs in other neurological disorders has not yet determined; further research examining song production in additional subjects with DAT and other brain damaged populations is needed. It was not until careful analysis of this music behavior was done that differential breakdown in song production was revealed. Therefore, future studies should emphasize detailed documentation of cases.

The relationship between song production and other aspects of music functioning should also be further explored. The functional selectivity of music disorders in persons with brain damage is currently being investigated by several researchers (Peretz, 1993b; Zatorre, 1984). The isolation of functionally relevant subsystems is a primary goal in cognitive neuropsychological studies of music (Peretz, 1993a; Sergent, 1993). The present case study documents how DAT can fractionate a cognitive function. In addition, the study of what components remain intact during different stages of DAT is also relevant to understanding the functional consequences of DAT. This perspective, thereby, holds that the progressive dementias are selective in their sites of pathology, and consequently, on cognitive functioning.

Acknowledgment

We wish to sincerely thank D.N. and her spouse for allowing us to spend more than 2 years of exploration. Without their collaboration, this type of research would not have been possible.

References

Assal, G. (1973). Aphasie de Wernicke sans amusie chez un pianiste. *Revue Neurologique, 129*, 251–255.

Bayles, K. A., & Kaszniak, A. W. (1987). *Communication and cognition in normal aging and dementia*. Boston: Little, Brown.

Beatty, W. W., Zavadil, K. J., Bailly, R. C., Rixen, G. J., Lavadil, L. E., Franham, N., & Fisher, L. (1988). Preserved musical skill in a severely demented patient. *International Journal of Clinical Neuropsychology, 10*, 158–164.

Benton, A. L., & Joynt, R. J. (1960). Early descriptions of aphasia. *Archives of Neurology, 3*, 109/205–126/222.

Borchgrevink, H. M. (1980). Cerebral lateralization of speech and singing after intracarotid amytal injection. In M. T. Sarno & O. Hook (Eds.), *Aphasia assessment and treatment* (pp. 186–191). New York: Masson Publishing.

Brain, W. R. (1941). Visual disorientation with special reference to lesions of the right cerebral hemisphere. *Brain, 64,* 244–272.

Brandt, J., Spencer, M., McSorley, P., & Folstein, M. F. (1988). Semantic activation and implicit memory in Alzheimer disease. *Alzheimer Disease and Associated Disorders, 2,* 112–119.

Claire, A. A., & Bernstein, B. (1990). A preliminary study of music therapy programming for severely regressed persons with Alzheimer's-type dementia. *Journal of Applied Gerontology, 9,* 299–311.

Crystal, H. A., Grober, E., & Masur, D. (1989). Preservation of musical memory in Alzheimer's disease. *Journal of Neurology, Neurosurgery, and Psychiatry, 52,* 1415–1416.

Dietsche, L. M., & Pollman, J. N. (1982). Alzheimer's disease: Advances in clinical nursing. *Journal of Gerontological Nursing, 8,* 97–100.

Dowling, W. J. (1973). Rhythmic groups and selective chunks in memory for melodies. *Perception and Psychoacoustics, 14,* 37–40.

Dowling, W. J., & Harwood, D. L. (1986). *Music cognition.* New York: Academic Press.

Folstein, M. F., Folstein, S. E., & McHugh, P. R. (1975). Mini-mental state. A practical method for grading the cognitive state of patients for the clinician. *Journal of Psychiatric Research, 12,* 189–198.

Gardner, M. F. (1982). *Test of visual-perceptual skills (non-motor).* Seattle, WA: Special Child Publications.

Geschwind, N., Quadfasel, F. A., & Segarra, J. M. (1968). Isolation of the speech area. *Neuropsychologia, 6,* 327–340.

Goodglass, H., & Kaplan, E. (1983). *The assessment of aphasia and related disorders.* Philadelphia: Lea & Febiger.

Gordon, H. W., & Bogen, J. E. (1974). Hemispheric lateralization of singing after intracarotid sodium amylobarbitone. *Journal of Neurology, Neurosurgery, and Psychiatry, 37,* 727–738.

Gott, P. S. (1973). Language after dominant hemispherectomy. *Journal of Neurology, Neurosurgery, and Psychiatry, 36,* 1082–1088.

Grimes, A. M., Grady, C. L., Foster, N. L., Sunderland, T., & Patronas, N. J. (1985). Central auditory function in Alzheimer's disease. *Neurology, 35,* 352–358.

Handel, S. (1989). *Listening.* Cambridge, MA: The MIT Press.

Heilman, K. M., Tucker, D. M., & Valenstein, E. (1976). A case of mixed transcortical aphasia with intact naming. *Brain, 99,* 425–426.

Hodges, J. R., Salmon, D. P., & Butters, N. (1991). The nature of the naming deficit in Alzheimer's and Huntington's disease. *Brain, 114,* 1547–1558.

Jackson, J. H. (1871). Singing by speechless (aphasic) children. *Lancet, 2,* 430–431.

Jellinek, A. (1956). Amusia. On the phenomenology and investigation of central disorders of the musical functions. *Folia Phoniatrica, 8,* 124–149.

Jossmann, P. (1927). Die Beziehungen der motorischen Amusie zu den apraktischen Störungen. *Monatschrift für Psychiatrie und Neurologie, 63,* 239–274.

Kaplan, E., Goodglass, H., & Weintraub, S. (1983). *The Boston naming test.* Philadelphia: Lea & Febiger.

Kast, A. (1885). Über Störungen des Gesangs und des musikalischen Gehörs bei Aphasikern. *Intelligenzblatt, 21,* 624–641.

Kempler, D. (1991). Language changes in dementia of the Alzheimer type. In R. Lubinski (Ed.), *Dementia and communication* (pp. 98–114). Philadelphia: B. C. Decker.

Knoblauch, A. (1890). On disorders of the musical capacity from cerebral disease. *Brain, 13,* 317–340.

Li, E. C., & Williams, S. E. (1991). An investigation of naming errors following semantic and phonemic cueing. *Neuropsychologia, 29,* 1083–1093.

Lipe, A. W. (1991) Using music therapy to enhance the quality of life in a client with Alzheimer's dementia: A case study. *Music Therapy Perspectives, 9,* 102–105.

Lowenstein, D. A., D'Elia, L., Guterman, A., Eisdorfer, C., Wilkie, F., LaRue, A., Mintzer, J., & Duara, R. (1991). The occurrence of different intrusive errors in patients with Alzheimer's disease, multiple cerebral infarctions, and major depression. *Brain and Cognition, 16,* 104–117.

Luria, A. R., Tsvetkova, L. S., & Futer, D. S. (1965). Aphasia in a composer. *Journal of Neurological Sciences, 2,* 288–292.

Mann, L. (1898). Casuistische Beitrage zur Hirnchirurgie und Hirnlocalization. *Monatschrift für Psychiatrie und Neurologie, 63,* 239–274.

Marin, O. S. (1982). Neurological aspects of music perception and performance. In D. Deutsch (Ed.), *The psychology of music* (pp. 453–477). New York: Academic Press.

McKhann, G., Drachman, D., Folstein, M., Katzman, R., Price, D., & Stadlan, E. M. (1988). Clinical diagnosis of Alzheimer's disease: Report of the NINCDS-ADRDA work group under the auspices of the department of health and human services task force on Alzheimer's disease. *Neurology, 34,* 939–944.

Mohr, E., Cox, C., Williams, J., Chase, T. N., & Fedio, P. (1990). Impairment of central auditory function in Alzheimer's disease. *Journal of Clinical and Experimental Neuropsychology, 12,* 235–246.

Monahan, C. B., & Carterette, E. C. (1985). Pitch and duration as determinants of musical space. *Music Perception, 3,* 1–32.

Morgan, O. S., & Tilluckdharry, D. H. (1982). Preservation of singing function in severe aphasia. *West Indian Medical Journal, 31,* 159–161.

Nebes, R. D. (1989). Semantic memory in Alzheimer's disease. *Psychological Bulletin, 106,* 377–394.

Norberg, A., Melin, E., & Asplund, K. (1986). Reactions to music, touch and object presentation in the final stage of dementia. An exploratory study. *International Journal of Nursing Studies, 23,* 315–323.

Olderog-Miller, K. A., & Smith, F. M. (1989). The influence of group singing therapy on the behavior of Alzheimer's disease patients. *Journal of Music Therapy, 26,* 58–70.

Peretz, I. (1993a) Auditory agnosia: A functional analysis. In S. McAdams & E. Bigand (Eds.), *Thinking in sound: The cognitive psychology of human audition* (pp. 199–230). New York: Oxford University Press.

Peretz, I. (1993b). Auditory atonalia for melodies. *Cognitive Neuropsychology, 10,* 21–56.

Pricket, C. A., & Moore, R. S. (1991). The use of music to aid memory of Alzheimer's patients. *Journal of Music Therapy, 28,* 101–110.

Polk, M., & Kertesz, A. (1993). Music and language in degenerative disease of the brain. *Brain and Cognition, 22,* 98–117.

Reisberg, B., Ferris, S., DeLeon, M. J., & Crook, T. (1983). The global deterioration scale for assessment of primary degenerative dementia. *American Journal of Psychiatry, 139,* 1136–1139.

Salmon, D. P., Heindel, W. C., & Butters, N. (1991). Patterns of cognitive impairment in Alzheimer's disease and other dementing disorders. In R. Lubinski (Ed.), *Dementia and communication* (pp. 37–46). Philadelphia: B. C. Decker.

Schwartz, M. F. (Ed.) (1990). *Modular deficits in Alzheimer-type dementia.* Cambridge: The MIT Press.

Sergent, J. (1993). Mapping the musician brain. *Human Brain Mapping, 1,* 20–38.

Shallice, T. (1990). *From neuropsychology to mental structure.* New York: Cambridge University Press.

Sloboda, J. A., & Parker, H. H. (1985). Immediate recall of melodies. In P. Howell, I. Cross, & R. West (Eds.), *Musical structure and cognition* (pp. 143–167). New York: Academic Press.

Smith, A. (1969). Nondominant hemispherectomy. *Neurology* (Minneapolis), *19*, 442–445.

Ulatowska, H., Allard, L., & Donnell, A. (1988). Discourse performance in subjects with dementia of the Alzheimer type. In H. Whitaker (Ed.), *Neuropsychological studies of non-focal brain damage* (vol. 4) (pp. 108–131). New York: Springer-Verlag.

Ulatowska, H. K., & Chapman, S. B. (1991). Discourse studies. In R. Lubinski (Ed.), *Dementia and communication* (pp. 115–132). Philadelphia: B. C. Decker.

Ulatowska, H. K., North, A. J., & Macaluso-Haynes, S. (1981). Production of narrative and procedural discourse in aphasia. *Brain and Language, 13,* 345–371.

Wertheim, N., & Botez, M. I. (1959). Plan d'Investigation des fonctions musicales. *Encephale,* 48, 246–254.

Yamadori, A., Osumi, Y., Masuhara, S., & Okubo, M. (1977). Preservation of singing in Broca's aphasia. *Journal of Neurology, Neurosurgery, and Psychiatry, 40,* 221–224.

Zatorre, R. J. (1984). Musical perception and cerebral function: A critical review. *Music Perception, 2,* 196–221.

Appendix A
Example of Song Text

Amazing grace how fine the word
Amazing grace how sweet the sound

And goust here come we sing
That saved a wretch like me

Twas love that brought ...(hums)...
I once was lost but now am found

And love will bring me home
Was blind but now I see

The text sung by the subject is in italics. The original song text is below. Portions of the second verse can be seen in phrase three and four:

Twas grace that taught my heart to fear
And grace will lead me home.

THE EFFECTS OF STRUCTURED MUSIC WORKSHOPS ON THE COMMUNICATIONS SKILLS, MUSICAL ABILITY, AND SELF-PERCEPTION OF MILDLY AND MODERATELY MENTALLY HANDICAPPED INDIVIDUALS

Raymond A. R. MacDonald and Patrick J. O'Donnell

Abstract

This paper investigates the benefits of a 10-week music course involving structured group situations for a population of 40 adults resident at mental health institutions. MacDonald, O'Donnell and Wallace (1993) reported significant gains in communication skills and musical ability. The present paper replicates a former study and also addresses two methodological issues raised by the first investigation, that is, the removal of the possibility of an experimenter effect, and also the measurement of subjects' self-perception of their musical ability. It was suggested that participation in the experimental group would produce significant improvements in musical ability, communication and self-perception. Results show significant gains on these variables. More specifically, the developmental gains observed in the first study were replicated.

Introduction

This study examines a specific type of music intervention that is somewhat different from the conventional music therapy (M.T.) approach. M.T. is normally defined as a one to one intervention conducted by a professionally qualified music therapist that focuses upon the clinical therapeutic process (Alvin, 1978; Nordoff & Robbins, 1992). The evaluation of music therapy thus defined has tended to be through the reporting of clinical cases, for example, Bunt (1984) and Salas (1990) However it is suggested here that music interventions that do not fall under this definition of "music therapy" may also have therapeutic potential (Sanger & Kippen, 1987). The workshops involved in this study were primarily aimed at increasing the participants' musical abilities, and it is suggested that various aspects of the workshop environment may produce therapeutic benefit as secondary gains (MacDonald, O'Donnell & Wallace, 1993). Whether the intervention utilizes the conventional music therapy approach or other means, the need for quantitative, empirical evaluation is paramount (Gfeller, 1990).

Controlled evaluation studies have begun to show generally positive effects of music therapy intervention (Bunt & Hoskyns, 1987; Pavlicevic, 1989). Hoskins (1988) used musical activities to enhance the language capacity of developmentally delayed children and found improvements on a specific language test. Hines (1989) investigated the effects of music therapy on self-esteem levels of emotionally disturbed adolescents. Although the objective measures showed no significant effects, there were impressionistic pieces of evidence to suggest that music therapy worked better than the control condition verbal therapy. Barker (1991) looked at the effects of music and relaxation techniques on the pain levels of patients suffering from severe burns and found that the combination of music and relaxation techniques had a significant positive effect. Also, Stein (1991) discovered that music reduced the anxiety of patients undergoing caesarean section, and Metzler & Berman

(1991) showed that music helped reduce anxiety as a result of a bronchoscopy procedure. Pavlicevic and Trevarthen (1990) demonstrated that music therapy had a positive effect on a chronic schizophrenic group compared with a no treatment control group. The index group showed improvements in the levels of engagement with the therapist and on objective psychiatric measures.

With specific reference to the special needs population that is of interest in the present study, several studies warrant attention. Oldfield & Adams (1990), dealing with a population of profoundly handicapped individuals, compared music therapy with play therapy in the achievement of specific objectives. Music therapy on a range of measures proved to be superior to play therapy. The aims of the study were not to teach subjects to play a musical instrument or to entertain subjects but rather to "use music towards the achievement of nonmusical aims" (Oldfield & Adams, 1990, p. 107) that were the development of communication, the control of movement and the expressing of emotions. Video tapes of the treatment sessions were analyzed using a time sampling method to record the occurrence of behavior indicating the achievement of the particular treatment objectives.

A similar study was conducted by Whyte (1991) and demonstrated improved communication and motor functioning skills in profoundly mentally handicapped adults. The experiment reported significant improvements in the number of eye contacts, vocalizations and hand movements in the experimental group. The study concluded that music therapy may help improve certain aspects of communication and motor functioning skills. Walker (1972) reported the effects of administering 12 daily music therapy sessions to an experimental group who made better progress at acquiring a number of functional words than a control group who were given daily talking sessions.

Anecdotal accounts of improved self-esteem have also been reported by researchers in this field (Nordoff & Robbins, 1992). Tyson (1981), in a review of music interventions, highlights the two most commonly shared goals of practising music therapists: "1. The establishment and reestablishment of interpersonal relationships; 2. The bringing about of self-esteem through self-actualization" (Tyson, 1981, p. 9). Several other studies have also reported improved self-esteem levels as a result of a music intervention. An instructional music therapy approach was found to improve self-esteem in a group of disadvantaged problem students (Michael & Martin, 1970). Ragland & Apprey (1974) reported that a community choir program aimed at recognizing and rechannelling disturbed behavior patterns was found to foster the development of decision-making skills and to increase self-esteem. Levels of self-esteem improved in a study by Singer (1962), where private music lessons were given in a cottage treatment centre. Gaston (1968) also discussed, without empirical evidence, the potential for music interventions to bring about self-esteem improvements. This concept is founded on the observation that musical participation may allow individuals an opportunity to communicate meaningfully when they have difficulty expressing themselves verbally (Nordoff & Robbins, 1992).

To summarize, there is suggestive evidence for the benefits of music therapy over a range of possible client groups. Definitive evidence is still lacking due to the absence of proper control in many of the experiments (Whyte, 1991; Bunt & Hoskyns, 1987). A second problem with the existing research literature is the focus on the conventional approach to music therapy. Further, the studies that deal with broad-based interventions utilize an observational and qualitative design such as that employed by Sanger and Kippen (1987). They reported a descriptive account of a particular musical and social event in which a Balinese Gamelan was used as part of a 2-week music course for the physically handicapped. By reporting their experiences and observations, the paper contributes to the body of information relating to the way in which people respond to musical stimuli. However, in order to evaluate the possible effects of music interventions, a more empirical and detailed account of the participants' experiences must be given, and this is one of the major issues addressed in the present study.

MacDonald, O'Donnell, and Wallace (1993) empirically examined the effects of a nonmusic therapy music intervention on a group of 40 mildly or moderately mentally handicapped individuals. They reported significant improvements in musical ability and communication skills. This music intervention was group-based as an organized course experience in playing the Javanese Gamelan.

Two important methodological issues were raised by this study. Firstly, a ceiling effect was obtained in the measurement of self-esteem using the *Khalid Semantic Differential technique* (Khalid, 1985) (see Appendix I). This questionnaire was chosen based upon the criticisms of other methods by Zetlin, Herriot and Turner (1985). Ten items were included in the scale with five possible responses for each item. These items were read aloud to compensate for any reading difficulties. Only the adjectives contained in the questionnaire were read to subjects, and no definition of those adjectives were given. The ceiling effect took the form of all subjects rating themselves as being at the top end of the scale during pretesting. In other words, they all felt very good, very friendly, very clean, etc. leaving no room for improvement. Secondly, both the pre- and posttesting was performed by the same experimenter, and this individual was also present at all the workshop sessions, introducing a potentially confounding variable in the form of the experimenter effect.

The present study is a replication of this original experiment and addresses the previously mentioned methodological issues, specifically:

1. Are the observed gains artifacts of a developing relationship between experimenter and subject? and

2. Is it possible to accurately measure subjects' self-perception of their musical ability before and after the experiment?

The aim of this study was to investigate whether there were any psychological and musical gains attributable to the music intervention across a range of measures. More specifically, the experimental hypothesis was that participation in the experimental group would produce significant improvements in musical ability, communication skills, and self-perception levels. These aspects of behavior were measured using either previously validated techniques or questionnaires designed and validated specifically for use in this study. One of the significant differences between this study and the first was that the experimenter in the posttest condition was unknown to the subjects, thus removing the possibility of experimenter effects influencing the results. Also, a self-perception visual analogue question was developed in the hope of assessing the participants' perceptions of their own musical development over the 10-week workshop period. This question was included for two reasons: Firstly, as an alternative to the *Khalid technique* (Khalid, 1985); and secondly, as a potential starting point in the development of a new self-esteem measure for use with this population.

Strathclyde Orchestral Productions

The organizational vehicle for delivery of the musical intervention was Strathclyde Orchestral Productions (S.O.P.), a music and theatre company that draws most of its musicians from within the special needs sector (in this instance, the term "special needs" refers to any individual with a mental or physical handicap). The company encourages musicians to develop their skills to the highest standard and ultimately aims to challenge existing views of disability. S.O.P. conducts music workshops where the emphasis is on every member of the group being involved and not on individual performance. In this study, the musical instrument used to meet this objective was a Javanese Gamelan.

The previously discussed review of literature has provided evidence that various types of music intervention can result in communication and self-esteem developments. However, the experience of musicians with special needs working with S.O.P. suggests that certain musical developments can also take place. Several musicians, after working with S.O.P., are now performing in a professional capacity with music and theatre companies. The conventional music therapy approach does not view musical developments as a concern (Alvin, 1978; Nordoff & Robbins, 1992), resulting in a lack of research literature in this area. It is suggested, given the educational emphasis of the S.O.P. approach, that musical developments are a possible outcome for participants in this study. Other British music companies, for example, "The Drake Music Project" also employ musicians with special needs in a professional capacity.

The Gamelan

Gamelan is a generic name for a complement of percussion instruments consisting of tuned gongs, metallophones, cymbals, and drums. These can be found throughout Malaysia and Indonesia and range in size from 4 to 40 instruments (Lindsay, 1989).

In Gamelan music, there is no conductor present and all communications are accomplished by musical means with one drum player leading all the other musicians. Effort is therefore required by everyone to follow the variations in tempo that occur. With specific reference to its use within the special needs sector, the most important feature of the Gamelan is accessibility; complicated digital dexterity is not required to commence playing the instrument. Given these particular characteristics, the Gamelan allows for all levels of ability and emphasis is placed on group based communication. The Gamelan is therefore an ideal instrument to use for therapeutic applications of music. This use for the Gamelan was outlined by Sanger and Kippen (1987). An additional feature of the Gamelan is its relative obscurity in Western culture. This feature allows people to approach the instrument without preconceived stereotypes. This aspect appears particularly relevant for people with special needs who may have experienced previous "failure" with music instruction in music groups.

Method

Design

This was a two-group design incorporating pre- and posttest subject assessment techniques. The experimental group received the music intervention, while the control group received no intervention.

Subjects

Forty subjects took part in this study. These participants were either mildly or moderately mentally handicapped individuals attending Adult Training Centres (A.T.C.'s) in the Glasgow area, or individuals attending the Occupational Therapy Department at Lennox castle Hospital, Glasgow. The experimental group contained 13 males and 7 females with a chronological age range of 17–55 and a mean age of 41.1 years. The control group contained 9 males and 11 females with a chronological age of 21–47 and a mean age of 38.1 years.

One criteria for inclusion in the study was that severe behavioral problems (which may have disrupted group dynamics) were not exhibited by the subjects. While it is recognized that such individuals may have benefited from this intervention, it was decided, as this was the second study of a long term project, that the effects of the workshops may have been diminished by their inclusion. This decision was made in consultation with the head of the Occupational Therapy Department. A future study is proposed to investigate the benefits of music workshops for a population of adults with mental handicaps and severe behavioral problems. Subjects who met the criteria were randomly assigned to either the experimental or control group.

Apparatus

A Javanese Gamelan was used to provide the musical focus for the experiment. All the subjects were interviewed and tested using the following assessment tools:

1. The *Rossi test of musical ability* (MacDonald, O'Donnell & Wallace, 1993).
2. Section 4 from the *Communication assessment profile for adults with learning difficulties (C.A.S.P.)*, (van der Gaag, 1988).
3. A visual analogue self-perception question (see Appendix II).

Procedure

The pretesting procedure, which utilized the previously mentioned assessment tools, and took the form of one to one consultations between experimenter and subject.

The *Rossi test of musical ability* (MacDonald, O'Donnell & Wallace, 1993) was designed and validated specifically for use during this project. Validation procedures carried out during the development of this test provided test retest reliability acceptable at 75.6% for simple rhythm production, and 88.4% for instrumental rhythm production. Inter-rater reliability was acceptable at 78.9% for simple rhythm production, and 82.8% for instrumental rhythm production. The development of this test was influenced by the work of Mills (1988), in particular her *Group tests of musical abilities*, and also the work of Bentley (1985), notably his *Measures of musical abilities.*

The test has two separate sections, which are detailed below:

1. Simple Rhythm Production (S.R.P.)

The first section was a clapping exercise. Subjects were asked to reproduce 15 rhythms as clapped by the experimenter, paying attention to the various tempos and stresses. The experimenter rated performance on each item on a three-point scale. Two points for the correct response, one point for a response that contains only minor errors (e.g., correct number of beats but with the wrong stresses) and 0 points for a completely erroneous response. The maximum score possible was 30.

2. Instrumental Rhythm Production (I.R.P.)

This test makes use of a Saron Barung, which is a single octave metallophone with a trough resonant. It is struck with a wooden mallet and forms part of the Gamelan. Subjects were asked to reproduce a rhythm played by the experimenter. This was scored on the same three-point scale as the rhythm test and contained a maximum score of 30.

Section 4 from the *C.A.S.P.* involved the identification of everyday objects and a brief description of their use. This section was chosen because it was simple to administer and contained less complex communication tasks than the other sections that were not relevant to this study. Van der Gaag (1989; 1990) reported detailed validation assessments of the various different sections contained within *C.A.S.P.*

The self-perception of participants was rated using a visual analogue question (see Appendix II). Subjects were asked to put an X on the scale to indicate their own Gamelan ability. They were then asked to put another X on the scale to indicate an expert's ability. The expert in this instance was the workshop leader. The distance between subjects' perceptions of themselves and their perceptions of an expert was recorded as the measurement of self-perception. After all individuals were pretested, the 20 subjects who formed the experimental group attended weekly workshops for 10 weeks.

These workshops lasted approximately 1 hour and began with warm-up and rhythm exercises. The purpose of the warm-up session was to relax the group and help set up cohesive group dynamics that are essential to the success of any workshop. The rest of the time was usually given over to playing the Gamelan.

Various methods were employed by the workshop leader when communicating the musical ideas to the subjects. Participants were initially asked to repeat a rhythmic pattern being played on one of the Sarons. More complex patterns were played as the workshop progressed, and there was opportunity for improvisation within the context of any piece of music. It was important to allow for the individual needs of each participant. In certain cases, a tutor (either an occupational therapist or a professional musician) would hold an individual's hand and perform the rhythms with the subject. After this support and encouragement, many individuals were able to play unaided with the rest of their group. Participants were also given the opportunity to play a chosen part of the Gamelan. The emphasis was on group involvement and rhythmic awareness through musical participation. Since the completion of this study, the institutions involved have introduced weekly music workshops. All control group subjects had the opportunity to participate musically in these activities.

Following the 10 weeks of workshops, all subjects were retested on the assessment measurements. However, unlike the original study, a different experimenter (who was unknown to the subjects) was used to carry out the posttesting.

Results

The experimental hypothesis stated that improvement in musical ability, communication skills and self-perception should be observed in the experimental group after the 10-week course of workshops.

The pretest score was subtracted from the posttest score on all measures for each subject. Thus difference scores were calculated for each subject between the pre- and posttest conditions. These difference score summarized changes in individual performance at the end of the experiment. The difference scores were then analyzed using the *t*-test procedure. There were significant improvements in instrumental rhythm production, simple rhythm, *C.A.S.P.*, and self-perception. These results are summarized in Table 1 and Figures 1 and 2.

Table 1. *Difference between Pre- and Posttest Scores on Musical and Communication Tests*

	Control Gp. mean	Exp. Gp. mean	t	p
Simple Rhythm Production	-0.44	5.57	-5.75	< .01
Instrumental Rhythm Production	-0.19	7.52	-5.52	< .01
C.A.S.P.	-0.56	5.21	-5.16	< .01

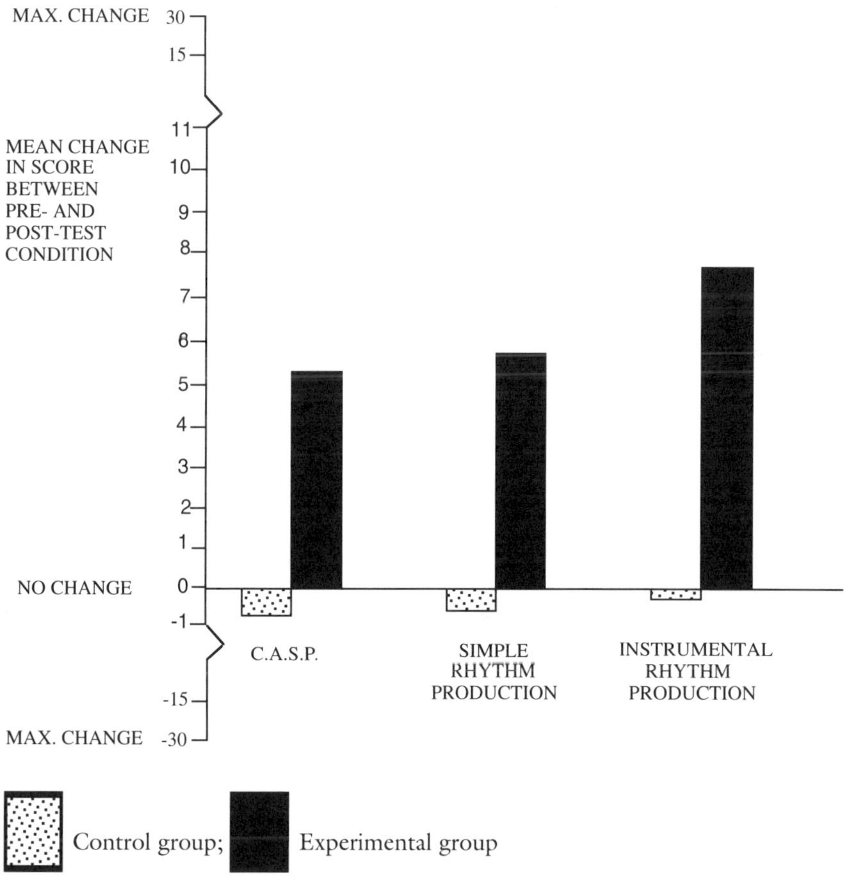

Figure 1. Changes in Musical and Communication Scores

Figure 1 shows the changes in scores for the experimental and control group across the musical and communication measures. The vertical axis displays the total difference between the pre- and the posttest scores. For example, the experimental group had a posttest mean of 24.79 and a pretest mean of 19.58 on *C.A.S.P.* The difference of 24.79 - 19.58 = 5.21 is the difference that is plotted on the graph. The horizontal axis displays the different measures employed for both groups. The figure shows negligible changes in the control group but significant changes in the experimental group.

A *t*-test comparison of the pre- and posttest self-perception scores also produced significant differences, $t(49) = 4.167$, $p = < .01$, in subjects' own perceptions of how they performed (see Figure 2).

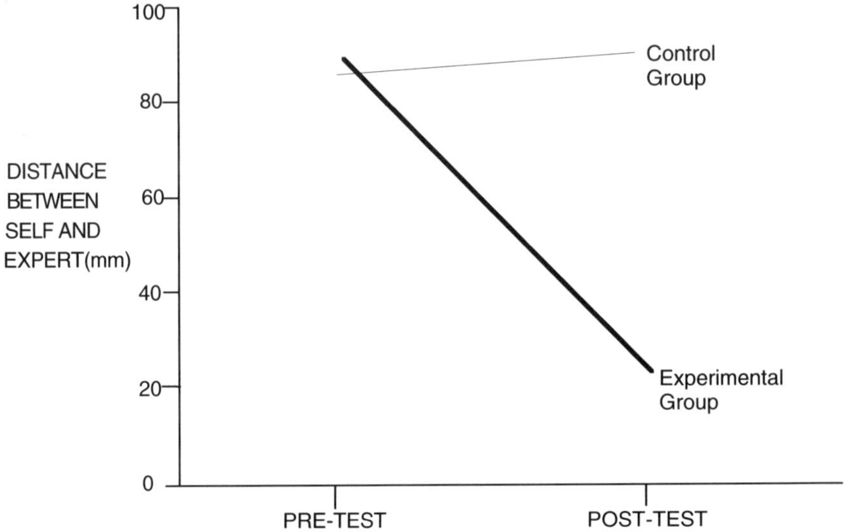

Figure 2. Change in Subjects' Self-perception of Musical Ability

Figure 2 summarizes the changes in self-perception for both control and experimental groups in the pre- and posttest conditions. The y-axis measures the difference between subjects' perceptions of their own Gamelan ability and that of an expert. Subjects were asked to put an X to indicate their own ability and an X to indicate an expert's ability. The distance between these two points was measured and this figure summarizes the results in the pre- and posttest conditions. That is, the distance between the two points in the pretest condition is much larger than the distance between the points in the posttest condition for the experimental group. Also, the control group shows negligible changes in self-perception of Gamelan ability. It can therefore be concluded that, for the experimental group, there is a significant increase in subjects' self-perception of Gamelan ability.

Finally, the difference scores for the first study were compared with the difference scores for the second study, and no significant differences, ($p < .05$), were found for any of the measures (see Figure 3).

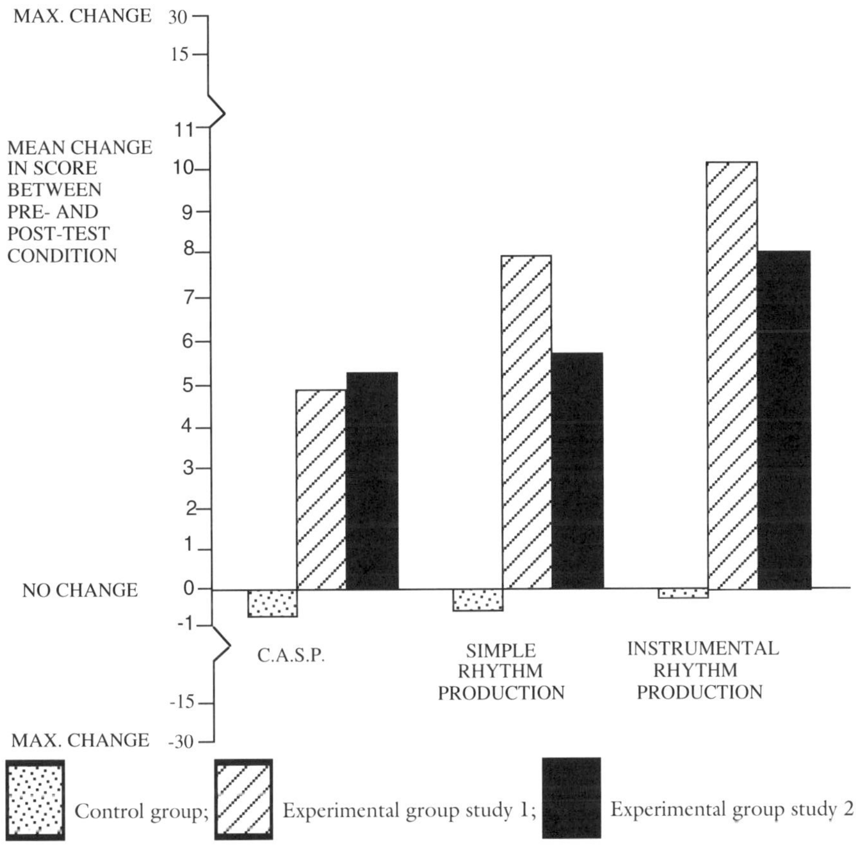

Figure 3. Comparison of Changes in Musical and Communication Scores between Studies 1 & 2

Figure 3 displays selected results from the two studies, showing negligible changes in the control group but significant changes in both experimental groups in the first and second studies. It is important to note the difference between experimental groups one and two for the musical scores. The raw data suggest an experimenter effect; however, this difference is statistically insignificant (see Table 2).

Table 2. *Differences between Musical and Communication Measures for Experimental Groups in Studies 1 and 2*

Musical and Communication Measures	t	p
I.R.P.	1.61	< .12
S.R.P.	1.92	< .07
C.A.S.P.	0.21	< .84

Discussion

The aim of this study was to investigate whether there were any psychological and musical gains attributable to the music intervention across a range of measures. It is clear that the intervention produces significant improvements in these measures for the experimental group.

It was argued that the experience of forming a developing relationship with the experimenter (who not only tested the subjects but also attended the workshops) may, in itself, produce significant improvements on the measurement scale. The fact that these gains remain when the posttest experimenter is unknown to the subjects suggests that the efficacy of the intervention is connected with the workshop environment. Given that there is evidence to support the efficacy of the musical intervention, future research must investigate in more detail which aspects of the experience produce these developmental gains. It is also important to note that the music may not be the main factor in producing these outcomes. The experience of communicating in a group situation, without a musical environment, may be an influential factor in producing the kind of developmental gains found in this study.

Future Research

In an attempt to answer this question, the research currently in progress attempts to examine more precisely what aspects of the workshop environment have facilitated these gains. The study examines the communication developments and self-perception changes that occur in a group of 20 individuals. The subjects are participating in an activity that involves a similar group communication environment to that found in the music workshop. However, the main difference between this particular study and the Gamelan studies is that there is no music present at the sessions. The workshops are focused not on musical awareness but rather on the development of either communal cooking or artistic skills. Future investigations may involve assessing the developments that take place after a music course that contains no group involvement, that is, a course that incorporates one-to-one teaching practices. It is also important to note that subjects who participated in the first study were retested to investigate whether the developmental gains made had remained after a 6-month period where there was no musical intervention. The results show that the initial gains have remained even in the absence of the ongoing musical environment, suggesting the existence of a maintenance effect.

Acknowledgments

We would like to thank Gillian M. Ferrier for her support and time, which was vital in the completion of this paper. Thanks also to Jean Cherry and Isabel Murdoch of the Occupational Therapy Department at Lennox Castle Hospital, Glasgow for their continuing encouragement and guidance. The constant administrative and musical input of Strathclyde Orchestral Productions was a major factor in the success of this study. This project also received support from The Greater Glasgow Health Board and The Strathclyde Regional Council, Scotland.

References

Alvin, J. (1978). *Music for the handicapped child.* London: Oxford University Press.

Barker, L. W. (1991). The use of music and relaxation techniques to reduce pain of burn patients during daily debridement. In C. D. Maranto (Ed.), *Applications of music in medicine* (pp. 124–139). Washington, DC: National Association of Music Therapy.

Bentley, A. (1985). *Measures of musical ability.* London: Nfer-Nelson.

Bunt, L. (1984). Research in music therapy in Great Britain. Outcome research with handicapped children. *British Journal of Music Therapy, 15*(3), 2–8.

Bunt, L., & Hoskyns, S. L. (1987). A perspective on music therapy research in Great Britain. *Journal of Music Therapy, 1*(1), 3–5.

Coopersmith, S. (1967). *The antecedents of self -esteem.* San Francisco: W. H. Freeman.

Gaston, E. T. (1968). Man and music. In E. T. Gaston (Ed.), *Music in therapy* (p. 26). New York: Macmillan.

Gfeller, K. (1987). Music therapy theory and practice as reflected in the research literature. *Journal of Music Therapy, 25*(4), 178–194.

Hines, J. H. (1989). The effects of music therapy on the self-esteem of emotionally disturbed adolescents. *Music Therapy, 8(*1), 78–91.

Hoskins, M. C. (1988). The use of music to increase verbal response and improve expressive language abilities of pre-school language delayed children. *Journal of Music Therapy, 25(*2), 73–84.

Khalid, R. (1985). *A comparative study of the self-esteem of the Pakistani minority and the indigenous children in Scotland.* Unpublished doctoral dissertation thesis, Department of Psychology, University of Glasgow, Glasgow.

Lindsay, J. (1989). *Javanese gamelan. Singapore*: Oxford University Press.

Michael, D., & Martin, D. (1970). Music and self-esteem research with disadvantaged problem boys in an elementary school. *Journal of Music Therapy, 7*(4),124–127.

MacDonald, R. A. R., O'Donnell, P. J., & Wallace, J. (1993, July). *Music as a catalyst for personal development.* Paper presented at the 5th World Congress of Music Therapy, Vitoria Gastiez, Spain.

Metzler, R. K., & Berman, T. (1991). The effects of sedative music on the anxiety of bronchoscopy patients. In C. D. Maranto (Ed.), *Applications of music in medicine* (pp. 163–175). Washington, DC: National Association of Music Therapy.

Mosey, A. C. (1986). *Psychosocial components of occupational therapy.* New York: Raven Press.

Mills, J. (1988). *Group tests of musical ability.* London: Nfer-Nelson.

Nordoff, P., & Robbins, C. (1992). *Therapy in music for handicapped children.* London: Victor Gollancz.

Oldfield, A., & Adams, M. (1990). The effects of music therapy on a group of profoundly mentally handicapped adults. *Journal of Mental Deficiency Research, 34,* 107–125.

Pavlicevic, M. (1989). A musical assessment of psychiatric states in adults. *Psychopathology, 22,* 315–334.

Pavlicevic, M., & Trevarthen, C. (1990). *Putting music therapy on the map.* Unpublished manuscript, Department of Psychology, University of Edinburgh, Edinburgh.

Piers, E., & Harris, D. (1969). *The Piers-Harris children's self-concept scale.* Nashville, TN: Counsellor Recordings and Tests.

Ragland, Z., & Apprey, M. (1974). Community music therapy with adolescents. *Journal of Music Therapy, 11*(3), 147–155.

Salas, J. (1990). Aesthetic experience in music therapy. *Music Therapy, 9*(1), 1–15.

Sanger, A., & Kippen, J. (1987). Applied ethnomusicology: The use of the Balinese Gamelan in recreational and educational music therapy. *British Journal of Music Education, 4*(1), 5–16.

Singer, S. (1962). Music therapy: Its application to emotionally disturbed children in a cottage treatment centre. *Journal of Music Therapy, 11*(3), 19–22.

Stein, A. M. (1991). Music to reduce anxiety during caesarean births. In C. D. Maranto (Ed.), *Applications of music in medicine* (pp. 7–23). Washington, DC: National Association of Music Therapy.

Tyson, F. (1981). *Psychiatric music therapy: Origins and developments* (p. 9). New York: Creative Arts Rehabilitation Center.

van der Gaag, A. (1988). *The communication assessment profile for adults with a mental handicap.* London: Speech Profiles.

van der Gaag, A. (1989). Joint assessment of communication skills: Formalisation of the role of the carer. *British Journal of Mental Subnormality, 25*(1), 22–28.

van der Gaag, A. (1990). The validation of a language and communication assessment procedure for use with adults with learning difficulties. *Health Bulletin, 48*(5), 254–260.

Walker, J. (1972). The use of music as an aid in developing functional speech on the institutionally mentally retarded. *Journal of Music Therapy, 9(1),* 1–12.

Weldin, C., & Eagle, C. T. (1991). An historical overview of music medicine. In C. D. Maranto (Ed.), *Applications of music in medicine* (pp. 7–23). Washington, DC: National Association of Music Therapy.

Whyte, C. M. (1991). *The effects of music therapy on communication and motor functioning in a group of profoundly handicapped people.* Unpublished M.A. thesis, Department of Psychology, University of Glasgow, Glasgow.

Zetlin, A., Heriot, J., & Turner, J. (1985). Self-concept measurement in mentally retarded adults: A micro analysis of responses. *Applied Research in Mental Retardation, 6,* 113–125.

Appendix I
Semantic Differential Scale*

GOOD :_____: :_____: :_____: :_____: :_____: BAD

CHEERFUL :_____: :_____: :_____: :_____: :_____: GLOOMY

FRIENDLY :_____: :_____: :_____: :_____: :_____: UNFRIENDLY

CLEVER :_____: :_____: :_____: :_____: :_____: STUPID

POPULAR :_____: :_____: :_____: :_____: :_____: UNPOPULAR

LOVELY :_____: :_____: :_____: :_____: :_____: UGLY

NICE :_____: :_____: :_____: :_____: :_____: HORRIBLE

KIND :_____: :_____: :_____: :_____: :_____: UNKIND

CLEAN :_____: :_____: :_____: :_____: :_____: DIRTY

SLIM :_____: :_____: :_____: :_____: :_____: FAT

*From Khalid (1985)

Appendix II
Self Perception Question

The workshop leader plays the Gamelan every day. He is a professional Gamelan Player.

On the following scale how would you rate his ability to play the Gamelan?

How would you rate your own ability to play the Gamelan?

NO SKILL	VERY HIGHLY SKILLED

EFFECTS OF MUSIC LISTENING AND BIOFEEDBACK INTERVENTIONS ON CARDIAC CHRONOTROPIC CONTROL OF WOMEN IN CHILDBIRTH

Jill Petersen Lex, Rosalie Rebollo Pratt, Hans-Henning Abel, and Ralph Spintge

Introduction

Birth is emotionally and physically stressful on women. Unfortunately, additional stress is placed on the mother when she is removed from active involvement in childbirth through the use of modern medical technologies, and the lack of communication regarding hospital procedures (Hodnett & Abel, 1986). This transfer of control to health care providers has left women powerless because they no longer supply the caregiver with information about themselves or the baby (McKay, 1991). As a result, the birthing process has become biologically safe, yet psychologically dehumanizing, unsatisfying, and disempowering (Leventhal, Leventhal, Shacham, & Easterling, 1989). Learning to take control of the birthing environment will permit women to experience more control in labor, to decrease stress, and to create positive attitudes about the childbirth experience.

Another important stress and anxiety reducing element in childbirth is to relieve the parturient of pain without putting the fetus at risk and without creating a disempowering birthing environment. There is some evidence that analgesia may be an inhibitor of the natural birthing process by extending the labor period, increasing the use of instrumental birth, and removing the mother from direct involvement with the birth of her child (McKay, 1991; Hodnett & Osborn, 1989; Hodnett & Abel, 1986; & Gregg, 1978). This suggests a need for alternative methods to reduce the pain associated with labor and birth. Women who choose to have unmedicated childbirth should be allowed to access to several nonpharmaceutical options in efforts to minimize their pain.

There are several reports in the literature that music has been effective in helping women to relax and to fortify themselves with coping techniques in preparation for childbirth and throughout labor. Most of them used a methodical approach that consisted of psychological questionnaires and self-reports, but not physiological measurements.

Hanser, Larson, and O'Connell (1983) showed that the birthing environment is positively affected when music is used in the hospital. Mothers, labor coaches, and hospital personnel have reported that music encouraged endurance and made the room feel more like home. Livingston (1979) stated that music also helped to block out other activity in the room. In addition, when music was present, hospital work could be carried out with less distraction to the mother. Stevens (1992) reported that the presence of music for the birthing woman established some control of the environment for the mother because she was able to personalize it with her choice of pieces. Halpaap, Spintge, Droh, Kummert, and Kogel (1985) and Hanser et al. (1983) played individually selected music for women during labor. Their results showed that, in the music group, ACTH, a stress hormone, was significantly reduced, and beta endorphin levels were significantly increased compared to the control group.

Studies on biofeedback training, a technique used to learn how to control involuntary emotional states with the aid of electronic devices, are confusing as to their actual effects on women in gestational and birthing environments. Most studies report that the women enjoyed the experience, that it helped them during labor, and that it created other positive effects. However, there are no objective data to substantiate these reports.

Gregg (1978) studied women who used electromyograph (EMG) and galvanic skin response (GSR) biofeedback training at home and in the labor room. The women in the biofeedback group spent significantly less time in labor, used diminished doses of sedatives and analgesics, and also required less physician time in the labor room than the women in the control group. Contrary to Gregg's (1978) findings, the biofeedback training session measurements of the study of St. James-Roberts, Chamberlain, Haran, and Huchingson (1982) suggested that the EMG was more effective than the GSR in training women before delivery and that women who trained with biofeedback experienced longer labor and used more anesthesia than the control group. However, these results are diminished because the data collected during labor and birth were collapsed—for statistical reasons—into two groups, a biofeedback group and a control group. Bernat, Woolrige, Marecki, and Snell (1992), who studied biofeedback-assisted relaxation for labor in Lamaze classes, used peripheral skin temperature readings along with autogenics as a dual biofeedback intervention to reduce stress in labor. The authors suggested that nursing goals promoting healthier and less stressful labor may include biofeedback-assisted relaxation, although there were no significant differences found between the experimental and control groups. Segal (1981) also studied the effects of EMG biofeedback training with Lamaze classes and found that the biofeedback training group showed significantly lower muscle tension and anxiety levels during and after training than did the Lamaze only group. The women in the experimental group experienced significant time reductions in the first stage of labor and overall length of labor, and they had less need for supplementary assistance. Lebowitz (1989) studied biofeedback-assisted relaxation training during first pregnancy, and the implications for childbirth in the postpartum period. At the postpartum interview, the greatest decrease in overall anxiety was experienced by the biofeedback group, which also showed decreased length in labor, less perception of pain, and more babies willing to nurse, in comparison to the control group.

Analysis of the chronotropic control of the heart constitutes an appropriate tool for the examination of the functional state of the central autonomic nervous system during different states of activity (Abel, Klüssendorf, Koralewski, Krause, & Droh, 1992). Therefore, results of heart rate pattern analysis, which include the analysis of variability and rhythmicity in the time series of heart beats, can be used for the determination of the balance between the activities of the parasympathetic and sympathetic parts of the autonomic nervous system. A rise in the central nervous activity during behavior is accompanied by increased sympathetic activity and a decrease in parasympathetic innervation of the heart, the so-called ergotropic functional state of the autonomic nervous system; a fall in central nervous activity during behavior is accompanied by a decreased sympathetic and an increased parasympathetic innervation of the heart, the so-called trophotropic functional state of the autonomic nervous system (Jung, 1986).

Parasympathetic chronotropic control of the heart can be mathematically quantified by an analysis of heart rate variability (Katona & Jih, 1975; Akselrod, Gordon, Ubel, Shannon, Barger, & Cohen, 1981). Consequently, distinct changes in the parasympathetic-sympathetic balance of the autonomic nervous activity that can be expected to occur during stress-reducing procedures can be detected by an analysis of heart rate variability.

Unfortunately, much of the data produced from studies in music listening or biofeedback training for childbirth has not been substantially validated. Prior research has either not contained control groups or has lacked the physiological measures necessary to provide objective data.

The purpose of this study was to determine the effects of (a) biofeedback training combined with selected music listening, (b) selected music listening alone, and (c) no intervention, on the heart rate and its variability of women during childbirth.

Method

Description of Subjects

Initial contact with the Ss, who were patients of the Nurse-Midwives, was made by means of a flyer placed at the Nurse-Midwives' office at Orem Community Hospital in Utah. The Ss were married, nullipara or multipara, pregnant women planning term vaginal births from April through December 1993 (see Table 1). Ss of the biofeedback and music group (B+M) and of the music group (M) were randomly assigned. Those of the control group (C) were recruited at a later time, and they received a stipend of $50.00. The Ss were asked to read and sign the formal Consent Form of the study.

Table 1. *Demographic Data*

	n	Age [yrs]	Height [cm]	Weight pre [kg]	Weight deliv [kg]
Biofeedback + Music	8	25 (22, 28)	170 (152, 173)$^{+}$	54.9 (47.6, 70.3)	68.9 (62.1, 76.6)
Music	8	24 (21, 27)	163 (160, 168)	59.9 (54.0, 73.9)	71.7 (64.9, 97.5)
Control	9	25 (21, 29)	173 (163, 178)	66.2 (47.6, 80.3)	84.1 (59.4, 91.6)

Median with minimum and maximum; Kruskal-Wallis test, $\alpha = 0.05$, $^{+}$: $p < 0.05$

Experimental Design

Prenatal Training. B+M Ss and M Ss participated in 6 weekly prenatal training sessions of about 30 minutes duration each. These sessions were conducted in the Biofeedback Research Lab located in the Department of Music, Brigham Young University. The lab was illuminated by a halogen lamp to eliminate artifact. The Ss were seated in an E-Z Boy lounger chair and maintained control of the angle at which the chair reclined. Most women opted to place the chair in a horizontal position with their feet partially elevated.

The decision to give each woman six training sessions was because (a) this is the standard number for prenatal classes, (b) this is the accepted minimum number considered effective for biofeedback training, and (c) the time and resources of the study were limited.

At the beginning of the first session, the women were asked about experiences they might have had with previous births as well as any worries or concerns they might have about the study. Each of the consecutive sessions started with a 5-minute discussion about the general well-being of the woman. In this way, sessions were individualized toward the particular woman and her needs.

The Ss were then asked to complete the *State Trait Anxiety Inventory (STAI),* which contains two 20-item scales that take about 5–10 minutes to complete. The test, which was corrected by hand during each of the six sessions yielded two scores, one for State anxiety and one for general Trait anxiety.

The next step in the first session was for the Subject to choose her individual music audiotape. To allow for personal taste and preference, the audiotapes in the Lab music library represented a broad spectrum of musical genres and styles, including classical, popular, folk, and meditation music. Ss were also encouraged to bring favorite music from their personal collection. The Ss listened to four or five selections and then made a final choice of one audiotape that was played throughout the sessions and during labor. The tape was played through a Pillow Phonix™, a stereo device designed so that a regular hospital bed pillow or the headrest of the lab chair could be placed between the two covered speaker, thereby giving the woman the option of listening to the music close to her without the nuisances of headphones or wires.

The B+M Ss were introduced to the biofeedback equipment during the first session, which consisted of the Autogenic System's AT33 Portable EMG and the PST-100 peripheral Skin Temperature unit. The subject was told that she would be able to see the digital readouts on both the Portable EMG and temperature units, and that the goal of the biofeedback training was to lower the EMG readings and to raise the peripheral skin temperature readings. The Subject then experimented with the equipment until any remaining questions were answered or anxieties abated. At each session for women in the Biofeedback group, skin temperature and EMG measures were taken.

Five relaxation scripts developed for the remaining sessions, focused on breathing awareness, body awareness, visualization of concrete ideas, visualization of abstract concepts, and positive self-talk during mock labor. They were used along with the music and lasted about 15–20 minutes, depending on the comfort status of the women.

The basic difference in treatment of the B+M and M Ss was that women in the B+M group received constant feedback on muscle tension and finger temperature readings, while the women in the M group had no such information. The C Ss received no relaxation interventions, no music listening, and no biofeedback before labor.

Delivery room protocol. When the subject was ready to go to the hospital, she contacted the investigator by beeper. The investigator then met the subject and her husband at one of the two hospitals serviced by the Certified Nurse-Midwives.

The first step was to attach the EKG electrodes to the proper sites on the woman's chest. If the woman was a subject in one of the two groups in which selected music was used, the same music was played for her on either a tape recorder or a Walkman was plugged into a Pillow Phonix on which the woman's head rested. When the midwife advised the investigator that the woman had reached 4 cm dilation, the investigator began a 30-minute recording on the EKG. A similar procedure was followed during the periods in which the woman experienced 5 cm and 6 cm dilation. After these three recordings were taken, the investigator left the room for the final stage of delivery. On several occasions, the investigator was asked by the woman to remain until delivery had occurred.

Physiological parameters

Temperature recording. For women in the Biofeedback group, a PST-100 temperature sensor was attached with surgical tape to the right index finger. These readings were recorded manually.

EMG recording. For women in the Biofeedback group, an Autogenic Systems AT33 Portable EMG machine was used to record readings on the belly of the brachioradialis muscle of the right arm. Temperature and EMG measurements were recorded as a baseline, 2-minutes before the beginning of the session, at the start of the session, and then subsequently at 5, 10, 15, and 20 minutes. Each EMG value was reported as a rectified, low-pass filtered, integrated signal.

EKG recording. For women in all three groups, EKG readings were obtained by placing three sensors on the thoracic area. The EKG signal was fed into the data logger PhysioLog A. The time between two successive R waves of the EKG (R-R interval) was computed with a precision of 1 ms and stored beat-by-beat throughout each 30-minute recording. For each 30-minute recording, the mean value of R-R intervals (mean RR) and the mean value of the modulus of successive R-R interval differences (MSD), a measure of beat to beat variability were computed:

$$MSD = \frac{1}{n} \sum_{i=1}^{n} |(RR_{i+1} - RR_i)|.$$

Results

Subjects

Forty-one Ss were recruited for this study (B+M: n = 15; M: n = 14; C: n = 12). A total of sixteen women were dropped from the study for different reasons. Four Ss were removed from the study before completing training sessions, data for two of the Ss were not recorded properly, three Ss failed to contact the investigator before delivery, three Ss had labor periods so accelerated that it was impossible to even do one recording, one Subject gave birth during her first recording, and three Ss had a Cesarean procedure. This attrition rate resulted in a total sample of n = 25 (B+M: n = 8; M: n = 8; C: n = 9).

The results of the demographic data analysis confirm the fact that the Ss could not be randomized because of the low number of participants (see Table 1). There was a statistically difference in height among the three groups. The assignment of Ss to the two experimental groups was changed when Ss dropped from the study to ensure a balance of Ss in each group. Another statistically significant difference was that women in the control group were heavier than the Ss in both experimental groups (Wilcoxon test, $a < 0.05$). This could be attributed to the fact that these women chose to be in the control group for financial reasons and, therefore, might have had different characteristics in personality and lifestyle than the Ss in the other two groups.

STAI Inventory

There was no statistical difference in State and Trait anxiety among the women in the three groups.

Skin Temperature during Biofeedback Sessions

The first step was to calculate for each subject the median time course of the second to the sixth Biofeedback sessions for the parameter of finger temperature. The second step was to calculate the median time course of the eight subject time courses. The finger skin temperature showed a range of steady increase from 91.1 to 93.6 degrees Fahrenheit during the Biofeedback session (see Figure 1).

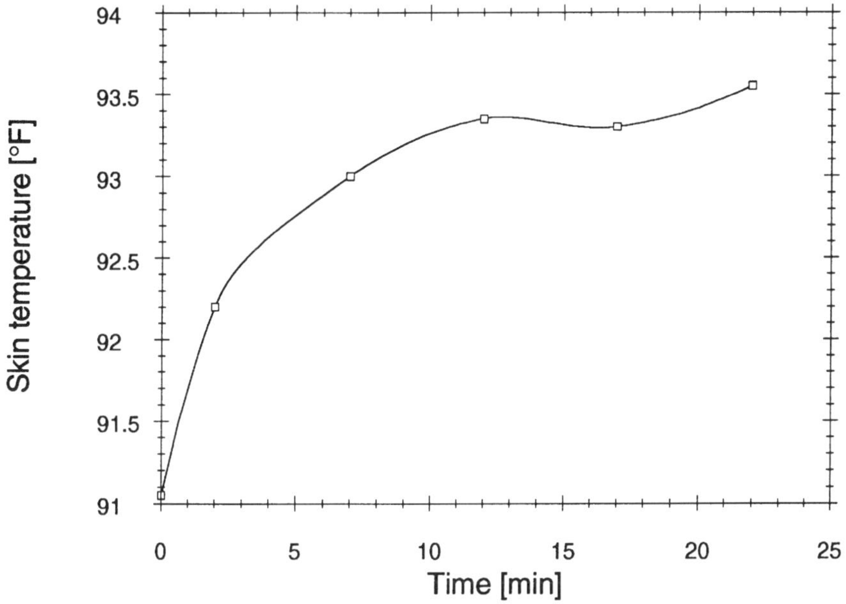

Figure 1. Intra-session Median Time Course of Ss' and Sessions' Averages of Finger Skin Temperature Scores Measured Six Times during the Biofeedback Session.

Brachioradialis EMG during Biofeedback Sessions

Before computing the median time courses, each raw EMG time course was mathematically transformed into a relative time course. The first EMG value of the time course constituted the reference and percentage changes were calculated for the values that followed. Then, the first step was to calculate for each subject the median time course of the second to the sixth Biofeedback sessions. The second step was to calculate the median time course of the eight subject time courses. The EMG activity showed a steady change up to -160% during the Biofeedback session (see Figure 2).

R-R Interval during Delivery

Analysis of the heart rate parameters of the first recording taken at 4 cm cervical dilation during delivery showed that B+M Ss experienced a 32% increase, and M Ss experienced 23% increase over the median beat-to-beat variability of the C Ss (see Figure 3). Differences in mean R-R interval were negligible.

During the course of delivery, certain differences between the experimental and control group Ss showed up involving the behavior of the parasympathetic chronotropic control of the heart. In comparison to 4 cm cervical dilation, at 5 cm dilation the M Ss showed a 24% increase in beat-to-beat variability (see Figure 4). In contrast, the B+M Ss and C Ss moved to a lower beat-to-beat variability. Again, changes in mean R-R interval were negligible.

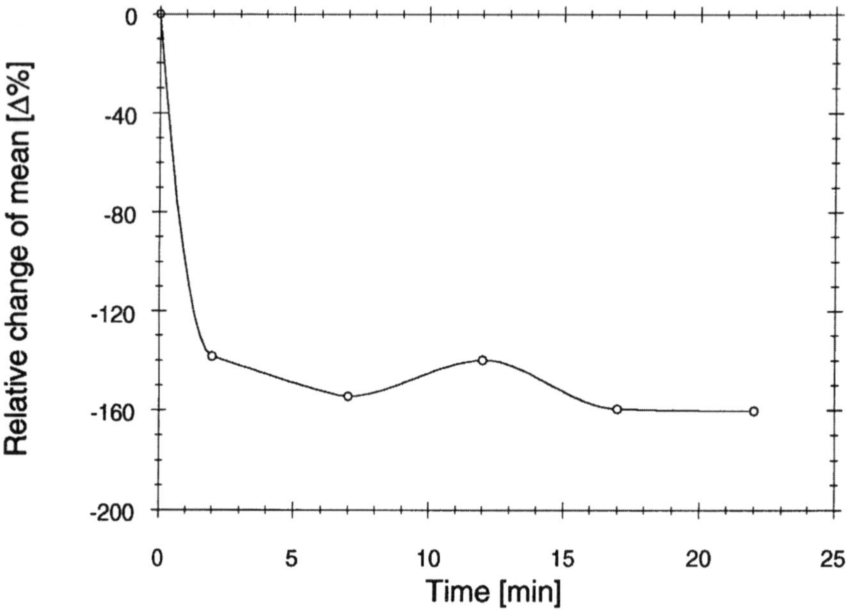

Figure 2. Intra-session Median Time Course of Ss' and Sessions' Averages of EMG Scores Measured Six Times during the Biofeedback Session.

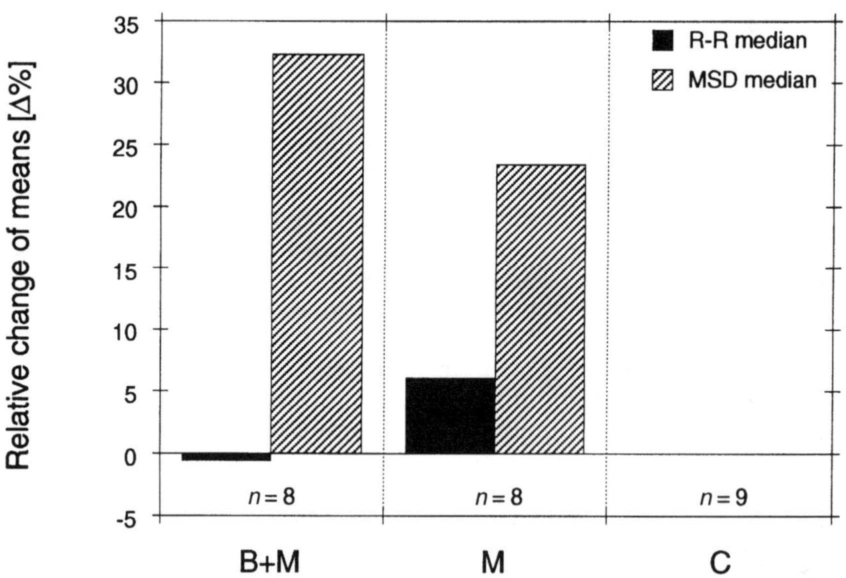

Figure 3. Percentage Differences of the Heart Rate Parameters R-R Interval (R-R) and Beat to Beat Variability of RR Intervals (MSD) in the B+M and M Group in Relation to the C Group at 4 cm Cervical Dilation during Delivery.

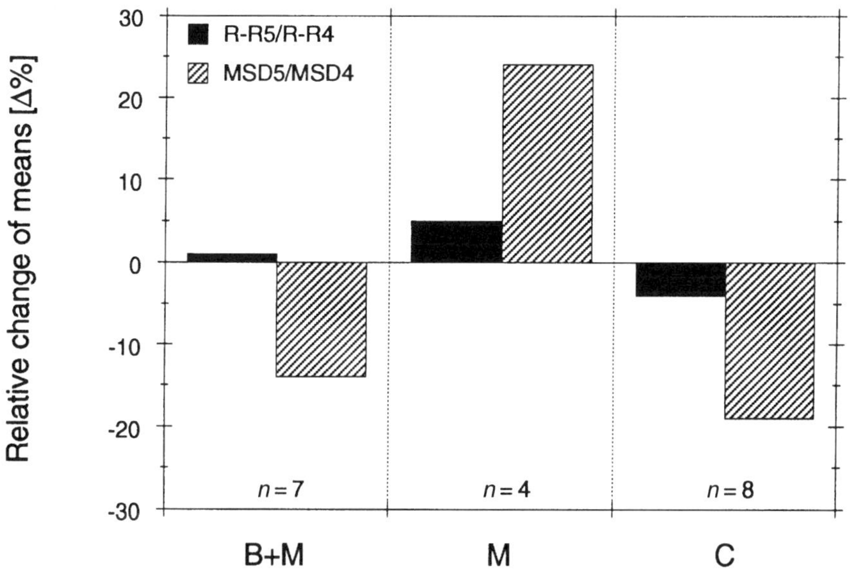

Figure 4. Percentage Differences of the Heart Rate Parameters R-R Interval (R-R) and Beat to Beat Variability of RR Intervals (MSD) between 4 cm and 5 cm cervical dilation during Delivery.

A comparison of heart rate parameters among the three groups at 6 cm cervical dilation were not performed because the total number of these recordings was 11. Missed recordings resulted from two problems: (a) Most of the Ss dilated quickly and were too close to giving birth to attempt another recording, and (b) one of the Ss experienced complications and the investigator was asked to leave the room before the recordings could be completed.

The results of the analysis of those Ss who completed the study (B+M: n = 3; M: n = 2; C: n = 6) showed that B+M and M Ss experienced a slight increase in their individual time courses of mean R-R interval and beat to beat variability during the ongoing delivery, whereas the C Ss showed a more opposite behavior in their R-R interval parameters.

All changes were not statistically significant, probably because of the high interindividual and intraindividual differences of the heart rate parameters, the differences of the demographic data, and the low total number of Ss.

Discussion

As anticipated, women during the course of the biofeedback sessions showed a steady increase in finger skin temperature and a steady decrease in muscle activity. The increase in temperature may reflect a decrease in the activity of sympathetic nerves, which innervate the smooth muscles in skin vessels. The activity in these sympathetic efferents as well as the activity in motor efferents depends, among other things, on the arousal state, emotional behavior, and temperature regulation demands. Although the change in skin temperature and muscle activity may have been due to the biofeedback intervention, it may also have been caused by diminution in the arousal state while relaxing in the reclining chair, or,

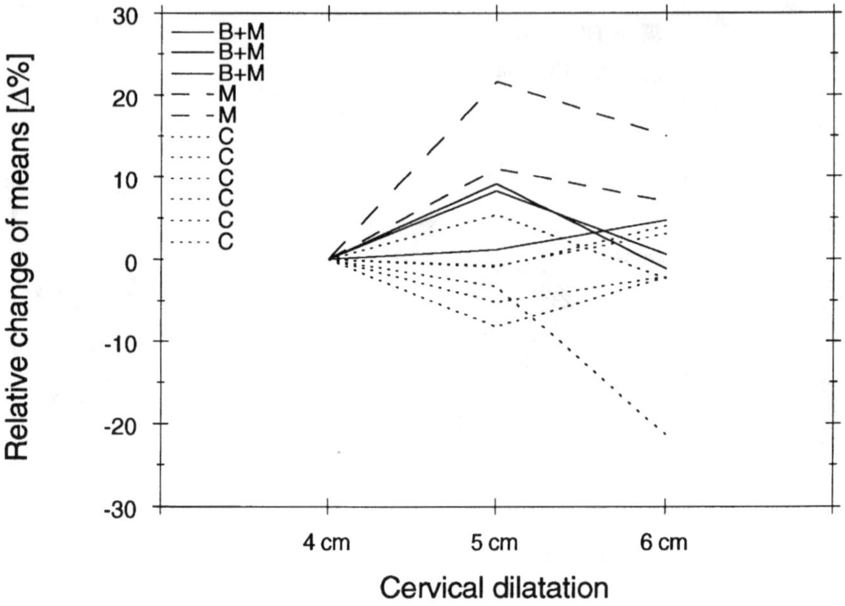

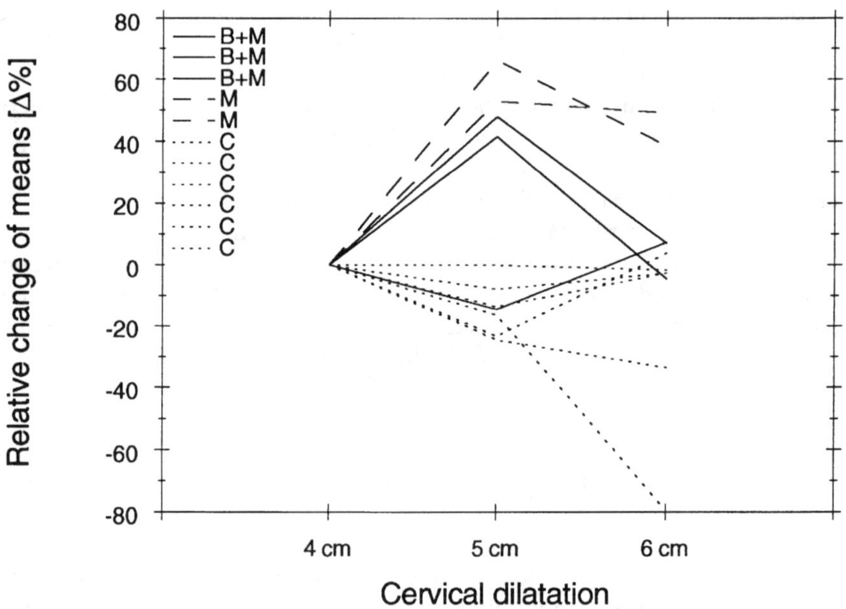

Figure 5. Individual Relative Time courses of Mean R-R Interval (see top of Figure 5) and Individual Relative Time Courses of Mean of successive Differences of R-R Intervals (see bottom of Figure 5) at 4, 5, ad 6 cm cervical dilation during delivery. Measures at 5, 6 cm were related to the 4 cm cervical dilation measure.

especially when the weather was cold, because the subject experienced relief from the cold. Nevertheless, these parameters indicate a diminution of the central nervous system activity, which may be interpreted as sedative state. It is not known whether the women in the music group might have experienced the same degree of temperature increase and muscle activity decrease as those in the biofeedback group. A future study should include physiological measures on subjects in all groups in order to determine the specific effects of biofeedback training, music listening, and no intervention on skin temperature and muscle activity.

Heart rate variability measures were taken in order to differentiate between ergotropic and trophotropic states of central autonomic nervous function. Beat to beat variability of the heart rate is closely related to the parasympathetic innervation of the heart. Therefore, it can taken as an indicator of the cardiac parasympathetic chronotropic control. During an ergotropic functional state (e.g., muscular work or mental task), heart rate variability decreases because of the decrease in parasympathetic nervous activity. A trophotropic state (e.g., rest, or slow wave sleep) is accompanied by an increased parasympathetic activity. In this situation, the heart rate variability is increased. Therefore, the clinical application of analysis of heart rate variability represents a tool to examine the autonomic functional state of women during childbirth. Usually, the delivery is accompanied by autonomic arousal, which, it was hypothesized, might be reduced by music listening and biofeedback training.

The reason for measuring heart rate variability at 4, 5, and 6 cm dilation was because these points are midway in the labor process, yet not at the final stage of labor and delivery. The women in the music listening group and biofeedback and music listening group showed a higher heart rate variability at 4 cm cervical dilation than the women in the control group. In comparison to the 4 cm cervical dilation, the women in the biofeedback and music listening group at 5 cm dilation evidenced a 14% decrease in heart rate variability, whereas the women in the music listening group showed a 24% increase in heart rate variability. The women in the control group showed also a decrease in heart rate variability. Individual time courses (of 4, 5, and 6 cm dilation) of the women in the different groups showed a certain variability that can be explained by individual differences in the reaction of the autonomic nervous system to the complex stimuli attendant to labor and delivery. At all cervical dilations, the women of the three groups showed only minimal changes in mean heart rate. This result is important because the parameter of beat-to-beat variability appears as a more sensitive measure than mean heart rate (Abel et al., 1992).

The changes in heart rate variability show that the women in the biofeedback training and music listening and the women in the music listening groups may have been in a more relaxed state than the women in the control group. Therefore biofeedback training and music listening alone may help to reduce stress in labor.

References

Abel, H.-H., Klüssendorf, D., Koralewski, H. E., Krause, R., & Droh, R. (1992). Spectral analysis of heart rate during different states of activity. In T. F. J. Schmidt, B. T. Engel, & G. Blümchen (Eds.), *Temporal variations of the cardiovascular system* (pp. 99–1166). New York: Springer Verlag.

Akselrod, S., Gordon, D., Ubel, F. A., Shannon, D. C., Barger, A. D., & Cohen, R. J. (1981). Power spectrum analysis of heart rate fluctuation: A quantitative probe of beat-to-beat cardiovascular control. *Science, 213*, 220–222.

Bernat, S. H., Wooldrige, P. J., Marecki, M., & Snell, L. (1992). Biofeedback-assisted relaxation to reduce stress in labor. *JOGNN, 21*, 295–303.

Gregg, R. H. (1978). Biofeedback relaxation training effects in childbirth. *Behavioral Engineering, 4*, 57–66.

Halpaap, B. B., Spintge, R., Droh, T., Kummert, W., & Kögel, W. (1985). Angstlösende Musik in der Geburtshilfe (Anxiolytic Music in Obstetrics). In R. Droh & R. Spintge (Eds.), *Music in Medicine* (pp. 145–54). Grenzach: Editiones Roche.

Hanser, S. B., Larson, S. C., & O'Connell, A. S. (1983). The effect of music on relaxation of expectant mothers during labor. *Journal of Music Therapy, 20*, 50–58.

Hodnett, E., & Abel, S. (1986). Person-environment interaction as a determinant of labor length variables. *Health Care of Women International, 7*, 345–356.

Hodnet, E., & Osborn, R. (1989). Effects of continuous intrapartum professional support on childbirth outcomes. *Research in Nursing & Health, 12*, 289–297.

Jung, R. (1986). The concepts of W. R. Hesse: Ergotropic and trophotropic somato vegetative coordination. *Journal of Autonomic Nervous System* (Suppl), 575–581.

Katona, P. G., & Jih, F. (1975). Respiratory sinus arrhythmia: Noninvasive measure of parasympathetic cardiac control. *Journal of Applied Physiology, 39*, 801–805.

Lebowitz, E. (1989). Biofeedback assisted relaxation training during first pregnancy: Implications for childbirth and the postpartum period (Doctoral dissertation, University of Maryland, 1980). *Dissertation Abstracts International, 49*, 2826B.

Leventhal, E., Leventhal, H., Shacham, S., & Easterling, D. V. (1989). Active coping reduces reports of pain from childbirth. *Journal of Consulting and Clinical Psychology, 57*, 365–371.

Livingston, J. C. (1979). Music for the childbearing family. *JOGNN*, 363–367.

McKay, S. (1991). Shared power: The essence of humanized childbirth. *Pre- and Peri-Natal Psychology, 5*, 283–295.

Segal, I. (1981). Biofeedback-assisted lamaze childbirth preparation: An analysis of variables and treatment effects (Doctoral dissertation, University of Alabama, Birmingham). *Dissertation Abstracts International, 42*, 2084B.

Stevens, K. M. (1992, September). My room – not theirs! A case study of music during childbirth. *Australian College of Midwives Incorporated Journal*, 27–31.

St. James-Roberts, I., Chamberlain, G., Haran, F. J., & Huchingson, C. (1982). Use of electromyographic and skin-conductance biofeedback relaxation training to facilitate childbirth in primiparae. *Journal of Psychosomatic Research, 26*, 455–462.

EFFECTS OF SELECTED MUSIC LISTENING ON CARDIOVASCULAR-RESPIRATORY PARAMETERS OF CHRONIC BACK PAIN PATIENTS

Hans-Henning Abel, Jens-Stefan Geier, Rosalie Rebollo Pratt, Ralph Spintge, and Roland Droh

Introduction

Human experience shows that music is much more than just an acoustic phenomenon. In addition to being a particular kind of human behavior (Gaston, 1968, p. 7) music is also, as clearly articulated in the Affektenlehre of the Baroque period, a vehicle for emotional expression as well as a way to bring on certain emotions.

The therapeutical use of music involves psychical and somatic processes that are interdependent and form, so to speak, a sensitive balance, that is mutually affected by change on either side. Therefore, physical conditions are affected by psychical influences, and vice versa. J. P. Hubert (1983) sums up the advantages and benefits of music listening in postoperative medical treatment with a series of relaxation techniques he calls "sophronisation-training technique": reduction of premedication; distinct reduction of postoperative pain; decreased occurrence of edema and hemorrhage; avoidance of postoperative shocks; increase of quality and acceleration of the healing process; and considerable reduction of the risks pertaining to circulation (Hubert, 1983, p. 689).

From a psychological standpoint, the following points may be made: 1. Soft music can induce relaxation if it is melodically conjunct, has slow harmonic changes, and is without extreme dynamics. The effects of relaxation on the soul and body were commented on by Aristotle (fl. 4th c. B.C.) and Boethius (fl. 6th c.). 2. In addition to reducing the anxiety of the patient, music may reduce the anxiety of the therapist who may be confronted with his or her own fears during sessions. Music listening may prove relaxing to both patient and therapist when anxiety and even panic have become projected into the session. This kind of relaxation may be termed psychopharmacological. 3. Music can induce suppressed emotions and affects. Through an immediate associative potential, it may have a direct influence on psychological and physiological processes (Hubert, 1983, p. 686).

The harmonic structure of a piece of music is an especially important affective factor; one might say that it is the emotional "personality" of music. Emotions, which can be defined as a modulation of psychical processes, are influenced, however, by cognition. It becomes even more problematic when one examines the psychomusicological literature and data to discover that a work of art can evoke different and inconsistent emotions throughout one listening. Therefore, the general ambiguity of psychomusicological experiments lies in the reliability of the experimental procedure as well as the cognitive interpretation of an aesthetic process.

The terms "tonal" and "atonal" imply a vast panoply of aesthetic principles, personal as well as objective responses and perceptions, and different musicological, philosophical, and social ideas. The terms "consonant" and "dissonant" are relative. As Lundin (1967, pp. 88–89) and Farnsworth (1969, pp. 37–41) have said, response to harmony is a cultural phenomenon. Listeners respond with the tools of their own experience and, therefore, their own harmonic expectations. This helps the listener "make sense of the music" (Meyer,

1967, pp. 288–293). Meyer (1967) has stated that the central thesis of the psychological theory of emotions is that "emotion or affect is aroused when a tendency to respond is arrested or inhibited" (p. 14). Therefore, when the listener does not find what he knows or can understand, and cannot respond, he is aroused.

It is difficult to isolate any one parameter of the musical triangle, melody, harmony, and rhythm, as the dominant part in the emotional perception of music. Although the musical complex itself is inseparable, there are constant transfers of emphasis within the musical process, for example, the melodical (Saint-Saëns' *Le Cygne*, from the *Carnéval des animaux*) or the rhythmical (Ravel's *Bolero*), or even harmonic (J. S. Bach's *Das wohltemperierte Klavier*).

The review of the scientific literature shows little controlled and rigorous study of physiological measures of heart rate and respiratory responses in patients treated with music therapy. Hodges (1980) and Standley (1986) pointed out the differences in research methodology and lack of rigor in many music therapy studies. Many studies indicate that music interventions reduced blood pressure, respiratory rate, heart rate, and electrodermograph level, while other studies reported the opposite results (Hodges, 1980). Other reasons for mixed results could be attributed to medications administered for control of blood pressure and heart rate, interruptions during interventions, environmental noise levels, severity of patients' illnesses, and the like. It is clear that more rigorous and strictly controlled physiological research measures must be used in future studies.

While there is nothing in the literature concerning the effects of music on physiological measures of chronic back pain patients, the frequent reporting of effects of music on physiological measures of cardiac patients may be due to the great interest in this population. Bonny (1983) found that music was very effective in improving mood states, reducing heart rate, pain, and anxiety levels. Davis-Rollans and Cunningham (1987) studied the effects of music on coronary care patients. Patients, assigned either to the experimental or control group, showed that music had positive effects on mood states. Statistically significant, but not clinically significant changes were found in decrease of heart rate. Zimmerman, Pierson, and Marker (1988) found no significant differences among subjects randomly assigned to music, "white noise", and control groups for dependent measures of heart rate, skin temperature, and blood pressure. When the groups were combined, however, significant differences were found in systolic and diastolic blood pressures, heart rate, and skin temperature. Guzzetta (1989) reported increased peripheral temperatures and reduced heart rates among Coronary Care Unit patients in a music listening and relaxation group compared to subjects in the control group. A study by White (1992) suggested that respiratory rates, heart rates, and state anxiety levels of randomly assigned myocardial infarction patients were significantly reduced in music listening group subjects compared with control group subjects.

We assume that the chronic condition of pain patients puts them in an ergotropic functional state. The question then arises as to whether is it possible to change this presumed ergotropic state to a more trophotropic state by means of a musical model that might be classified as tonal. On the other hand, would a presumed ergotropic state be exacerbated by music that might be classified as atonal? The research question of this study is as follows: Does the tonal or atonal structure of a piece of music influence the functioning of the cardiovascular-respiratory system?

Method

Description of Subjects

The subjects included 17 females and 12 males between 23–60 years of age, who were suffering from chronic back pain and were currently being treated with Bupivacaine 3 times a week applied by means of a peridural injection. All measurements were done on a therapy-free day. Exclusionary criteria included professional musicians and persons with a distinct verbal aversion to classical piano music.

Table 1. *Demographic Data*

	n	Age [yrs]	Weight [kg]	Height [cm]	Therapy [days]
Male	12	47.5 (31, 60)$^{+}$	81 (71, 96)$^{++}$	174 (165, 188)$^{+}$	7 (6, 10)
Female	17	34 (23, 53)	70 (54, 95)	168 (152, 179)	6 (2, 10)

Median with minimum and maximum; Mann-Whitney U test, $\alpha = 0.05$, $^{+}$: $p < 0.05$, $^{++}$: $p < 0.01$

Questionnaire

An investigator-generated questionnaire that asked 60 subjects in the validation phase to operationally define consonant and dissonant, and verbal descriptors for preferred music and for disliked music was taken to obtain information about the subjective perception of the two test pieces of music. Validated terms were used as semantic differentials (for example calming – disquieting) in a polarity profile (Figure 1). The questionnaire was completed by the subjects immediately after the end of data recording.

Protocol

The research design was an independent measures procedure. The subject was given 15 minutes to acclimate to the laboratory ambiance and temperature. During this time, the appropriate electrodes, sensors, and transducers were applied to the body surfaces.

Two pieces of music with contrasting structures, one tonal, and the other atonal, were chosen: a piano transcription of Johann Sebastian Bach's choral BWV 659 *Nun komm der Heiden Heiland*, and *Klavierstück I*, by Karlheinz Stockhausen. A jazz ballad by Dexter Gordon, *Darn that dream*, was the reference music.

First the subject listened to 5 minutes of the Gordon piece, which served as the sound segment that filled the resting period in which the subject became used to sound. Then, the piano transcription of the choral BWV 659 by J. S. Bach was presented followed by the Stockhausen piece. The Bach piece was played for 5 minutes and the Stockhausen piece for 3:40 minutes. All three sound segments were separated by 1-minute breaks. To avoid order effects, the Bach and Stockhausen pieces were rotated in sequence from subject to subject.

Equipment

Electrodes were attached on the rib cage to record the Electrocardiogram (Siemens Sirecust 402); a source of light on one side and a sensor sensitive to light on the opposite side were placed at the tip of the fourth finger to record the Photoplethysmogram (Satlite);

"I experienced music selection 1/2 as:"

item no.			
1	calm	☐ ☐ ☐ ☐ ☐	restless
2	relaxed	☐ ☐ ☐ ☐ ☐	tense
3	orderly	☐ ☐ ☐ ☐ ☐	chaotic
4	unharmonious	☐ ☐ ☐ ☐ ☐	harmonious
5	aggressive	☐ ☐ ☐ ☐ ☐	balanced
6	loud	☐ ☐ ☐ ☐ ☐	soft
7	varied	☐ ☐ ☐ ☐ ☐	boring
8	beautiful	☐ ☐ ☐ ☐ ☐	unpleasant
9	harsh	☐ ☐ ☐ ☐ ☐	gentle
10	violent	☐ ☐ ☐ ☐ ☐	peaceful
11	calming	☐ ☐ ☐ ☐ ☐	exciting
		1 2 3 4 5	*degree of choice*

"While listening to piece 1/2 I felt:"

item no.			
1	tense	☐ ☐ ☐ ☐ ☐	relaxed
2	restless	☐ ☐ ☐ ☐ ☐	calm
3	hectic	☐ ☐ ☐ ☐ ☐	composed
4	insecure	☐ ☐ ☐ ☐ ☐	secure
5	happy	☐ ☐ ☐ ☐ ☐	unhappy
6	extroverted	☐ ☐ ☐ ☐ ☐	introverted
7	satisfied	☐ ☐ ☐ ☐ ☐	dissatisfied
8	angry	☐ ☐ ☐ ☐ ☐	joyful
9	stressed	☐ ☐ ☐ ☐ ☐	tranquill
10	aggressive	☐ ☐ ☐ ☐ ☐	balanced
		1 2 3 4 5	*degree of choice*

Figure 1. Questionnaire Containing Semantic Differentials in a Polarity Profile (Five Different Degrees of Choice). Top: "I experienced piece A/B of music as…"; bottom: "While listening to piece A/B of music I felt…".

and a Thermistor (Siemens) was placed at the oryphis of the nose for recording respiration related temperature changes in the airflow. All parameters were measured continuously and digitized with a sample rate of 1 ms for data analysis during each 16-minute recording session.

Analysis

A computerized analysis of the three parameters was done for each 16-minute recording (Figure 2). The electrocardiogram was computed by means of an algorithm that detected the R-wave of each QRS-complex and calculated the time between two successive R-waves. The result was a sequence of R-R intervals. For each piece of music the mean value of R-R intervals (mean RR), its standard deviation S.D. RR, and the mean value of the modulus of successive R-R interval differences (mean $|\Delta RR|$) were calculated (Formula 1). The variable mean $|\Delta RR|$ represents a simple measure of beat-to-beat variability that is very closely correlated to the parasympathetic innervation of the heart. For each heart beat, correlated deflexion of the finger plethysmogram was computed for the maximum and minimum scores; the difference between the two scores for each heart beat was calculated as amplitude A. For each piece of music the mean value of As (mean A), its standard deviation S.D. A, and the mean value of the modulus of successive A differences (mean $|\Delta A|$) were calculated. The variable mean $|\Delta A|$ represents a measure of amplitude-to-amplitude variability (Formula 2) that depends on the modulation of sympathetic mediated vasomotion. From the thermistor signal of the respiratory airflow the time between the maxima of two successive breaths was computed as the respiratory cycle time (TT). For each piece of music the mean value of TTs (mean TT), its standard deviation S.D. TT, and the mean value of the modulus of successive TT differences (mean $|\Delta TT|$) were calculated. The variable mean $|\Delta TT|$ represents a measure of breath-to-breath variability (Formula 3).

For statistical analysis the Friedman test and the Wilcoxon signed ranks test were used with a level of significance of 0.05.

$$(1)\quad \text{mean } |\Delta RR| = \frac{1}{n}\sum_{i=1}^{n} |(RR_{i+1} - RR_i)|$$

$$(2)\quad \text{mean } |\Delta A| = \frac{1}{n}\sum_{i=1}^{n} |(A_{i+1} - A_i)|$$

$$(3)\quad \text{mean } |\Delta TT| = \frac{1}{n}\sum_{i=1}^{n} |(TT_{i+1} - TT_i)|$$

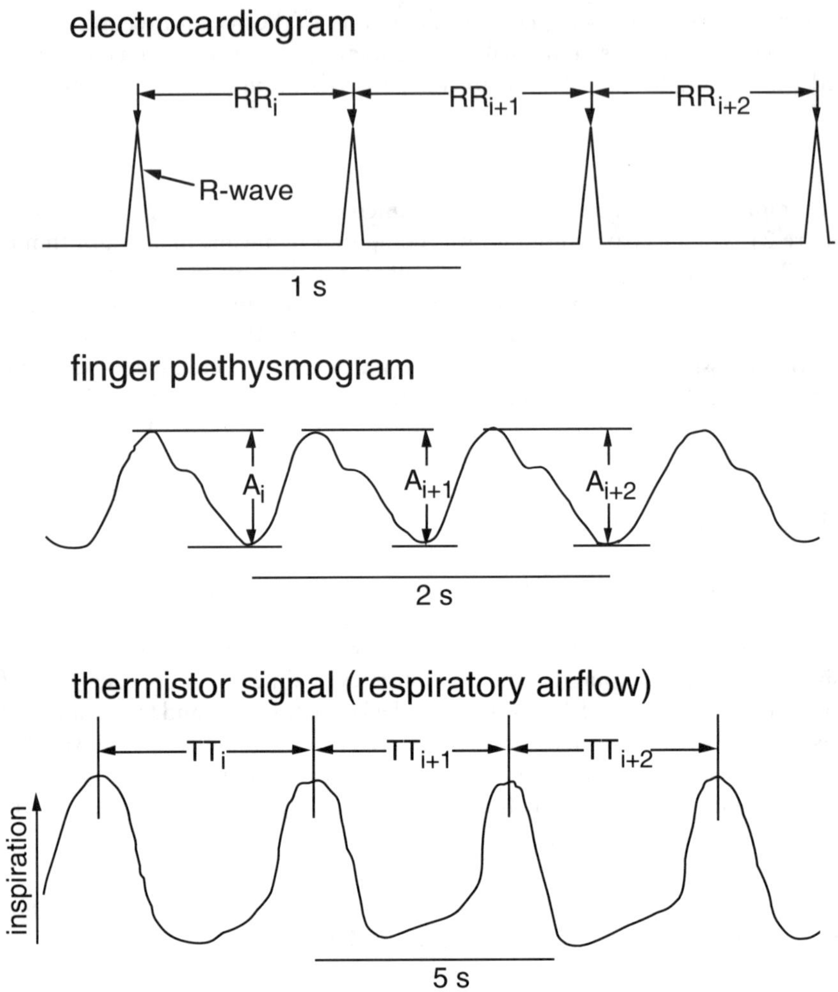

Figure 2. Scheme of the Analysis of Electrocardiogram, Finger Plethysmogram, and Thermistor Signal. For further explanation see text.

Results

In general, the individual time series of the instantaneous (event-to-event calculated) heart rate, amplitude of the finger plethysmogram, and respiratory rate of the studied subjects showed a pronounced variability of all parameters in the course of the 16-minute recording session (Figure 3). The instantaneous heart rate is 60/RR [bpm] and the instantaneous respiratory rate is 60/TT [cpm]. This event-to-event variability is a characteristic phenomenon of cardiovascular-respiratory variables. The raw data showed no obvious changes that could be related to the different pieces of music. Thus, a statistical analysis was performed to differentiate among cardiovascular-respiratory patterns related to different types of music.

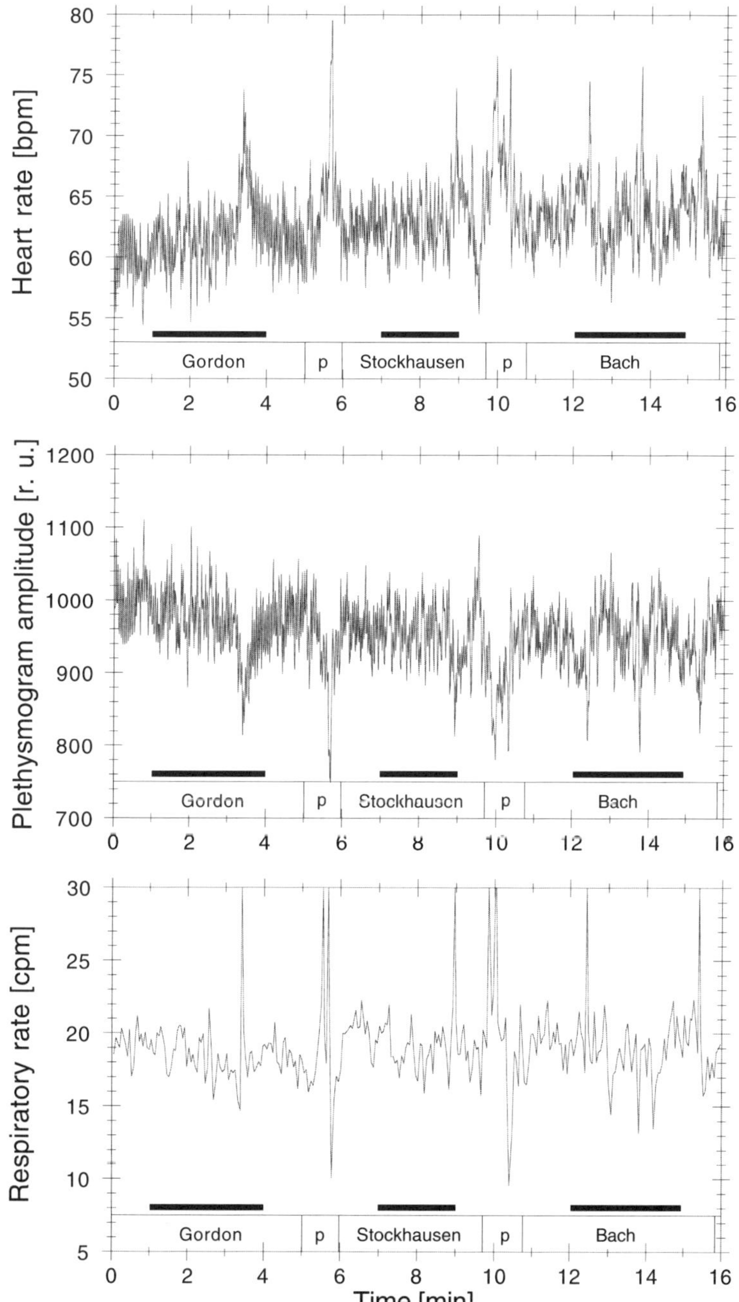

Figure 3. Individual Time Series of Instantaneous Heart Rate, Amplitude of Finger Plethysmogram, and Respiratory Rate of the Whole 16-minute Recording Session. Note the Pronounced Event-to-Event Variability of All Cardiovascular-Respiratory Variables.

The variable mean RR showed very small differences among listening responses to Gordon (median: 815 ms), Stockhausen (819 ms), and Bach (822 ms; Friedman test: p = 0.87). Similar insignificant differences occurred with the variable mean TT among listening responses to Gordon (median: 3.64 s), Stockhausen (3.42 s), and Bach (3.48 s; Friedman test: p = 0.87). However, the variable mean A showed more pronounced changes compared to the variables mean RR and mean TT. In comparison to listening responses to Gordon, the variable mean A decreased around 12% (median) during responses to Stockhausen and around 8% during responses to Bach (Figure 4). The conclusion can be drawn that during listening to both experimental pieces of music a vasoconstriction of finger vessels occurred, with a greater extent, however, during the Stockhausen than during the Bach.

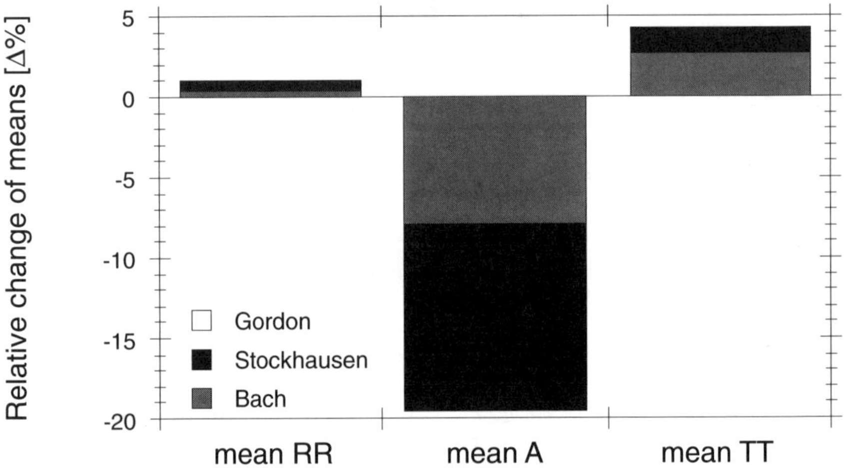

Figure 4. Changes of the Variables Mean R-R Interval (Mean RR), Mean Amplitude of Finger Plethysmogram (Mean A), and Mean Respiratory Cycle Time (Mean TT) during Listening Responses to Stockhausen and Bach. The Median of Percentage Changes Compared with the Listening Responses to the Values for the Gordon is Presented.

The analysis of variability was done using two approaches: 1. the standard deviation (S.D.) of the mean value and 2. the mean value of the modulus of successive value differences (mean |Δvalue|) calculated for each piece of music. The variable S.D. represents the overall variability and depends on trends of the raw values, whereas the variable mean |Δvalue| is extremely independent of trends and represents the extent of variation between two successive values.

Therefore, as expected, different results of the analysis of variability were obtained (Figure 5). Comparing the effects of the two pieces of music on heart rate variability, no substantial differences were obvious regarding the variables S.D. RR and mean |ΔRR|.

However, the variable S.D. A was increased around 13% (median) during listening responses to the Bach compared to the Gordon. This percentage change was significantly higher compared to the negligible increase in S.D. A during listening responses to the Stockhausen. The described change in variability pattern of the finger plethysmogram amplitude has to be related to an occurrence of trends and not to an increased amplitude-to-amplitude variability. On the other hand, the insignificant change in variability pattern during the listening responses to the Stockhausen was based on a 5% decrease in amplitude-to-amplitude variability and not on changes in the variable S.D. A.

The analysis of the variability of respiratory cycle times exhibited an overall decrease during listening responses to the Stockhausen in comparison to the Gordon. The 13% decrease (median) in the variable S.D. TT during listening responses to the Stockhausen

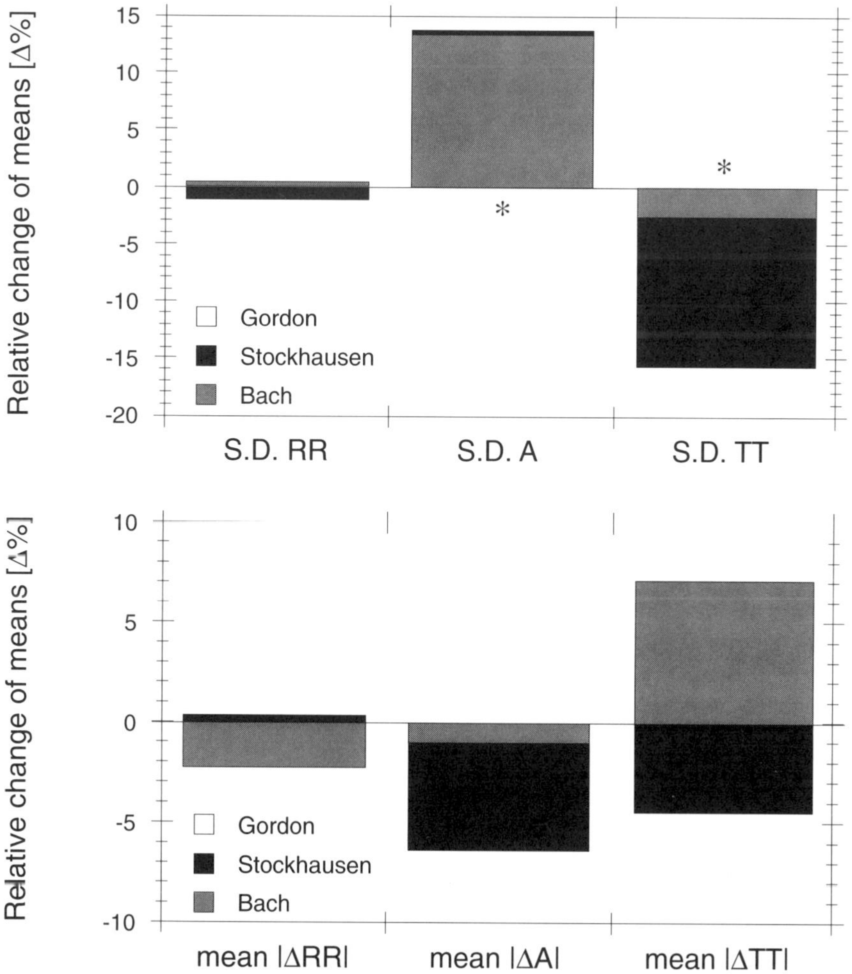

Figure 5. Changes of the Variables Standard Deviation R-R Interval (S.D. RR), Standard Deviation Amplitude of Finger Plethysmogram (S.D. A), and Standard Deviation Respiratory Cycle Time (S.D. TT), top, and Changes of the Variables Beat-to-Beat Variability (Mean |ΔRR|), Amplitude-to-Amplitude Variability (Mean |ΔA|), and Cycle-to-Cycle Variability (Mean |ΔTT|), bottom, during listening responses to the Stockhausen and the Bach. The Median of Percentage Changes Compared with the listening responses values to the Gordon Listening is Presented.

was significant compared to its small 3% decrease during the Bach. The variable mean $|\Delta TT|$ showed a different behavior during the listening responses to the Stockhausen and the Bach. Compared to Gordon, the mean $|\Delta TT|$ decreased around 4% during the listening responses to the Stockhausen but increased around 7% during the Bach. Thus, in contrast to Stockhausen, listening responses to the Bach were accompanied by an increased variation of the differences between successive respiratory cycle times.

The evaluation of the questionnaires showed that the tested subjects perceived the Stockhausen and Bach pieces in entirely opposite ways and their reported affective responses during listening to these pieces were also quite different (Figure 6).

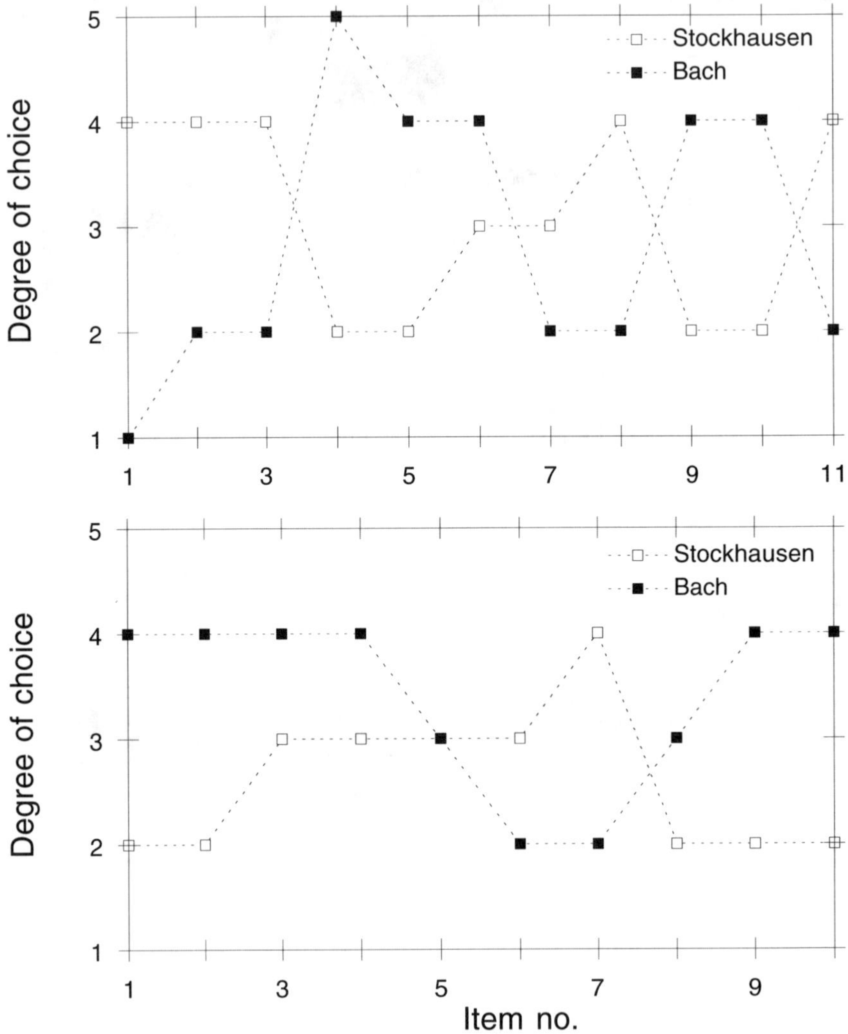

Figure 6. Evaluation of the Questionnaire Containing Semantic Differentials in a Polarity Profile "I perceived piece A/B of music as..."; "During listening to piece A/B of music I felt...". See Figure 1.

Discussion

The results show that listening to the selected musical pieces was accompanied by changes in the cardiovascular-respiratory parameters. The most striking results are changes in the variability of cardiovascular-respiratory parameters and not changes in their mean values. This specific pattern was also found in heart rate parameters when subjects expected a mental test (Abel, Klüßendorf, Koralewski, Krause, & Droh, 1992). One week before performing the Raven test, the heart rate variability was decreased in the experimental group compared to the control group, whereas there were no apparent differences in mean R-R interval between both groups. This was a remarkable result because normally there is a positive correlation between mean R-R interval and its variability parameters, for example, during physical rest and mental and muscular work (Abel et al. 1992).

A particularly notable result of this study is the lack of change in heart rate pattern during selected music listening. We found only very small and therefore insignificant differences in the heart rate variables of mean R-R interval, standard deviation of the mean value, and mean beat-to-beat difference. Therefore, chronic back pain patients showed a constant heart rate pattern during the 16-minute period of listening to different types of musical pieces. These findings contradict the hypothesis that a more trophotropic state could be induced by means of a musical model that might be classified as tonal. On the other hand, a more ergotropic state could also remain unheightened by music that might be classified as atonal. Consequently, we conclude that, since the parasympathetic part of the autonomic innervation of the heart is primarily responsible for changes of the mean R-R interval and its variability in a physically relaxed condition, it is clear that none of the selected musical pieces-which are, in fact, different in structure and expression—led to a change of the parasympathetic control of the heart.

However, there were statistically significant differences between responses to the Bach and Stockhausen compared to response to the Gordon in the analysis of the two other parameters, plethysmogram amplitude and respiratory cycle time. During listening to tonal (Bach) and atonal (Stockhausen) music, a diminution in the mean amplitude of the finger plethysmogram was observed. This result must be interpreted as a vasoconstriction of finger blood vessels caused by an increased sympathetic vasomotor innervation. Compared to the negligibly small differences in mean R-R interval, the more pronounced but not significant differences in mean plethysmogram amplitude are assumed to be physiologically significant. On this assumption, we have to conclude that listening to Bach and Stockhausen was accompanied by a dissociation of sympathetic innervation: increase in activity of sympathetic neurons, which supply the blood vessels of the finger, and no change in activity of neurons supplying the heart. This conclusion is supported by the different findings regarding heart rate variability and plethysmogram amplitude variability.

It is remarkable that the statistically significant changes concerned variability parameters of the plethysmogram amplitude and respiratory cycle time and not the mean value of these variables. The conclusion is obvious that listening to the tonal and atonal pieces was accompanied by a significant change in the modulation of sympathetic activity and in the modulation of respiratory timing determining mechanisms. The increase in vascular-respiratory variability during listening to the Bach piece can be interpreted as an indicator for a change of central autonomic nervous function in a direction toward a trophotropic state because of the well known enhancement of autonomic variability at physical rest (trophotropic state) in comparison with increased physical activity, for example, muscular work (ergotropic state). On the other hand, the decrease in vascular-respiratory variability during listening to the Stockhausen piece can consequently be interpreted as an indicator for a change in direction toward an ergotropic state.

Since it is known that the analyzed heart rate parameters usually react sensitively to external or internal stimuli, there are two possible interpretations for the lack of change in heart rate pattern during both tonal and atonal music listening periods:

1. The analysis of the polarity profile shows clearly that the Stockhausen piece was distinctly regarded as dissonant, a view that correlates—if we look at the results of the items validation—with stress, negative emotions, and musical aversions. By contrast, Bach was regarded as very consonant, a view that correlates widely with relaxation, positive emotions, and the personal music concept. Thus, it can be concluded that the two pieces led to subjective variations in emotional state. However, the musical stimuli were too weak to evoke distinct reactions in mechanisms controlling the sympathetic-parasympathetic balance in the chronotropic control of the heart.

2. A more plausible explanation is that the patients were not completely relaxed, evidenced by the relatively high resting heart rate of 74 bpm (median). This could be explained by the physical and psychical stress they were experiencing, together with the chronic pain and the "unnatural" life situation in a hospital. Therefore, because of the guaranteed level of arousal evoked by environmental stimuli, the musical stimuli were too weak to cause changes of the sympathetic-parasympathetic balance in the chornotropic cardiac control.

We assume that the observed differences of the analyzed cardiovascular-respiratory variables in response to the music listening can be explained by a threshold concept (Hess, in Jung, 1986). Heart rate variables have a low threshold, which means that, in terms of these variables, the above-mentioned environmental stimuli are strong enough to reach the threshold before the music listening begins, and, therefore, the applied musical stimuli exert no further effect. On the other hand, when compared with heart rate variables, vasomotor and respiratory variables have a higher threshold since they respond to musical stimuli added to the environmental stimuli.

In summary, listening to a tonal and an atonal piece of music did not produce any change in mean heart rate and heart rate variability, although there was a verbally reported distinction between the two pieces as far as expressed emotional feeling of patients suffering from chronic back pain. On the basis of Hess' concept (Jung, 1986), it has to be concluded that—contrary to our expectation—the different musical stimuli could induce neither a trophotropic nor an ergotropic state of central autonomic nervous function. Nonetheless, the striking vascular-respiratory changes were noted as an increase in variability of both the plethysmogram amplitude and the respiratory cycle time during the listening period to the Bach piece, while there was a decrease in variability of these parameters during listening to the Stockhausen (when compared to the Gordon work). Thus, autonomic responses to both pieces, the Bach and the Stockhausen, reflect different emotionally colored perceptions of tonal and atonal music.

References

Abel, H.-H., Klüssendorf, D., Koralewski, H. E., Krause, R., Droh, R. (1992). Spectral analysis of heart rate during different states of activity. In T. F. H. Schmidt, B. T. Engel, & G. Blümchen (Eds.), Temporal variations of the cardiovascular system (pp. 99–116). Berlin: Springer-Verlag.

Aristotle. (fl. 5th c. B.C.). *Politics* 8. 1340a. 5.

Boethius. (fl. 6th c.). *De institutione musica* 1. 1. 13–15.

Bonny, H. L. (1983). Music listening for intensive coronary care units: A pilot project. *Music Therapy, 3*(1), 4–16.

Clynes, M. (1980). The communication of emotion. Theory of sentics. Emotion-theory, research and experience. In R. Plutchik & H. Kellerman (Eds.), *Theory of emotion,* vol. 1 (pp. 271–300).

Davis-Rollans, C., & Cunningham, S. G. (1987). Physiological responses of coronary care patients to selected music. *Heart & Lung, 16*(4), 370–378.

Farnsworth, P. R. (1969). The social psychology of music. 2nd ed. Ames, Iowa: The Iowa State University Press.

Gaston, E. T. (Ed.). (1968). *Music in therapy.* New York: Macmillan.

Guzzetta, C. E. (1989). Effects of relaxation and music therapy on patients in a coronary care unit with presumptive acute myocardial infarction. *Heart & Lung, 18*(6), 609–616.

Harrer, G. (Ed.). (1975). *Grundlagen der Musiktherapie und Musikpsychologie.* Stuttgart: Fischer Verlag.

Hodges, D. A. (1980). Appendix A: Physiological responses to music. In D. A. Hodges (Ed.), *Handbook of music psychology* (pp. 293–400). Maryland: National Association for Music Therapy.

Hubert, J. P. (1983). La Rélaxation en Pratique Privée. *Actualités Odonto-Stomatologiques, 144*, 686–689.

Jung, R. (1986). The concepts of W. R. Hess: Ergotropic and trophotropic somato-vegetative coordination. *Journal of the Autonomic Nervous System* (Suppl), 575–581.

Meyer, L. B. (1967). *Emotion and meaning in music.* Chicago: University of Chicago Press.

Lundin, R. W. (1967). *An objective psychology of music.* New York: Ronald Press.

Osgood, C. E., Duci, G. J., & Tannenbaum, P. H. (1957). *The measurement of meaning.* Urbana: University of Illinois Press.

Standley, J. M. (1986). Music research in medical/dental treatment. Meta-analysis and clinical applications. *Journal of Music Therapy, 23*(2), 56–122.

Weber, K. (1994). *The effects of live music on heart rate, blood pressure, and skin temperature of cardiac patients.* Unpublished M. A. thesis, Department of Music, Brigham Young University, Provo, Utah.

White, J. M. (1992). Music therapy: An intervention to reduce anxiety in the myocardial infarction patient. *Clinical Nurse Specialist, 6*(2), 58–63.

Zimmerman, L. M., Pierson, M. A., & Marker, J. (1988). Effects of music on patient anxiety in coronary care units. *Heart & Lung, 17*(5), 560–566.

RELAXATION, IMAGERY, AND MUSIC AS ADJUNCT THERAPY TO NARCOTIC ANALGESIA IN THE PERIOPERATIVE PERIOD

Maureen Patricia Reilly

Abstract

The experience of pain in the perioperative period is often treated solely by the use of pharmacologic agents. The client becomes the passive recipient of these medications, often left with no coping mechanism for the overall pain experience. This study examined the use of relaxation, imagery and music as adjuncts for pain control in a population of 18–40-year-old male clients with lower limb injuries. A quasi experimental design used in this pilot study included experimental group subjects who received instruction in the use of relaxation and imagery with music on a prerecorded audio tape in addition to the traditional anesthetic plan of medications. Control group subjects received the traditional anesthetic plan of medications only. The groups were then compared by counting frequency and route of narcotic administration in the immediate post operative period. A decrease in frequency in oral postoperative medications was noted in the experimental group. In postoperative interviews, all subjects in the experimental group reported a decrease in the sense of anxiety in the preoperative holding area when listening to music. This was an unexpected finding and not part of the hypothesis in the initial proposal. The trend illustrated by this pilot indicates the usefulness of these modalities as adjuncts to anesthesia and should be explored in diverse populations in larger studies.

Introduction

Pain has been described as subjective, characterized as a psychological state resulting in an unpleasant experience. Pain has been further defined by the International Association for the Study of Pain as an unpleasant sensory and emotional experience associated with actual or potential tissue damage, or described in terms of such damage (Weisenberg, 1984).

Pain or discomfort is a problem addressed in most nursing plans of care for the hospitalized client. The problem poses a challenge to the professional nurse both in the traditional roles of the nurse as well as the expanded role of the Nurse Anesthetist. Central to the role of the Nurse Anesthetist is the assessment of pain and discomfort in the perioperative client. The Nurse Anesthetist must correctly diagnose the client's needs to experience a stress-free operative course. Practicing within a holistic health care paradigm, the Nurse Anesthetist can deliver care to the client on both physiological and psychological planes (Keegan, 1987).

The purpose of this paper is to examine visual imagery, relaxation, and music as effective adjunct therapies to narcotic analgesia for the male perioperative client undergoing lower limb surgery. Pain is said to have two components, a physical one, and a psychological one. In her report on pain assessment, Gaston-Johansson (1984) has divided pain into sensory and reactive components. Many factors influence the reactive component of pain that deal with emotions, anxiety, learned experiences, coping mechanisms, and cultural background.

The sensory component of pain experienced in the perioperative period is controlled by the administration of pharmacologic agents and the method of anesthetic delivery. The choice of anesthetic method specifically addresses the anatomic location and physiologic intensity of the pain that is caused by the surgical intervention. The anesthetist may decrease client discomfort in the perioperative state by also directly dealing with the reactive component of pain. By increasing the repertoire of coping mechanisms, the anesthetist affords the client increased comfort in the perioperative period.

Visual imagery has been discussed as a coping mechanism in chronic pain control in the opinions expressed by Griffin (1986) in her article examining imagery as a technique used in her practice with elderly clients. Little or no documented research deals with the use of visual imagery in the arena of acute pain control (Griffin, 1986).

Relaxation and music have been used as adjuncts to anesthesia in a pilot study described by Bonny and McCarron (1984). Little other published research is available documenting these three modalities as a combined approach to decrease the acute pain experience.

Relaxation refers to deep progressive isometric relaxation. The client is directed through an orderly progressive exercise system that increases the intensity of muscular relaxation. Visual imagery is the use of the client's active participation in the creation and involvement of a mental picture that either puts the client in control of the pain sensation or removes the client mentally from the actual pain environment. The client is motivated to first take part and then gradually create and participate in the visual image. Music is the modality that intensifies and unifies the relaxation and imagery experience.

The need for a study of this type is clear. Research into the subject of acute pain control is sparse, and the major body of research has focused on imagery as a coping mechanism in chronic pain rather than acute postoperative pain. Relaxation and music have also been primarily the focus of chronic pain experience in the past. The results of this study may be applied to additional populations and applied to clinical practice of the Anesthetist in the area of pain management of the perioperative client with a limited coping repertoire for pain.

Literature Review

A study by Tollinson, Kreigel, and Downie (1985) supports the view that reactive pain behaviors are not a direct result of organic tissue damage and may be successfully dealt with by the use of several therapies including relaxation therapy. A component of the relaxation therapy used was visual imagery. The use of the two therapies was reported as a single instrument and individual components were not considered. Coping mechanisms for post-surgical pain have been examined by Scott and Chumm (1984). The results of their study support the view that differing personality types will respond differently to increased coping skills. They describe individuals as being either avoiders (those who respond by blocking and denial), or sensitizes (those who are more vigilant, overly anxious, and alert to threat). Sensitizes appear to be more responsive to the relaxation therapy that was introduced as an independent variable in this study.

Self concept and illness attitudes have also been examined as an explanation for patients reactive response to pain. The object of a study (Large, 1985) to encourage the patient to manage pain with less reliance on the medical system supports the notion that alteration in illness attitudes is an effective tool in pain management.

Further support for the effectiveness of added coping mechanisms as a tool in pain management is reported by Gross (1986). The major finding of this study stated that the use of particular coping mechanisms related to the relief of pain. The study did not, however, support the idea that teaching patients cognitive strategies would be useful; rather it supports focus on loss of control experienced by the patient. The Gross study illustrates that increasing coping mechanisms may be utilized as a successful strategy in pain management.

Zeimer (19830 explored information as another method of postsurgical pain management. She hypothesized that increased information will directly increase postsurgical coping. Again, the effect of information is that the information becomes part of the pain therapy by increasing postsurgical coping. Her discussion and conclusions note the need for further research with stronger interventions to be indicated.

As stated previously, the positive effect of relaxation therapy has been demonstrated in studies by Lawliss (1985), and specifically by Tollinson (1985), who used visual imagery in the Pain Therapy Center study. Lawliss, Shelby, Hinant, and McCoy (1985) reported a decrease in Demerol usage by more than 50% in relaxation groups, and a decrease in hospitalization by an average of 2 days. In a master's thesis presented to University of Texas Health Science Center, San Antonio, Texas, Miller (1984) examined the relationship of visual imagery as an effective tool in coping with the pain association with burn therapy. In this pilot study, results supported the original hypothesis that visual imagery was effective in reducing reactive pain in the burn therapy patient.

Wells (1982) reported that relaxation training appears to reduce the psychological component of pain in patients undergoing abdominal surgery. Muscle tensions were objectively measured by surface EMG and showed no significant differences in pre- and post-session levels. The interpretation of data, which reported significantly lowered perceptions of pain, was attributed to increased cognitive coping mechanisms.

The use of music as an anxiolytic and analgesic tool was studied by Bonny and McCarron (1984) in a study of 25 perioperative patients. The results showed a subjective description by patients of decreased anxiety while listening to music. In an extensive review of research literature, Bechler-Karsch (1993) chronicled 14 reports made since the early 70s. The study particularly describes the concept of audioanalgesia and provides a brief description of studies in various populations using music as a particular model for decrease in perceived pain. Studies describe diverse populations consistently reporting improvement of patient outcomes as a result of music being added to treatment regimens.

In summary the literature search reveals a multitude of studies dealing with pain management, with controversy surrounding the methods and means of significant measures for intervention. The effect of increasing coping strategies represented a strong trend in enhancing patient outcomes in all literature reviewed. Many studies were vague in statistical review of subjects but reported consistent trends indicating favorable patient outcomes.

Most of the reviewed literature suggests that an effective tool is relaxation therapy as a pain management technique, specifically in chronic pain control. The definition of relaxation therapy differs from study to study, with the basic and constant core concept of an active patient participation in cognitive invocation of a relaxation response. What the literature does not disclose in the majority of cases is whether or not visual imagery—if specifically employed—would be effective. There is a particular scarcity of research dealing with visual imagery as a coping mechanism in acute postsurgical pain. Visual or guided imagery is also consistently described as an active cognitive strategy employed by the study participants.

Finally, music is acknowledged as an effective tool in management of pain and anxiety in previous studies. The type, duration, and method of introduction of music into the therapeutic regimen differs from study to study, but the core concept of using music as an active coping strategy is consistent throughout the review. The literature does not show studies using the combination of relaxation, visual imagery and music as an adjunctive methodology for analgesic effect in the perioperative patient.

Purpose and Rationale

The purpose of this study was to examine the use of visual imagery, relaxation and music as an adjunct to narcotic analgesics in the perioperative period. The research question posed by the present study is: Does the use of these therapies reduce the total doses of narcotic analgesics needed to control pain in the population under study?

Conceptual Framework

The conceptual framework of this study may be termed a concert of mind and body, since holism guides the study. The concept of holism is central to the nursing theory espoused by Nightingale in her works written over 100 years ago. In her work *Notes on nursing*, Nightingale (1859) discusses the holistic concept of bringing both mind and body into a single unit to be cared for by the nurse. This concept of a holistic paradigm gives this study its central focus. The role of the anesthetist is in the core concept of a care-versus-cure model. The extended role of the anesthetist is an example of the care model in a holistic framework. The goal of care is stress-free anesthesia. Keegan (1987), in her work on holistic nursing, describes the resurgence of holism in health care delivery in the late 1970s. She expresses the view that nursing can lead the way in integrating whole health concepts in modern technological nursing. She describes the works of Nightingale on holism as current and relevant in today's health care arena.

The works of Pelletier (1979) on holistic health and medicine also provide a primary conceptual framework for this study. The role of the nurse anesthetist is an interdependent role that borrows many of its technical aspects from the physician. Pelletier has however assumed a theory similar to the theory espoused by Nightingale over 100 years ago. This can be viewed as collegial acceptance of a method of practice common to the nursing profession.

Fernandez defines a cognitive strategy to include the characteristics of self initiation, thought, cognition, and private events. He describes and defines the elements of what should be included in the visual imagery strategy. Visual imagery is classified as four specific types, dependent on the type of image manufactured. Images may be incompatible, translated, stimulus transformative, and response transformative (Fernandez, 1986). These elements of visual imagery provide specific types of information that will be utilized as guidelines for the initiation and implementation of this research.

The use of relaxation and imagery combined with the acoustic stimulation of music as a holistic therapy regimen form the central concepts of the model for implementation of a study of this nature.

Alternative Hypotheses

It was hypothesized that there would be a significant difference in the amount of narcotic analgesics used by the control group versus the experimental group in the study. It was further hypothesized that the group experiencing the independent variable, the visual imagery, relaxation and music sessions, would have a significantly lower use of narcotic analgesics in the postoperative period. The level of significance was originally set at $p < .05$.

Research Design and Methodology

Implementation of the pilot study employs a quasi-experimental research design. The sample is a convenience sample of male patients at a single hospital in the catchment area of one Medical Department Facility in the continental United States.

Variables

The independent variable in the study was the implementation of visual imagery, relaxation, and music as cognitive coping strategies. Confounding variables included the type of medications ordered by the physicians in the postoperative period as well as unknown previous experiences with pain encountered by the clients in the control group.

Sample

The patient population consisted of young healthy males, aged 18–40, admitted for surgical repair of a new onset lower limb injury. The particular group had no history of prior hospitalizations or chronic pain problems. This segment of the population was chosen for several reasons. A preliminary review of the literature demonstrated that the bulk of research had focused on older chronic pain patients and a younger population had not been previously studied. Secondly, this population constituted the most frequent admission to the proposed study facility. These clients were hospitalized for elective surgical treatment of a lower limb injury that required more than outpatient surgical revision. The clients were on the orthopedic service of the hospital.

The initial proposed number of subjects was 100, equally assigned to control and experimental groups. The actual number of subjects was 24, with an analysis of 17 cases. The project was prematurely cut short due to a major deployment of the study population to the Mideast during Operation Desert Shield. The study was then relegated to the status of a pilot project.

It was assumed that the patients who underwent the pilot study were free of known prolonged narcotic analgesic use. It was also assumed that patients willingly participated as volunteers. Even though the study was conducted in one facility, the variety of ethnic and cultural backgrounds of subjects increased the application of the results of the study, The subjects were randomly assigned to either the control or experimental group. Both groups consisted of patients who were given a short briefing as to the intent of the study and then a written informed consent was obtained from each subject. The control group consisted of patients demographically matched to the experimental patient group. These charts were reviewed for the number of narcotic doses administered to the patient in the 24 hours immediately following surgery.

Acknowledged limitation of the study was the size of the population, which was smaller than originally proposed for study. The military hospital still maintains a ward setting, and this lack of privacy might decrease compliance with the practice sessions. The size of the population necessarily limits the report to that of a pilot study.

Implementation

After approval by appropriate Clinical Review Boards, the project was implemented in April 1990. The total number of subjects was 24, consisting of an experimental group (n = 12), and a control group (n = 12). The experimental group was provided with a tape-recorded dialogue and instructions for its use. Informed consent was obtained at the time of the original interview from all subjects.

The surgical team was aware of the ongoing study and was briefed on the details of added conversation that may occur between the nurse anesthetist and the patient during the surgical procedure. The surgical ward staff was not briefed on the patients involved in the procedure in order to prevent unintended interference with pain medication administration postoperatively. The patients underwent various anesthetic techniques including general anesthesia and regional technique. The patients were reassured that there would be no medication withheld from patients in the study.

The experimental group was matched to predetermined demographics. Once the client consented to voluntary participation in the study during preoperative interview, they were randomized to the control or experimental group by a number assignment. The basic concepts of relaxation and visual imagery were discussed with the patient. Both groups were reassured that the standard of care for medication administration would be maintained for all study participants. During the preoperative interview, each patient in the experimental group was introduced to progressive isometric relaxation and guided visual imagery. These patients received an audiotape of a prerecorded relaxation exercise followed by a guided imagery exercise with soft music that set a basic atmosphere and time limit for the guided imagery. The music chosen was an acoustically recorded Celtic harp composition. The piece was selected because it would be unfamiliar to participants and would not draw undo attention from the relaxation and imagery dialogue. The music provided a quiet peaceful environmental background filtering out the noise of the holding area, operating suite, and ward. Review of the literature revealed diverse opinions on the choice of music. Each of the patients in the experimental group was provided with a cassette player for use during the hospitalization. These cassette players were approved through the biomedical department for safe use in the Operating Room. Preop sedation was standardized for participants in both groups. Sedation was limited to Midazolam with the dose calculated by body weight The client was taught progressive relaxation by the use of Isometric Squeeze Relation (Appendix I) (Smith, 1985). The client was then introduced to the actual guided imagery, which was a personal experience and differed for each client. The client was asked to practice the technique at least three times during the preoperative period. During the induction phase of anesthesia, the patient was again encouraged to participate in the Isometric Relaxation and Guided Imagery. The background music was played during the induction to further the relaxation and guided imagery experience. The music was utilized to enhance the effect of the cognitive modification methodology. Finally the client was instructed to utilize the tape recording in the postoperative period. The patient was given the tape recording on discharge in order to assist with the relaxation and imagery in the post discharge period.

Results

Data Collection and Interpretation

To insure confidentiality, the patient was asked to select an arbitrary number that was used to record individual data for each patient actively participating in the study. Specific data collected was the frequency (defined as occurrences), route, and dosage of medication administered for the first and second postoperative days. Prospective records were reviewed that recorded the same information as noted above. These records were retrieved from a time period simultaneous with that of the experimental group. These records were matched as noted previously.

Simple descriptive statistics were used and scatter plot graphs were used for reporting of results. Differences between the groups were analyzed by means of a comparison of total numbers of doses per client and then per group. These totals were to be analyzed by means of chi square and simple t test. The chi square is appropriate for use in nominal data such as dose recency in comparing two independent samples. The groups are independent; one group experiencing a variable, the other classified as the retrospective review group. This statistical review will be reported but, because of the attrition of records, the analysis may be viewed properly as a trend and indication for replication of this study in larger populations. The hypothesized functional relationship was that the decreased use of narcotics within the experimental group is a function of the relaxation, imagery and music.

Validity and Reliability

To insure reproducibility and consistency within this study, an accepted dialogue (Appendix I) was used by a single investigator. The dialogue is an isometric relaxation exercise from Smith's (1985) work *Relaxation dynamics: Nine work approaches to self relaxation.* The subjects who met selection criteria and volunteered for the study were provided with an instruction sheet concerning the study as noted in the attached Appendix. All data were maintained in a confidential manner with random numbers assigned for the purpose of recording data.

Data Analysis

Twenty-four subjects met sample criteria. Data retrieval was complicated by difficulty in locating hospital files of eight of the subjects. Seventeen records were located, with the greater number being those of subjects in the control group. The uneven distribution of records lead to an uneven distribution of surgical procedures. More anterior cruciate ligament repair surgeries were clustered in the experimental (n = 3) versus the control group (n = 1). Since this type of surgery is not comparable to a simple arthroscopy, these subjects were excluded from final analysis. Attrition from the study also resulted from the unexpected deployment of a number of the study participants, and then a marked drop in population on the test site, also secondary to this prolonged unexpected deployment.

The final analysis of statistical data based on the control group (n6) and the experimental group (n5) is given in Table 1.

Table 1

	CONTROL	EXPERIMENTAL
Size	6	5
	TOTAL DOSE FREQUENCY	
Mean	1.66	1.4
Variance	.51	.3
PO number	10	6
IM number	3	3

Chi square and *t*-tests showed a significant difference exceeding the stated level of difference of 0.5; *t* distribution was 3.55, needed level to exceed 1.82 for statistical difference. As discussed earlier, these figures represent a much smaller number than originally needed, so they are viewed as a trend rather than strong statistical evidence of the interventions. Since the number of patients in the final analysis does not represent a large sample, these reports must be considered as preliminary and the need for replication of the study with a larger group necessary. Table 2 shows the distribution of doses. Anesthetics included a distribution of general endotracheal anesthesia, subarachnoid block, and epidural.

Table 2

GETA	1
SAB	8
Epidural	3

Discussion

Group size was limited by the deployment of active duty forces from the test site, but the size of the group was sufficient for the purpose of a pilot study. In the experimental group, results showed a significant difference in the number and frequency of doses of oral pain medications in the postoperative period. This difference in requirements for oral pain medication may indicate that these strategies are particularly effective at the level of moderate pain. The request for, and administration of, intramuscular injections is usually intended for pain that is of greater intensity, creating profound levels of discomfort that would not be relieved by oral medications.

Postoperative interviews with the members of the experimental group disclosed positive experience by all subjects, with one subject reporting no difference in pain control with the use of the tape. All patients in the experimental group reported a perceived decrease in anxiety with the use of the tape. This was an unexpected result, since the original hypothesis was a measure of the variable of pain experience only. During these interviews, additional data were obtained regarding experience in the pre- and postoperative holding area being influenced by the use of the tapes. The subjects reported that feelings of anxiety were greatest in the holding area, which is a small congested area in the front of the operating suite, holding as many as six patients (each with a significant other) at one time. The patients reported that, at this particular time, the tape was helpful in coping with the anxiety. Patients also reported that use of the tape the evening before surgery was helpful as a measure to decrease preoperative anxiety. In the postoperative period, the patients reported that the tapes were helpful while waiting for pain medication or as an aid to decreasing the anxiety that they experienced from the postoperative pain. The patients reported that the tapes assisted them in "relaxing and making the pain not feel as bad".

Limitations of this study included the inability to retrieve all the postoperative records as well as the size of the group. Application of this study to a larger population as well as the use of different surgical procedures would add to the statistical significance of the results of this study.

Application to practice is obvious. It is the intent of anesthetists to provide a stress-free anesthetic experience. The implementation of the combination of these strategies affords an economical method of providing the patient with a more pleasant, less anxious anesthetic experience. An additional strength of this methodology is the fact that the patient can continue to use these new coping strategies beyond the perioperative experience. The serendipitous finding regarding the decreased anxiety perceived by the patient on the evening before surgery and in the preoperative holding area only add to the support of the use of the techniques of relaxation, visual imagery, and music as an effective adjunct to narcotic analgesics in the perioperative period.

The combination of Imagery, Relaxation and Music as adjunctive pain measures provides a cost-effective and quality nonchemical adjunct to traditional pain therapies in the immediate postoperative period. The use of these methodologies may be easily taught to those caring for the patient and, most importantly, learned by the patient himself. It is recommended that this study be replicated in more diverse populations and in larger numbers to add to the body of evidence attesting to the effectiveness of the treatments.

References

Bechler-Karsch, A. (1993). The therapeutic use of music. *The Online Journal of Synthesis of Nursing Knowledge, 1*(4), 1–21.

Bonny, H., & McCarron, N. (1984). Music as an adjunct to anesthesia in operative procedures. *Journal of the American Association of Nurse Anesthetists, 52*(1), 55–57.

Fernandez, E. (1986). A classification system of cognitive coping strategies for pain. *Pain, 26,* 141–149.

Griffin, M. (1986). In the mind's eye. *American Journal of Nursing, 7,* 804–806.

Gross, A. (1986). The effect of coping strategies on the relief of pain following surgical intervention for lower back pain. *Psychosomatic Medicine, 48*(3/4), 229–241.

Keegan, L. (1987). Holistic nursing. *AORN, 46(*3), 499–506.

Johansson, F. (1984). Pain assessment: differences in quality and intensity of the word pain, ache and hurt. *Pain, 20,* 69–76.

Large, R. (1985). Self-concepts and illness attitudes in chronic pain. A repertory grid study of a pain management program. *Pain, 23,* 113–119.

Lawliss, G. F., Selby, D., Hinnant, D., & McCoy, C. E. (1985). Reduction of postoperative pain parameters by presurgical relaxation instructions for spinal pain patients. *Spine, 10*(7), 649–561.

Miller, C. (1984). *An investigation of the effectiveness of imagery-based relaxation on the pain associated with burn therapy: A pilot study.* Unpublished master's thesis. University of Texas, Health Science Center, San Antonio, TX.

Nightingale, F. (1859). *Notes on nursing*. London: E Stern.

Pelletier, K. R. (1979). *Holistic medicine*. New York: Delacorte Press.

Scott, L. E., & Chum, G. A. (1984). Examining the interaction effects of coping style and brief interventions in the treatment of postsurgical pain. *Pain, 20,* 279–291.

Smith, J. C. (1985). *Relaxation dynamics: Nine world approaches to self-relaxation*. Illinois: Research Press.

Tollison, C., Kreigel, M., & Downie, G. (1985). Chronic low back pain: Results of treatment at the Pain Therapy Center. *Southern Medical Journal, 78*(11), 1291–1295.

Weisenberg, M., Aviram, O., Wolf, Y., & Raphaeli, N. (1984). Relevant and irrelevant anxiety in the reaction to pain. *Pain, 20,* 341–383.

Wells, M. (1982). The effect of relaxation on postoperative muscle tension and pain. *Nursing Research, 31*(4), 236–238.

Zeimer, M. (1983). Effects of information on postsurgical coping. *Nursing Research, 32*(5), 282–287.

Appendix

Isometric Relaxation
(Smith, 85)

Script: First, rest both arms in your lap. Now, gently shrug your shoulders. Pull them up or back, whatever feels better. Squeeze the muscles more and more until the squeeze feels most complete and pleasurable. Now, release the tension. Let your shoulders hang. Let the tension begin to flow out. Notice how you can create both feelings of tension and relaxation in your shoulders. For about 30 seconds let your shoulders relax more and more and attend to the pleasant sensations.

In this exercise we are going to relax by letting our minds dwell on a relaxing scene or setting.

PAUSE

Make sure you are seated upright in a comfortable position.

PAUSE

Are your feet flat on the floor?

PAUSE

Are your hands resting comfortably in your lap?

PAUSE

Now gently close your eyes & let yourself settle into a position that is comfortable.

PAUSE

For the next minute or so let your body become and more quiet.

PAUSE 1 MINUTE

Let yourself begin to settle down and relax as you remain still.

PAUSE

And now attend to your body.

PAUSE

Let your breathing be calm and even.

PAUSE

Let every outgoing breath carry away any tension you might feel.

PAUSE

Let yourself feel more and more comfortably relaxed.

PAUSE
And now quietly ask yourself "What scene or setting is most relaxing to me at the moment?"
PAUSE 10 SECONDS
You might want to picture a quiet beach, or a grassy plain, or a cool mountain top, or a peaceful pond.
PAUSE 10 SECONDS
Whatever scene or setting is most relaxing to you, let it come to you in whatever way it wishes.
PAUSE 10 SECONDS
And now, quietly let your mind dwell on this scene for the next few seconds.
PAUSE 15 SECONDS
Let the scene become as vivid and real as possible.
PAUSE 10 SECONDS
How does it look?
PAUSE 10 SECONDS
Can you see the sky?
PAUSE
Can you feel the wind brushing against your skin?
PAUSE
Can you smell the gentle, cool air?
PAUSE
Can you feel the warm sunlight or perhaps the cool night air?
PAUSE
Involve all of your senses.
PAUSE
What do you see?
PAUSE
What do you hear?
PAUSE
What is touching your skin?
PAUSE
Can you taste or smell anything?
PAUSE
And let the scene grow in whatever way is most relaxing to you.
PAUSE 10 SECONDS
Perhaps words come to your mind that describe the scene.
PAUSE
If words or phrases come, simply let them repeat over and over like echoes.
PAUSE
Try not to force these words to change or make sense. Simply let them repeat over and over very peacefully and quietly.
PAUSE
Let it change and evolve on its own.
PAUSE 15 SECONDS
If your mind wanders or is distracted, that's OK.

PAUSE
Quietly and gently return to your relaxing scene.
PAUSE 10 SECONDS
If you find yourself engaged in thinking about something or trying to figure something out, that's OK.
PAUSE
Quietly and gently return to your relaxing scene.
PAUSE 15 SECONDS
Let yourself sink deeper and deeper into a pleasant state of relaxation.
PAUSE
From time to time let yourself quietly repeat whatever words or pictures suggest deeper, more complete, and more satisfying relaxation.
PAUSE
You might think words "I am sinking deeper and deeper," or "I am letting go more and more," or "There is nothing for me to do but let go," or "I am more fully aware."
PAUSE
Let the deepening suggestions come to you in whatever way feels more satisfying and relaxing.
PAUSE
Again and again, every time your mind wanders or is distracted, gently return to your pleasant, relaxing scene.
PAUSE
And now, continue attending to your scene for about 10 minutes. See where it leads you. See how it deepens. See how it grows and becomes more relaxing for the next 10 minutes.
PAUSE 10 MINUTES
And now, very gently let go of what you are attending to.
PAUSE 5 SECONDS
When you are ready, gently open your eyes.
PAUSE 5 SECONDS
Take a breath.
PAUSE 5 SECONDS
And stretch.
PAUSE 5 SECONDS
This completes the thematic imagery exercise.

MUSIC AND MUSIC VIBRATION FOR PAIN RELIEF: STANDARDS IN RESEARCH

Donald E. Michel and Kris S. Chesky

Introduction

Our interest in the topic of this paper was originally stimulated by the recent research of Chesky (1992) that dealt with the use of music with music vibration to relieve pain in patients with rheumatoid arthritis and, more recently, from a national survey inquiring about music for pain relief utilization (Michel & Chesky, 1993, in press). From the research reviewed and the survey responses, it is apparent that there needs to be more scientific rigor in current research in this area of music and pain relief.

Our literature review revealed developments in the fields of music medicine, nursing, and algology (study of pain) that suggested the need for more stringent future research. While the complexities of pain perception and relief as well as the complexities of perception of music and its effects on human behavior are recognized, it is not the intent of this paper to deal with these issues. Nor is it the intent to rationalize or conceptualize the use of music and music vibration for pain relief that has already been reported in recent articles (Brown, Chen, & Dworkin, 1989; Chesky & Michel, 1991; Eagle & Harsh, 1988; Chesky, Michel, & Kondraske, 1994). Rather it is our purpose here only to review critically (a) recent studies of music used for pain relief, (b) recent studies of music and vibration in pain relief and other similar uses, and (c) to suggest how future studies may be improved with more attention given to adherence to scientific and medical standards.

Background

A recent survey of National Association of Music Therapy (NAMT) members ($n = 348$) serving the elderly, medical, neurologically impaired, and physically disabled populations asked respondents about strategies, techniques, and evaluations of the use of music for pain relief (Michel & Chesky, 1993, in press). Results indicated that approximately 45% of the respondents are currently using music therapy specifically for pain management in their practice. Many who were not using music therapy for pain relief indicated difficulty in justifying such potential applications. Most therapists, both those using and those not using music for pain relief including music and vibration, indicated a desire to learn more about rationales and protocols of music therapy in pain management.

Writers in the fields of algology and nursing promote a multidisciplinary approach to pain management that encourages the use of nonpharmacological and noninvasive strategies for pain management such as relaxation, biofeedback, psychological coping techniques, transcutaneous vibration and transcutaneous electrical stimulation (TENS). However, a writer for the Federal Drug Administration (Hecht, 1992) warned that "people... should be wary of products that offer 'special' or 'secret' formulas that promise quick or easy cures, and that are promoted by case histories and testimonials" (p. 1). Hecht concluded that "things that vibrate—chairs and mattresses for example—also have been 'hot' items but they certainly are not harmless" (p. 1). Interestingly, producers of some music vibration chairs and beds claim such "special" or "secret" formulas. Eakin (1993), producer of the Somatron™ recently wrote: "[other] efforts have been made to apply musical or other acoustic/sonic vibrations to more of the body than the ears. However, nobody besides the present inventor seems to understand that the degree of coupling between the musical or other acoustic vibrations and the body is critical, or how to accomplish it for the benefits sought" (p. 7). To date, no meaningful descriptions of the vibrations that the Somatron™ produces have been found. Promotional materials from other companies, such as NextWave's "Physioacoustic" device, claim that the amplitudes of the vibrations produced are of a "chosen" type to gain the desired effects but do not further describe them (Lehikoinen, 1991, 1993). Both of these examples seem to fit Hecht's uneasiness about 'secret' and unproved 'special' formulas.

A recent critique of music therapy by a physician highlights concerns about the field as a scientifically valid discipline. Newmark (1991) asked "...is music therapy clinically valid? It would seem that music therapy must be subject to the same sort of analysis that we as physicians routinely use to evaluate any other therapeutic modality" (p. 1). Newmark reviewed Standley's (1986) meta-analysis of music in medicine and dentistry, and both praised and questioned it in terms of the studies reported. He concluded that "study design must become (more) rigorous and focused to generate the data acceptable to those who are not music therapists" (p. 2). Spintge and Droh (1992) also emphasized the importance of valid/reliable research, stating: "...the reputation of music therapy/music medicine and its acknowledgment by the medical community depends on how it meets the scientific and therapeutic standards of state-of-the-art health care and science" (p. 347).

In the following paragraphs, research reports that discuss the use of music specifically for pain relief and music as or with vibrotactile stimulation will be reviewed. The focus of this examination is on the primary research concern of replication and reliability and adherence to the scientific standards expected in the field of medicine. Suggestions for future research will be provided.

Review of Studies

Music for Pain Relief

Standley's meta-analyses (1986, 1992) and other sources have reviewed music and pain studies. A review of 11 music therapy studies, specifically naming pain relief as a dependent variable, found that most investigations failed to provide titles of the prerecorded music used in the study. Some studies did list general categories of music with or without subject preferred selection procedures, and some listed modes or means of presentation to the subjects (Table 1).

The result of not naming specific selections of music used is that these studies are not completely replicable, which in turn jeopardizes their reliability. In Bonny's study for example (1983), the description of the music used in intensive care situations included general terms such as "popular" and "classical". Considering the enormous variety of music in each of these genres, it becomes futile to attempt even a close replication with such limited information. A list of specific music selections would facilitate replication in follow-up research, enable comparisons with other types of music and provide insights into possible causes for differing results in other studies.

Table 1. *Studies Using Music for Pain Relief*

AUTHOR	DATE	PATIENT TYPE	DESCRIPTION OF MUSIC
Studies reported in Standley's meta-analysis (1986, 1992a)			
Bonny	1983	cardiac	music described in general terms – no specific selections
Clark, McCorkle & Williams	1981	obstetric	"standardized group of 20 prerecorded selections varying in style, period, and characteristics"
Codding	1982	obstetric	no specific selections
Curtis	1982	cancer	no specific selections
Gardner & Licklider	1959	dental	white noise and music – no specific selections
Hanser, Larson & O'Connell	1983	obstetric	"individualized programs"
Jacobson	1957	dental	continuum of sedative instrumental selections in the "popular" idiom
Loscin	1960	dental	subject selected, mostly instrumental
Monsey	1985	dental	"audio analgesia", no specific music
Rider	1990	spinal cord injury	partly documented, but incomplete; some specific music used produced different EMGs
Gfeller, Logan & Walker	1990	adolescent dental	subject selected music – "from a tape library"
Studies not reported in meta-analysis			
Zimmerman, Pozehl, Duncan, & Schmitz	1989	cancer	"ten different types of instrumental tapes" or "Halpern 'Antifrantic' tape"
Kowler-Kerry, & Lander	1987	child injections	"a piece of music suitable for children"
Menagazzi, Paris, Kersteen, Flynn, & Trautman	1991	emergency room	selected from "50 available styles and artists"
Spintge	1991	perioperative	"anxiolytic music" – no specific selections
Whipple & Glynn	1992	experimental pain	titles included

In the cases of music used in childbirth situations such as Clark, McCorkle, and Williams (1981) and Hanser, Larson and O'Connell (1983), the importance of giving control to subjects by allowing them to choose their music is recognized. However, if we also recognize music as an important variable, there is a need to know what specific selections were used in each situation.

This applies to other studies where subjects' choice of music was part of the procedure, for example, Jacobson (1957), Monsey (1960), and Gfeller, Logan and Walker (1990) where music was used in dental treatments. Especially when the subject-selected procedure seemed to produce positive results, it is important to know what the specific music selections were. This missing information is the problem with most of the studies listed in Table 1.

One study, however, did report some differences in results that seemed attributable to the specific music selections (Rider, 1985). In this case, one composer's music seemed to be more effective than another in lowering EMG readings as a measure of tension and pain. In another study (Whipple and Glynn, 1992) about the effects of soothing and stimulating music on pain and tactile thresholds, results showed that soothing music significantly elevated pain but not tactile thresholds while stimulating music significantly elevated pain as well as tactile thresholds. Specific music selections were listed for this study, which can be replicated.

Studies that do not provide descriptive data on the music used imply that music is almost "generic" and that it does not matter, even for replication purposes. "Just use any music", or "use any music that the subjects choose" is the implied protocol. The efficacy of self-selection protocols is still an open question for future research.

When prerecorded music is used in research, descriptions should include at least the title and composer; title of recording (tape/CD/disc); length of excerpt(s) used; equipment used for playback (free-field or headphones); loudness levels used; and elapsed time between selections. Even more detailed acoustical analysis of the music might be useful.

Music and Vibration

The use of music as or with vibrotactile stimulation has been of increasing interest to several researchers (Table 2). In addition to music listening, protocols include the use of mechanical vibration generated from an acoustical energy source and applied to the body through some device, usually a chair, table or bed. Studies in algology, neurophysiology and neuropharmacology indicate that particular vibrations can prompt pain suppressive effects by stimulating particular mechanoreceptor systems. This body of knowledge provides a potent resource to justify and direct research using vibration with music. A conceptual model for applying musical vibration with music listening for pain relief, based within these constructs, has been reported by Chesky and Michel (1991), Chesky (1992), and Chesky, Michel, and Kondraske (1994).

Music with Vibration Studies

The purpose of this section is to review recent reports utilizing music with vibration. Discussions on whether or not the vibrations are described, as well as the problems of interpretation without descriptions of the vibration, will follow.

Reports by Skille (1989, 1992) claim general health benefits from applications of the "Vibroacoustic method". This method is described as the use of "special equipment and software" that emits "low frequency sound signals, sinus/pure tones between 30–120 Hz." mixed with "special audio cassettes".

Darrow (1992), Darrow and Goll (1989), Madsen, Standley, and Gregory (1991), Standley (1991, 1992b) and Clair and Bernstein (1993) used the Somatron™ to explore the effects of music and music vibration with hearing impaired, preschool children, healthy college age subjects and elderly persons with dementia. Marketing materials describe the vibrations emitted by the Somatron™ as "dense" while others have described them as "intense" (Standley, 1991).

Chesky (1992) reported statistically significant reductions of pain for rheumatoid arthritis patients attributable to music plus music vibration as compared to music alone or placebo using the Music Vibration Table (MVT™). The parameters of the vibrations used (amplitude, frequency, and spectrum) were selected to stimulate particular mechanoreceptor systems. The MVT™ was used to measure and control the vibrations while patients were being stimulated. Music selections were described in detail.

In Table 2, the above studies are listed with the descriptions of the music vibration as reported. Some studies did include basic descriptions of the actual music and the duration of treatment or exposure to the vibration stimulus but did not describe the vibration.

Table 2. *Studies using Music and Music Vibration*

AUTHOR	DATE	MUSIC/SOUND	TIME (min)	FREQUENCY OF VIBRATION	SPECTRUM OF VIBRATION	AMPLITUDE OF VIBRATION
Darrow & Goll	1989	8th + 16th notes*	?	?	?	?
Skille	1989	Special tapes w/sinus-tones 30–120Hz	?	?	?	?
Madsen, et al.	1991	included	10	?	?	?
Standley	1991	included	6.5	?	?	?
Chesky	1992	included	30	range 60–600Hz	instantaneous + average spectrums	range = 0–100μm, average = 26μm
Standley	1992 b	included	4.5 6.8	?	?	?
Darrow	1992	pitches**	?	?	?	?
Skille	1992	Special tapes w/sinus-tones 30–120Hz	?	?	?	?
Clair & Bernstein	1993	included	15	?	?	?

Note: The word "included" indicates descriptions were provided. The"?" symbol indicates no information given.

*The reference to the music/sound was "rhythm patterns" without reference to pitch, metronome marking, quality/timbre or loudness.

**There was no reference to duration, metronome marking, quality/timbre of sound, loudness, or time between sounds.

In studies where music vibration is not measured and reported, it is impossible to understand and interpret outcomes. Darrow (1992), working with hearing impaired subjects, reported improved perception of pitch change through vibration-enhanced sounds from the Somatron™ vibration bed. Without the vibrations being measured and controlled however, the subjects' perceptions of change can not be attributed to frequency factors of the vibration alone but must include possible responses to changes in amplitude (Sherrick, 1984).

Standley (1991) studied the effect of music versus the sound of a dental drill, paired with or without music vibration through the Somatron™ vibration bed and stated that the results were "rarely as predicted" (p. 132). It was found that "music alone without vibration... was... the most pleasurable condition of the experiment" (p. 132). In addition, "...58% of the subjects experienced anxiety, usually in responses to the sound of the dental drill, (and) the 'intense vibrations' of the Somatron" (p. 127). Perhaps the results of this study, including the increased anxiety and less pleasurable responses from the "intense vibrations", were related to a particular amplitude, frequency, or spectrum of the vibration, all of which were not reported. Standley hypothesized that a positive, comforting experience would result in a rise in skin temperature and that the vibrotactile stimulation would enhance the effects of the auditory stimuli. Results showed that instead, the ***aversive dental drill sound*** presented with vibration caused a rise in skin temperature, which contradicted the stated hypothesis. Another result was that the female subjects had, on average, lower skin temperatures on all readings and minimal change compared with male subjects. If the vibrations had been measured, the difference in average weights of females versus males might have been found to be a pertinent factor in the actual vibration amplitudes of each group. Several studies report that application of vibration on the skin causes changes in vasomotor activity and that resulting skin temperature changes are dependent on the amplitude and frequency of the vibration (Pyykko, & Hyvarinen, 1973; Skoglund, & Knutsson, 1985; and Skoglund, 1989). This could help explain the temperature differences found in Standley's subjects.

Medical Applications of Vibration

In contrast to not reporting vibration stimulus used in most music and music vibration studies is the detailed descriptions provided in all medical studies using vibration. In fact, vibration is treated as a potent experimental variable and can cause a wide range of possible effects which are dependent on the parameters of the vibration applied. See Chesky (1992) for a review of medical studies using vibration for pain relief.

In applications of music vibration, acoustical energy is generating the vibration in which the amplitude, frequency, and spectral qualities of the vibration change continuously over time. Measurement nomenclature for such activity require additional indexes including ranges of frequency and amplitude, as well as measures of spectral components. Michel and Chesky (1990), and Chesky, Michel and Kondraske (1994) have listed parameters for applications of music vibration that are similar to the dimensions provided in the medical literature. So far as is known, the MVT™ is the only device that provides measurements and control of musical vibration (Chesky & Michel, 1991). By adhering to standards used in medical applications of vibration, the MVT™ meets the "scientific and therapeutic standards of state-of-the-art health care and science" mentioned by Spintge and Droh (1992, p. 347).

Summary

In this paper we have not tried to present a comprehensive coverage of the problem of research in the music for pain relief and music vibration area, but only to review and critique recent published studies. In most of them we found incomplete descriptions of the music used so that exact replications of the studies are not possible, putting into doubt their reliability. In addition, we have found a lack of theory or rationale in some of the studies for their use of music or music vibration (in pain relief and in other areas) as well as incomplete or totally lacking descriptions of important measurements of the music vibration stimuli. In so noting these deficiencies we conclude that there is a strong need for closer adherence to standards which require precise measures in future research in these areas.

By pointing out this need, we certainly do not imply or support a simplistic approach to research, that is, "just follow these suggestions for good research." By noting the deficiencies, we are suggesting that future researchers pay more attention to providing all important details for replication of their research—always an important aspect of developing reliability. We fully acknowledge the complexities of research in this area of pain relief, including the assessment and prediction of subjects' perceptions of music and/or with music with vibration. Indeed, we see them as further challenges for our own continued research (the many variables yet to be tested), including subject-choice of music, the use of different styles of music, different amplitudes and frequency of vibration, the assessment of subject imagery and its use during treatment, and the variability of needs of clients with the many types of pain experienced with different illnesses/diseases. Then there are also the many variables of coping styles for persons suffering pain, which need to be considered, for example, how they may be influenced by music and music vibration. In addition, there is the problem of pain assessment and the possible role of music in it. We consider these to be very exciting challenges in the immediate future and hope that our enthusiasm may be shared with others.

Finally, our critiquing of these studies is not intended to diminish/denigrate their value as pilot, and sometimes "landmark" studies in some areas. We have undertaken this review to extend the challenge for more rigorous research methods. However, one thing we became aware of in this review was that the fields of music therapy and music medicine do not yet provide a regular mechanism for critiquing research and providing feedback for researchers. This is provided in other fields through their journals; for example, a study of music and pain relief reported by Whipple and Glynn (1992) was critiqued by McCaffery (1992) in the same issue of the journal, *Scholarly inquiry for nursing practice: An international journal.* Perhaps it is time for us to provide such stimulation/feedback for our own research.

References

Bonny, H. L. (1983). Music listening for intensive coronary care units: A pilot project. *Music Therapy, 3*(1), 4–16.

Brown, C., Chen, A., & Dworkin, S. (1989). Music in the control of human pain. *Music Therapy, 8*(1), 47–60.

Chesky, K. S. (1992). The effects of music and music vibration using the MVT™ on the relief of rheumatoid arthritis pain. *Dissertation Abstracts International, 53*(8), 2725B. (University Microfilms No. AAC 9300593).

Chesky, K. S., & Michel, D. E. (1991). The Music Vibration Table (MVT™): Developing a technology and conceptual model for pain relief. *Music Therapy Perspectives, 9*, 32–38.

Chesky, K. S., Michel, D. E., & Kondraske, G. V. (1994). *Developing methods and techniques for scientific and medical applications of music vibration.* Paper presented at the meeting of the V International Music Medicine Symposium, San Antonio, Texas.

Clair, A. A., & Bernstein, B. (1993). The preference for vibrotactile versus auditory stimuli in severely regressed persons with dementia of the Alzheimer's type compared to those with dementia due to alcohol abuse. *Music Therapy Perspectives, 11*, 24–27.

Clark, M., McCorkle, R., & Williams, S. (1981). Music therapy-assisted labor and delivery. *Journal of Music Therapy, 18*, 88–109.

Codding, P. A. (1982). An exploration of the uses of music in the birthing process. *Unpublished Master's Thesis*, The Florida State University.

Curtis, S. L. (1982). The effects of music on the perceived degree of pain relief, physical comfort, relaxation, and contentment of hospitalized terminally Ill patients. *Unpublished Masters Thesis*, The Florida State University.

Darrow, A. A. (1992). The effect of vibrotactile stimuli via the Somatron™ on the identification of pitch change by hearing impaired children. *Journal of Music Therapy, 29*(2), 103–112.

Darrow, A. A., & Goll, H. (1989). The effect of vibrotactile stimuli via the Somatron™ on the identification of rhythmic concepts by hearing impaired children. *Journal of Music Therapy, 26*, 115–124.

Eagle, C., & Harsh, J. (1988). Elements of pain and music: The aio connection. *Music Therapy, 7*(1), 15–27.

Eakin, B. (1993). Patent # 5, 216, 769. U.S. Patent & Trademark Office. Washington, D.C.

Fowler-Kerry, S., & Lander. J. R. (1987). Management of injection in children. *Pain, 30*, 169–175.

Gardner, W. J., & Licklider, J. C. R. (1959). Auditory analgesia in dental operations. *The Journal of American Dental Association, 59*, 1144–1149.

Gfeller, K., Logan, H., & Walker, J. (1990). The effects of auditory distraction and suggestion on tolerance for dental restorations in adolescents and young adults. *Journal of Music Therapy, 27*(1), 13–17.

Hanser, S., Larson, S. C., & O'Connell, A. S. (1983). The effects of music on relaxation of expectant mothers during labor. *Journal of Music Therapy, 20*(2), 50–58.

Hecht, A. (1992). Hocus-pocus as Applied to Arthritis. *Department of Health and Human Services*, Public Health Service, FDA. Rockville, MD.

Jacobson, H. L. (1957). The effect of sedative music on the tensions, anxiety and pain experienced by mental patients during dental procedures. In E. T. Gaston (Ed.), *Music therapy 1956: Book of proceedings of the National Association for Music Therapy, Inc.* (pp. 231–234). Lawrence, KS: NAMT.

Lehikoinen, P. (1991, 1993). The Physioacoustic Method. *Marketing Materials*, Next Wave, Inc. Kalamazoo, Mi.

Locsin, R. G. (1981). The effect of music on the pain of selected post-operative patients. *Journal of Advanced Nursing, 6*, 19–25.

Madsen, C., Standley, J., & Gregory, D. (1991). The effect of a vibrotactile device, Somatron™, on physiological and psychological responses: musicians vs. non-musicians. *Journal of Music Therapy, 28*(1), 14–22.

McCaffery, M. (1992). Response to "Quantification of the effects of listening to music as a non-invasive method of pain control". *Scholarly Inquiry for Nursing Practice: An International Journal, 6*(1), 59–62.

Menegazzi, J., Paris, P., Kersteen, C., Flynn, B., & Trautman, D. (1991). A randomized, control trial of music during laceration repair. *Annals of Emergency Medicine, 20*, 348–350.

Michel, D. E., & Chesky, K. S. (1990, November). *Music vibration and pain: Creative collaboration in multi-dimensional measurement.* Paper presented at the annual meeting of the National Association of Music Therapy, Washington, D.C.

Michel, D. E., & Chesky, K. S. (1993). *A survey of music therapists using music for pain relief.* Poster session presented at the annual meeting of the National Association of Music Therapy, Toronto.

Michel, D. E., & Chesky, K. S. (in press). A survey of music therapists using music for pain relief. *Arts in Psychotherapy.*

Monsey, H. L. (1960). Preliminary report of the clinical efficacy of audioanalgesia. *Journal of California Dental Association, 36*, 432–437.

Newmark, J. (1991). Music as medical therapy: What use is it? *Classical Overtones.* Cedar Knoll, NJ.

Pyykko, I., & Hyvarinen, J. (1973). The physiological basis of the traumatic vasospastic disease: A sympathetic vasoconstrictor reflex triggered by high frequency vibration. *Work, Environment and Health, 10*, 36–47.

Rider, M. (1985). Entrainment mechanisms are involved in pain reduction, muscle relaxation, and music mediated imagery. *Journal of Music Therapy, 22*(4), 183–192.

Sherrick, C. E. (1984). Basic and applied research on tactile aids for deaf people: Progress and prospects. *Journal of the Acoustical Society of America, 75*(5), 1325–1342.

Skille, O. (1989). Vibroacoustic therapy. *Music Therapy, 8*, 61–77.

Skille, O. (1992). Vibroacoustic research 1980–1991. In R. Spintge & R. Droh (Eds.), *MusicMedicine* (pp. 249–256). St. Louis, MO: MMB Music.

Skoglund, C. R. (1989). Vasodilatation in human skin induced by low-amplitude high-frequency vibration. *Clinical Physiology, 9*, 361–372.

Skoglind, C. R. , & Knutsson, E. (1985). Vasomotor changes in human skin elicited by high frequency low amplitude vibration. *Acta Physiologica Scandinavia, 125*, 335–336.

Spingte, R. (1991). The neurophysiology of emotion and its therapeutic applications in music therapy and music medicine. In C. Maranto (Ed.), *Applications of music in medicine* (pp. 59–72). Washington, DC National Association of Music Therapy.

Spingte, R., & Droh, R. (1992). Toward a research standard in music medicine/music therapy: A proposal for a multimodal approach. In R. Spingte & R. Droh (Eds.), *MusicMedicine* (pp. 345–349). St. Louis, MO: MMB Music.

Standley, J. M. (1986). Music research in medical/dental treatment: Meta-analysis and clinical applications. *Journal of Music Therapy, 23*, 56–122.

Standley, J. M. (1991). The effect of vibrotactile and auditory stimuli on perception of comfort, heart rate, and peripheral skin temperature. *Journal of Music Therapy, 28*, 120–134.

Standley, J. M. (1992a). Meta-analysis of research in music and medical treatment: Effect size as a basis for comparison across multiple dependent and independent variables. In R. Spintge & R. Droh (Eds.), *MusicMedicine* (pp. 364–378). St. Louis, MO: MMB Music.

Standley, J. M. (1992b). Research note. Preschoolers' response to auditory and vibroacoustic stimuli. *Psychology of Music, 20*, 80–85.

Whipple, B., & Glynn, N. J. (1992). Quantification of the effects of listening to music as a noninvasive method of pain control. *Scholarly Inquiry for Nursing Practice: An International Journal, 6*(1), 43–58.

Zimmerman, L., Pozehl, B., Duncan, K., & Schmitz. (1989). Effects of music in patients who had chronic cancer pain. *Western Journal of Nursing Research, 11*, 298–309.

DEVELOPING METHODS AND TECHNIQUES FOR SCIENTIFIC AND MEDICAL APPLICATIONS OF MUSIC VIBRATION

Kris S. Chesky, Donald E. Michel, and George V. Kondraske

Introduction

The purpose of this paper is to introduce several of the essential elements for developing medical and scientific applications of music vibration. A conceptual model for using music and music vibration for pain relief is reviewed, and scientific methodologies and nomenclature for such applications are identified. While few studies by professionals in music therapy and music medicine have yet been concerned with the development of new scientific tools to better utilize the power of music for pain relief, there is now interest in learning more about such applications (Michel & Chesky, in press).

Conceptual Model for Music and Music Vibration for Pain Relief

The conceptual model depicted in Figure 1 illustrates the application of music listening together with music-generated vibrotactile stimulation. Introduced as a *Two Pronged* approach (Chesky & Michel, 1991), this model was derived from Michel's (1976; 1985) concept of music used in therapy as a *Two-Edged Sword,* one edge being the physiological effects of music as sound itself, the other edge, the psychosocial effects of music experienced by most people.

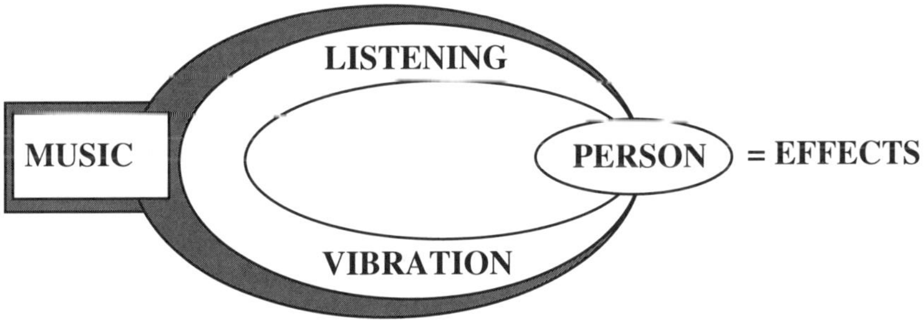

Figure 1. The *Two-Pronged* Approach. The *Two Pronged Approach* applies music listening and music vibration for pain relief and is conceptualized as engaging both psychological (music listening) and physiological (music vibration) processes to suppress pain. The two prongs represent (a) efferent neural suppressive effects and (b) afferent neural suppressive effects, as well as sensory integration for synergistic activity between the two. From Chesky and Michel (1991).

This model does not deny the physiological effects of music alone, nor the psychological effects of vibration. It is, however, a perspective that separates the two phenomena to better understand cause and effect relationships and to direct scientific methodologies for research and clinical application. By engaging psychological processes (music listening) together with physiological processes (transcutaneously applied music vibration), this approach activates pain suppressive efferent neural activity as well as pain suppressive afferent neural activity. In conjunction, the two prongs also integrate somatic and auditory neural activity that may provide for synergistic mechanisms in the central nervous system.

Prong 1 The Efferent System

Pain relief from efferent neural impulses is based on the fact that an enormous variety of psychological factors influences pain. Melzack (1973) stated:

> The evidence... shows that cognitive or higher central nervous system processes such as attention, anxiety, anticipation, and past experience exert a powerful influence on pain processes. It is also firmly established that stimulation of the brain activates descending efferent fibers that can influence afferent conduction at the earliest synaptic levels of the somaesthetic system. Thus it is possible for brain activities subserving attention, emotion and memories of prior experience, to exert control over the sensory input. (p. 160)

Anticipation, attention, suggestion, cognition and previous experiences are presumed to influence pain perception. Numerous psychological techniques, particularly cognitive coping strategies, have been developed to help pain patients help themselves (Chaves & Barber, 1974) and are effective when subcortical and direct cortical pain modulating systems in the central nervous system are activated (Turk, Meichenbaum, & Genest, 1983). A summary of this literature concludes that most strategies are designed to help the patient increase the internal locus of control by directing thoughts away from the pain. These methods fall into one of three broad categories: (a) imagery, (b) self-statements, and (c) attention-diversion techniques (Fernandez & Turk, 1989).

The use of music is often associated with pain relief. Although not typically a primary practice in professional music therapy, this application is receiving increased attention. Theoretical articles about music and music therapy for pain relief provide some basis for such utilization (Brown, Chen, & Dworkin, 1989; Chesky, & Michel, 1991; and Eagle, & Harsh, 1988) and a recent National Association of Music Therapy (NAMT) professional utilization survey (Michel & Chesky, 1994, in press) indicates that many music therapists are currently using (or are trying to justify the use of) music in pain management while treating patients with long term chronic pain. Research studies have reported positive outcomes from using music for pain relief. A critical review by Michel and Chesky (1993a), however, indicates that many studies about music for pain relief address acute pain but do not provide enough information for replication and are, therefore, suspect to issues of reliability.

Prong 2 The Afferent System

Following suggestions by Melzack and Wall (1965), many researchers have utilized methods involving large diameter afferent fiber stimulation for treating acute and chronic pain. Research has demonstrated that vibration is capable of raising experimental pain thresholds of cutaneous pain (Bini, Cruccu, Hagbarth, Schady, & Trebjork, 1984; Pertovaara, 1979; Sherer, Clelland, O'Sullivan, Doleys, & Canan, 1988), muscular pain (Billini, Duranti, Galletti, & Pantaleo, 1984; Duranti, Pantelo, & Billini, 1988; Pantaleo, Duranti, & Billini, 1986), and of tooth pain (Ekblom & Hansson, 1982; Ottoson, Ekblom, & Hansson, 1981). Experimental pain thresholds have also been raised using vibration with people experiencing various preexisting pain conditions (Lundeberg, Abrahamsson, Bondesson, & Haker, 1988). Specific transcutaneous vibration has also reduced pain in many chronic musculoskeletal and neurogenic conditions (Lundeberg, 1983; Lundeberg, 1984a; Lundeberg, 1984b; Lundeberg, Nordemar, & Ottoson, 1984). This research indicates that vibration is most effective when placed close to the area of pain, and that stimulation of 30–40 minutes is the most effective and efficient duration for long term relief (up to 8 hours). Stimulation of larger skin areas (up to 200cm^2) is more effective than smaller areas, but only vibration frequencies within the sensitivity range of the Pacinian Corpuscle are effective. (For a more extensive review of these studies, see Chesky, 1992.)

The Pacinian Corpuscle (PC) is a large mechanoreceptor located throughout subcutaneous tissue and in connective tissues around visceral organs and joints. PCs are very sensitive to vibrations in the frequency range from 60Hz up to 600Hz and transmit through large diameter afferent fibers (Quillian & Sato, 1955; Hubbard, 1958). The initiation, transmission and central processing of PC receptor information can cause pain suppressive effects. Pain is treated as a specific sensation with its own sensory channel (Perl, 1971; Willis, 1985; Besson, & Chaouch, 1987). Nociceptors (pain receptors), encapsulated nerve endings (Burgess & Perl, 1967), are found in the skin, joints and viscera and transmit to the dorsal horn of the spinal cord via small diameter afferent fibers. When pain signals enter the dorsal horn of the spinal cord, they transmit to nociceptive specific neurons, which then project information to higher levels (Figure 2).

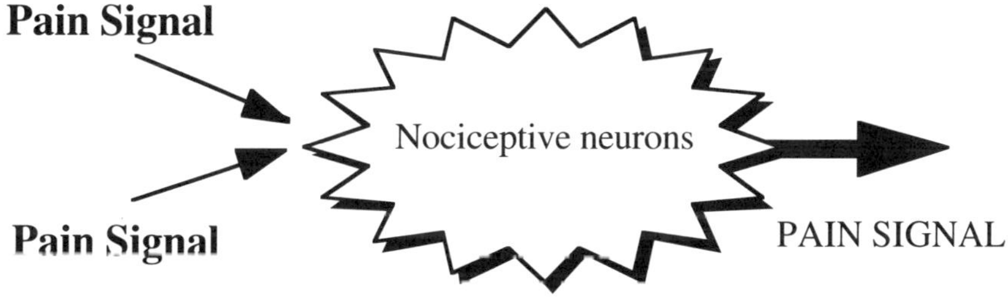

Figure 2. Nociceptive Neurons Activated by Pain Signals. Nociceptive signals enter the spinal cord and transmit to nociceptive neurons. The resulting output from the nociceptive neuron is projected to higher levels of the central nervous system.

PC receptor information entering the dorsal horn suppresses the firing rate of the nociceptive neurons (Fig. 3). This process is mediated by adenosine acting through PI-purinergic receptors (Salter & Henry, 1987). Adenosine has depressant effects upon excitatory synaptic transmission (Dunwiddle & Proctor, 1987) and is an important neuromodulator with effects on noxious sensory input (Goodman & Snyder, 1982). Adenosine-mediated inhibition of nociceptive neurons by vibration is the result of an inhibitory postsynaptic potential (IPSP) caused by a K+ conductance (De Koninck & Henry, 1988). ATP-sensitive K+ channels appear to mediate an inhibitory postsynaptic potential (IPSP) in dorsal horn neurons elicited by vibration stimulation (Salter, De Koninck, & Henry, 1992).

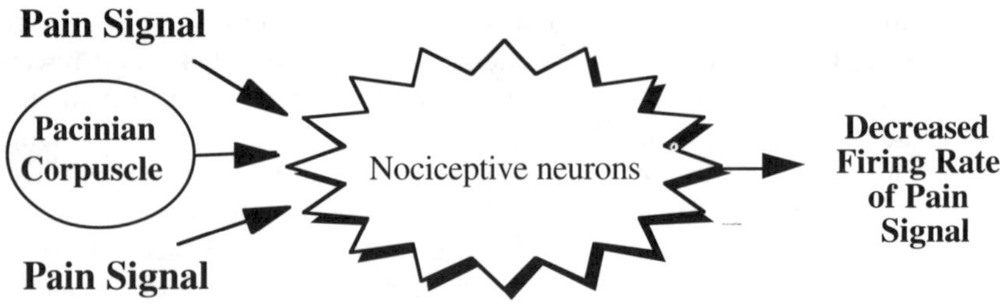

Figure 3. Input from Pacinian Corpuscles Decreases Nociceptive Activity. Vibration sensitive afferent activity, from Pacinian Corpuscles, decreases the firing rate of nociceptive neurons and suppresses pain.

Although the above-mentioned studies indicate that neuronal inhibition is involved in pain suppressive effects, they do not elucidate the causes for the long-term poststimulation pain relief latency period found in many studies. Some studies have suggested that met-enkephalins and beta-endorphins are not involved in these long-term poststimulation analgesic effects (Lundeberg, 1985; Guieu, Tardy-Gervet, Blin, & Giraud, 1992).

Music as vibration

Periods of vibration stimulation (at a single frequency and amplitude) quickly give rise to habituation and fatigue in vibrotactile sensitivity, transmission and central processing that may be attributable to changes in central vibration specific neurons or in synaptic processes associated with these central neurons. Percentage of decrease and rate of recovery have been shown to be functions of amplitude, frequency, and time of sustained excitation (O'Mara, Rowe, & Tarvin, 1988). Music provides the frequency bandwidth needed to excite PC receptors and can be transduced into mechanical vibration and applied to the body. Musically fluctuating vibration may increase the potential of vibration induced analgesia by lessening the degree of adaptation over time (Figure 4) and utilizes a range of frequencies within the sensitivity range of the PC to also offset adaptation and allow for greater vibration sensitive afferent activity (Figure 5).

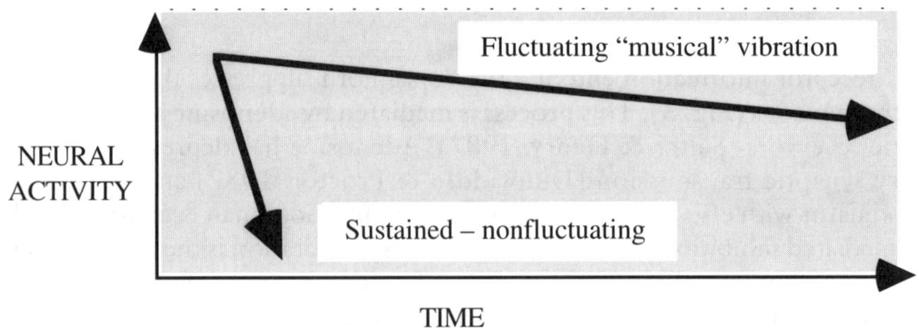

Figure 4. Music Vibration May Decrease Neural Response Decrements Associated with Single Frequency and Amplitude Vibration. Fluctuations (changes in frequency, amplitude and spatial distribution) may reduce habituation and fatigue and therefore increase vibration sensitive afferent activity over time.

In using music as the source for vibration, our model incorporates vibration stimulation of torso, arms and legs (the whole body excluding the head) so that PC receptors are activated over large surface areas of the body. Stimulation over multiple dermatomes creates inputs into multiple segments of the spinal cord.

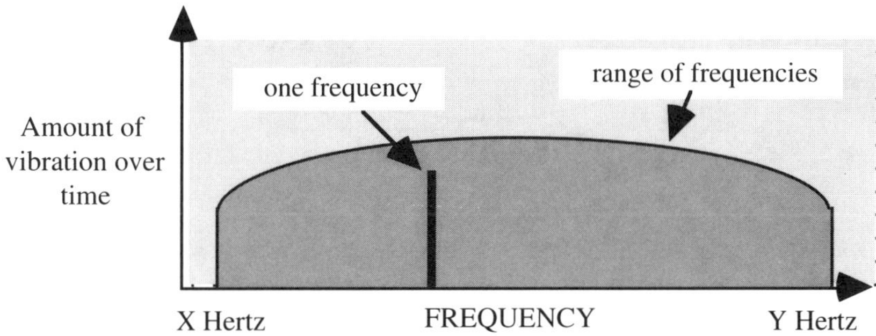

Figure 5. Comparison of One Frequency Stimulation to a Range of Frequencies Using Music. Music can provide for the production of vibration over a specified bandwidth utilizing a range of frequencies.

Nociceptive and PC fiber activity enter the spinal cord at levels representing particular dermatomes. Stimulation of large spatial areas recruits greater numbers of PC receptors and accommodates for many conditions where the pain is not necessarily localized in one area or dermatome of the body (e.g., Fibromyalgia).

Implementation of Music Vibration For Pain Relief

Many factors influence the ultimate effects of music and music vibration on the human system and must be considered regardless of whether the approach is for pain relief or some other benefit sought. As previously mentioned, music listening (top prong), alone or through a composed *therapy* process, has the pleonastic potential to prompt and maintain psychological activity while music vibration (bottom prong) must incorporate a means (technology) to transduce acoustical energy into mechanical vibration (Figure 6). Similar to electricity, inasmuch as it can cause a wide range of effects, the levels of vibration applied demands attention as an important factor in considering the effects of music vibration.

In the music therapy literature, some reports have described effects associated with applying music vibration (Clair, & Bernstein, 1993; Darrow, 1992; Darrow, & Goll, 1989; Madsen, Standley, & Gregory, 1991; Skille, 1989, 1992; Standley, 1991, 1992). A recent review of this literature (Michel, & Chesky, 1993a) points out that the vibration parameters used in these studies were not reported, which leaves the outcomes vulnerable in terms of understanding the effects. Nevertheless, many resources are available to help, describe, predict and understand outcomes associated with particular levels of vibrations. For example, most developed countries publish and continually update standards for nomenclature, evaluation, measurement, and risk determination associated with human vibration (Table 1). Analogous to standardizations and regulations of other sources of risk from exposure (e.g., chemicals, electricity, drugs), these conventions enable a reliable and valid means for describing vibrations.

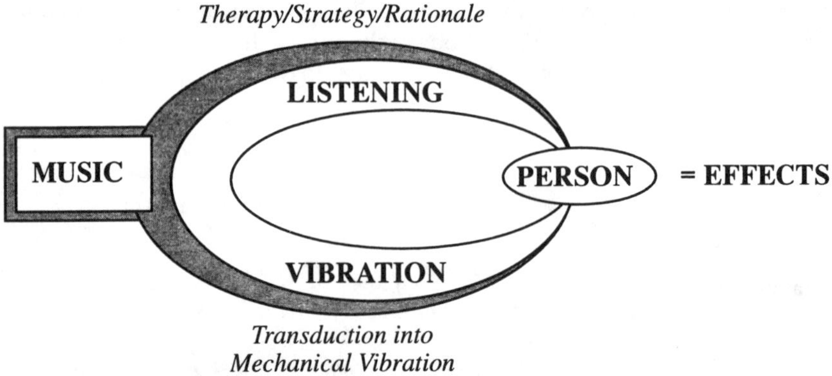

Figure 6. The *Two Pronged* Approach. The top prong incorporates a therapy, strategy, or rationale mediated by music, while the bottom prong utilizes a method of transducing acoustical energy to mechanical vibration.

The reports in Table 1 are primarily concerned with the potential ill-effects associated with vibration exposure. Other sources, as mentioned in the previous section, focus on basic neuroanatomical effects as well as the potential benefits including pain relief. One important aspect of all this literature is that, in all cases, the vibration is quantitatively described, which provides a basis for communication among professionals interested in medical and scientific applications of music vibration. This information is an important resource to direct development and justify applications of music vibration. For medical and scientific applications of music vibration to be acknowledged by the medical and scientific community, research and clinical practices must incorporate the factor of measure and a report must be given of the vibrations used. Accordingly, our research and development efforts follow the requirements (a) to conform to scientific international standards for quantitative measurement of vibration, (b) to use vibration parameters known to cause medically beneficial effects, (c) and have valid and reliable means to alter the vibration parameters for research.

Table 1. *Examples of National and International "Standards" for Human Vibration*

U.S.A. ANSI S3.18 (1979) "Guide for the evaluation of human exposure to whole body vibration"
Norway NS-ISO 2631/1 (1985) "Evaluation of human exposure to whole body vibration. General requirements"
France NF E 90–401 (1980) "Mechanical vibration. Guide for the evaluation of human exposure to whole body vibration"
International ISO 5805 (1981) "Mechanical vibration and shock affecting man – Vocabulary" ISO DP 9996 (1988) "Mechanical vibration and shock–Human exposure–Disturbance of human activity and performance–Taxonomy"

Vibration Parameters Reported in Medical Literature

Numerous vibration studies, representing many disciplines including physiology, algology and human factors engineering, describe vibration using a set of standard scientific nomenclature and include measures of vibration frequency and amplitude (Table 2). Changes in any of these vibration parameters has the potential to influence psychological, neurological, pharmacological, psychophysiological and autonomic effects (Dupuis & Zerlett, 1986; Ryan, 1981). Vibration parameter selection also influences specific pain relieving effects associated with transcutaneously applied vibration (Bini, et al., 1984; Lundeberg, et al., 1984; Lundeberg, et al., 1988; Panteleo, et al., 1986).

Music Vibration Parameters and Research

A set of parameters suggested for use in applications of music vibration (Table 3) was first presented at the 1990 National Association of Music Therapy conference (Chesky & Michel, 1990). These parameters represent parameters cognate to those used in medical and scientific applications.

Although it is possible to identify the parameters that should be measured and reported in medical and scientific applications of music vibration, it is difficult and technically challenging to obtain such measures because the stimulus is continuously changing. This is further complicated by interactive factors between the subject's weight/displacement and the vibrating medium. The coupling of a subject with a vibrating medium (all subjects being different) may change the required energy for vibration production of equal magnitude between subjects.

Table 2. *Scientific Nomenclature for Describing Vibration*

AMPLITUDE – Physical Displacement of Vibration – In Micrometers (μm)
FREQUENCY – Number of Cycles per Second of Periodic Motion – In Hertz (Hz)
WAVEFORM – Shape of Periodic Motion – Typically Sine Wave
DURATION – Time of Exposure to Vibration
SURFACE AREA – Body Location and Contact Area

Note: Vibration applied for pain relief is mono-directional, oscillating in one plane (x-axis) perpendicular to the surface of the skin.

Table 3. *Music Vibration Parameters Derived from Scientific Standards*

AMPLITUDE – Ranges and Averages – Physical Displacement
FREQUENCY – Ranges and Spectral Analysis
WAVEFORM – Shape of Periodic Motion
DURATION – Time of Exposure
SURFACE AREA – Body Location and Contact Area
SPATIAL DISTRIBUTION – Distribution of Vibration Energy over Surface Area

The only known study attempting to deal with these issues is the research completed by Chesky (1992) which was conducted within the Internal Medicine Department of the medical branch of The University of North Texas. A homogeneous pain population of persons with Rheumatoid Arthritis (*n* = 27) was exposed to music and music vibration, music alone (Table 4), or placebo. The same music was used for both music listening and music vibration production. This study utilized an early lab version of the Music Vibration Table™ (MVT™), which was designed and built by Chesky for this research.

Table 4. *Music Used for Both Listening and Vibration*

TITLE	COMPOSER(S)	COMPACT DISC	TIME
She Could be Mine	Don Grusin	Out of the Shadows	5:15
The Heart is a Lonely Hunter	Dave Grusin & Peggy Lee	One of a Kind	5:33
Dolphin Dreams	Lee Ritenour	On the Line	5:08
Birk's Works	John Gillespie	New Faces	6:26
Very Nice Indeed	Dave Valentine	Jungle Garden	3:50
Fountain of You	Chieli Minucci	Modern Matters	3:52

Music used for Group One (music with music vibration) & Group Two (music alone). The total elapsed time was 31 minutes. (from Chesky, 1992)

Scores from Visual Analogue Scales (VAS) and McGill Pain Questionnaires (MPQ) determined group differences in present pain intensity, amount of pain relief, and changes over the various dimensions of the pain experience as measured by the MPQ. Analysis of Variance (ANOVA) and post hoc analysis indicated that VAS scores from the music with music vibration condition were significantly greater than the music alone condition or placebo. MPQ scores also indicated larger percentages of change in pain perception for the music with music vibration condition (Table 5).

Table 5. *Amount of Pain Reduction as measured by the McGill Pain Questionnaire (MPQ)*

MPQ CATEGORIES	GROUP ONE MUSIC & VIBRATION	GROUP TWO MUSIC ALONE	GROUP THREE PLACEBO
Sensory	57%	26%	0%
Affective	73%	63%	-21%
Evaluative	55%	19%	0%
Miscellaneous	71%	-14%	12
Total	64%	24%	-2%

Subjects receiving music and vibration showed greater reductions in pain as compared to other groups. Negative percent means an increase in pain. (From Chesky, 1992)

Continuous vibration measurements were taken while persons were being stimulated. Reported measurements represented the whole vibrating surface during the entire treatment session.

Following positive outcomes from this research and a better understanding of the complexities inherent in vibration production, control and measurement, recent focus has included an intensive research and development phase in the MVT™ technology. The purpose of this effort was to research and develop the vibration production, selection, control and measurement capabilities of the MVT™ and to re-engineer the technology for future applications in a wide variety of clinical and research settings. These developments enable sophisticated experimental and clinical protocols to be conducted in most medical settings that will help researchers understand the effects of various parameters used in applications of music vibration.

MVT™ Design and Characterization Issues

In the previous section, Table 3 lists a set of parameters that are important to use to characterize any system used to deliver vibration stimuli derived from music in both research and clinical settings. While these parameters all have well-accepted meanings, the attachment of values to each is not always straightforward in practice. Any stimulus generation will consist of: (a) a source (music tape, CD, tone generator), (b) an amplifier, (c) an electrical to mechanical energy transducer (e.g., a speaker), (d) a membrane, and (e) a supporting structure and housing. In addition, it is likely that some form of padding will be used between the membrane and the subject to increase comfort during treatment. In this section, we discuss some of the key issues that must be considered in design that affect both the stimulus delivered and quantitative characterization of it.

Source and Transducers

To measure the stimulus amplitude in terms of the signal input characteristics (e.g., voltage) is inadequate. As noted, this parameter has units of displacement (e.g., micrometers) and thus some form of calibration is required that allows conversion. Due to the very small amplitudes involved, sensors with high frequency response that transduce displacement directly are difficult to obtain and use. Accelerometers can be employed, but it must be noted that the output of an accelerometer will increase if the amplitude of displacement is kept constant and only frequency is changed. This frequency dependence, however, is predictable and can be accounted for to achieve accurate measurements at different frequencies.

Membrane and Housing

Misleading numerical data can be obtained with regard to stimulus characterization or an undesirable stimulus can be delivered if the dynamic characteristics of the membrane and housing are not given careful consideration. Factors such as membrane geometry and dimensions, material properties (e.g., stiffness), and method used to mount the membrane to the housing combine in a relatively complex way to determine the resonant characteristics and vibrational modes. In this sense, the design of the MVT™ is much like that of a fine violin.

The influence of geometric and mechanical properties is illustrated in Figures 7 and 8. Both Figures contain similar plots made from recorded data obtained with an accelerometer placed at points on a grid mapped onto the surface of the membrane. The experimental MVT™ membrane used in Figure 7 was 18″ x 36″ x .063″ – #304 stainless steel anchored directly to a rigid frame with 16 fasteners.

As illustrated by the topographical pattern of nulls and peaks, misleading information would be communicated if a researcher selected only one location randomly on the membrane to calibrate the system for reporting stimulus amplitude. Note also, that a comparison of left and right plots shows that such effects are functions of frequency. This must be

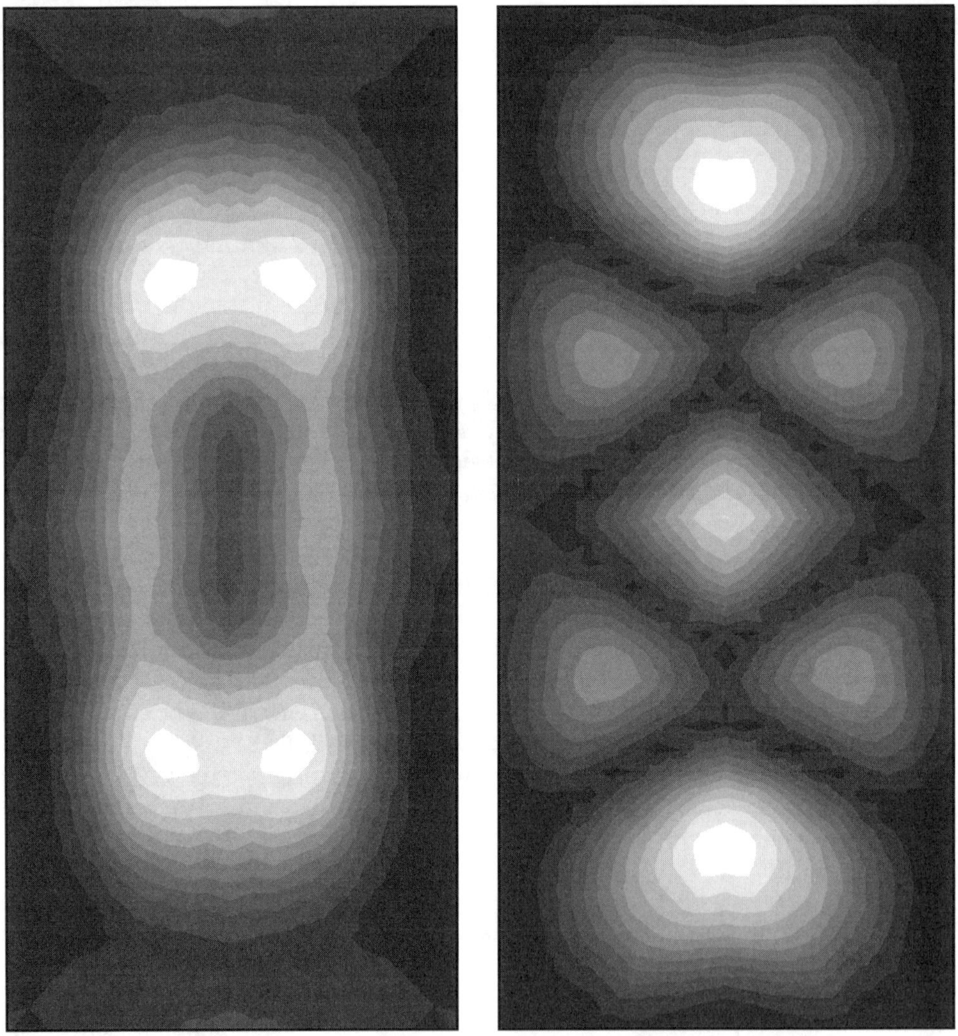

Figure 7. Vibrational Characteristics of MVT™ Test Membrane (St.-t1) at Two Frequencies. The two MVT™ test membranes (left = 125Hz; right = 175Hz) illustrate dramatically different spatial patterns. The membrane geometry, input voltages and the materials (stainless steal) are the same. The grey scale represents changes in amplitude (light = high amplitude, dark = low amplitude).

considered a significant complicating factor with both sinusoidal stimuli and stimuli derived from music sources.

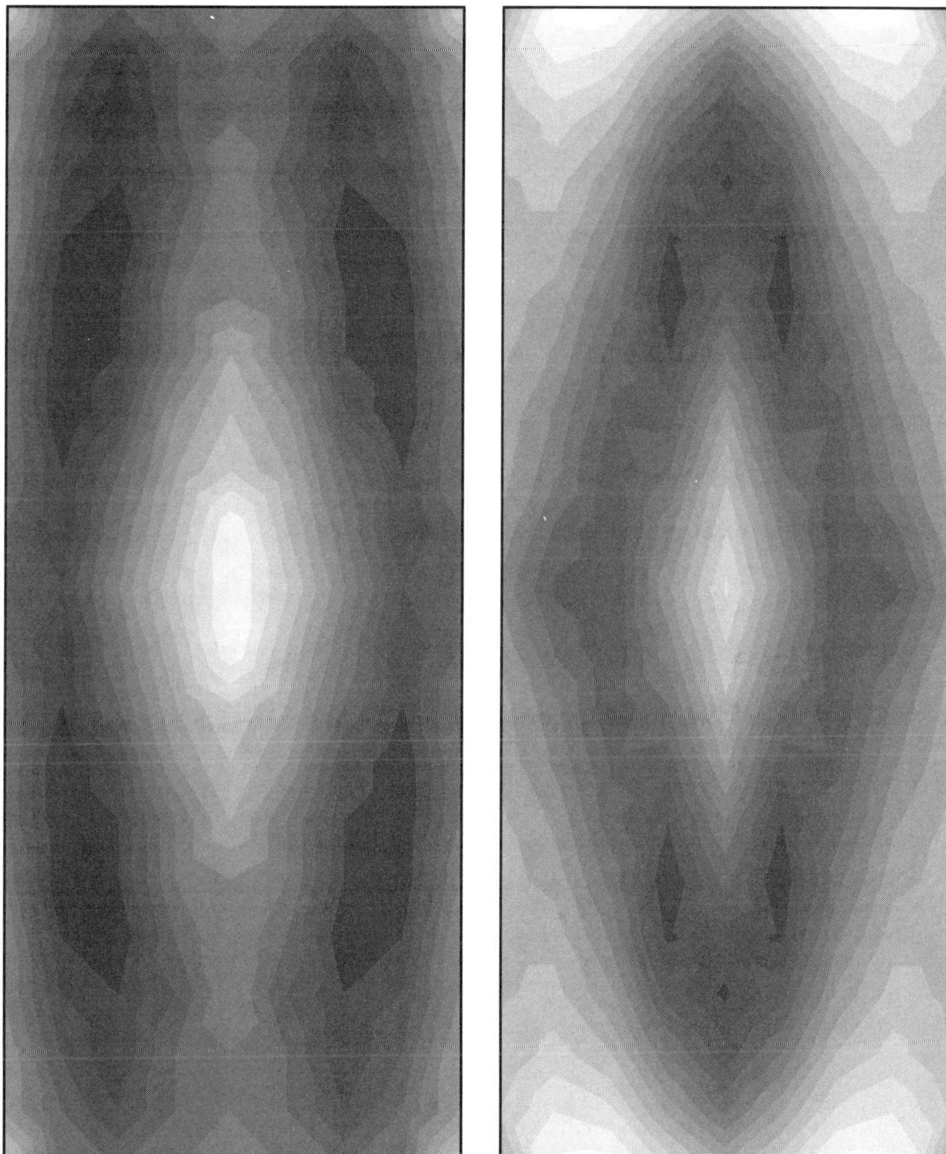

Figure 8. Vibrational Characteristics of MVT™ Test Membrane (A1-t2) at Two Frequencies. Two MVT™ test membranes (left = 125Hz; right = 175Hz) illustrate more even spatial patterns. The membrane geometry, input voltages and the materials (Aluminum Composite) are the same. The grey scale represents changes in amplitude (light = high amplitude, dark = low amplitude).

In attempts to improve the ability to characterize the stimulus delivered in accurate and simple terms, as well as to improve the spatial consistency, other experimental MVT™ membranes were fabricated and tested. One test membrane consisted of an aluminum panel (.09″ – 6061T6) attached to a special lightweight aluminum aircraft material (Figure 8). This material is constructed like cardboard (i.e., corrugated) and has a very high stiffness-to-mass ratio. The composite membrane was attached to the same frame and housing used in the previous tests with a rubber isolator (.25″ thick, 80 durometer rating) around the perimeter of the membrane. Experimental characterization of this membrane is illustrated in Figure 8 with noticeable improvement in the spatial consistency. The use of a single number to characterize amplitude is more acceptable in a system with a membrane that responds more consistently at different locations and at different frequencies across the range of interest.

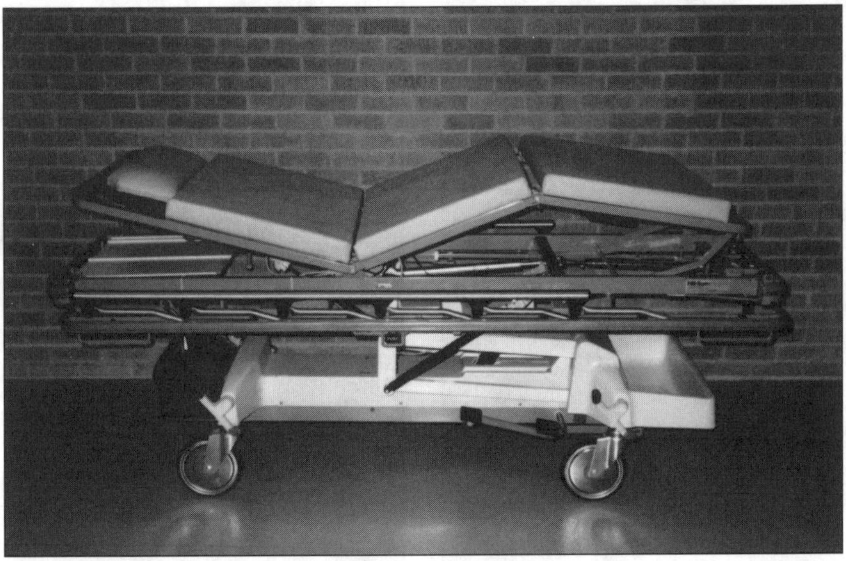

Figure 9. MVT™ Technology. Note: The current MVT™ consists of three independently controlled submodules and a single main control unit. The system is designed to implement a closed-loop adaptive control scheme that compensates for both variability in the frequency content of music sources and load variations on each submodule independently to produce a desired vibratory stimulation profile over the course of a treatment session. The internal microprocessor facilitates research, development, and testing of novel control algorithms to determine those that are most effective in achieving the desired clinical effects. The system has the ability to measure stimulus characteristics over time during a session.

In a system used clinically such as the MVT™ (Figure 9), it can be anticipated that foam padding and a cover would be incorporated for both aesthetics and comfort. These components affect the transmission of vibrations from the membrane to the subject receiving treatment. In research, if the inclusion of these components is set aside in experimental setups for convenience to the researcher, results reported in the literature may have limited use as a basis for determining desired stimulus characteristics. While it may be possible to develop engineering models that would allow one to estimate *post hoc* the equivalent stimulus that would be delivered from a given stimulus generator if a particular foam and cover were employed, experiments should be conducted with stimulus generation systems that contain all components envisioned to be required in a complete clinical version. Experiments such as those described above for the membrane alone, are recommended to characterize the composite "membrane + foam + cover" system that ultimately interfaces to the subject.

Summary and Discussion

The "Two Pronged" conceptualization of music and music vibration for pain relief implies some directions for those who would apply it clinically. Such clinicians may or may not be music therapists, even though music therapists should be well prepared by training to make such applications. A recent survey of music therapists already using music for pain relief indicates that many are interested and ready to learn new techniques (Michel & Chesky, 1993b; in press).

Whether or not future practitioners are music therapists or other health professionals, we think they would be well advised to be aware of the research cited in this paper. For example, the neuropharmacology of vibration, especially adenosine and the modifying effects of such stimulants as caffeine and other methylxanthines on the effectiveness of music vibration are worthy of notice by practitioners.

Another area of particular research interest is in determining exactly the type of vibration to be applied. For example, some current music vibration systems advertise the use of low frequency vibrations (below 60Hz) which is, in some studies, associated with possible ill effects. It also should be noted that there is conflicting usage of the term "vibration". Disciplines related to physiology and neurology describe stimuli greater than 60Hz as "vibration" and designate the term "flutter" for stimuli below 60Hz, which is based on the classification scheme of mechanoreceptors, which in turn is based on the most likely property of the stimulus for which they encode information. On the other hand, other reports utilize the term vibration to mean all oscillating mediums regardless of the frequency content. This is common practice in human factors engineering and ergonomics that are typically interested in industrial and work related environments.

What would seem to be important is the fact that before the MVT™ technology—or any new technology—is used is that it should be based on research to fit the specific needs of individual patients. This implies adequate assessment of the pain problems of such patients as well as careful application of remedial measures such as music and music vibration with the MVT™.

While methods and techniques for scientific applications of music vibration such as those provided by the MVT™ are still in a developing stage, the MVT™ is ready for applications in clinics where caregivers as well as "consumers" may find it beneficial—as well as challenging from a research standpoint. We certainly do not intend to infer that the MVT™ is a new magical "cure-all" device or treatment program; however, we are confident about future developments of all possible uses of music and music vibration in reducing pain and improving human health.

References

Besson, J. M. & Chaouch, A. (1987). Peripheral and spinal mechanisms of nociception. *Physiology Reviews, 76*, 67–186.

Billini, F., Duranti, R., Galletti, R., & Pantaleo, T. (1984). Variations in muscular pain thresholds and eyeblink response induced by vibratory stimulation. In B. Bromm (Ed.), *Pain Measurement in Man. Neurophysiological Correlates of Pain* (pp. 135–141). Amsterdam: Elsevier.

Bini, G., Cruccu, G., Hagbarth, K. E., Schady, W., & Trebjork, E. (1984). Analgesic effect of vibration and cooling on pain induced by intraneural electrical stimulation. *Pain, 18*, 239–248.

Brown, C., Chen, A., & Dworkin, S. (1989). Music in the control of human pain. *Music Therapy, 8*(1), 47–60.

Chaves, J. F., & Barber, T. X. (1974). Cognitive strategies, experimenter modeling, and expectation in the attenuation of pain. *Journal of Abnormal Psychiatry, 83*, 356–363.

Chesky, K. S. (1992). The effects of music and music vibration using the MVT™ on the relief of rheumatoid arthritis pain. *Dissertation Abstracts International, 53* (8), 2725B. (University Microfilms No. AAC 9300593).

Chesky, K. S., & Michel, D. E. (1991). The Music Vibration Table (MVT™) Developing a technology and conceptual model for pain relief. *Music Therapy Perspectives, 9*, 32–38.

DeKoninck, Y., & Henry, J. L. (1988). In vivo intracellular investigation of the vibration-induced depression of nociceptive dorsal horn neurons in the cat spinal cord. *Society of Neuroscience Abstracts, 14*, 697.

Dunwiddie, T. V. (1985). The physiologic role of adenosine on the central nervous system. *International Review of Neurobiology, 27*, 63–139.

Dunwiddie, T. V., & Proctor, W. R. (1987). Mechanisms underlying physiologic responses to adenosine in the central nervous system. In E. Gerlach and B. F. Becker (Eds.), *Topics and perspectives in adenosine research: Proceedings of the 3rd international symposium on adenosine* (pp. 499–508). New York: Springer.

Dupuis, H., & Zerlett, G. (1986). *The effects of whole body vibration*. Berlin: Springer-Verlag.

Duranti, R., Pantelo, T., & Bellini, F. (1988). Increase in muscular pain threshold following low frequency-high intensity peripheral conditioning stimulation in humans. *Brain Research, 452*, 66–72.

Eagle, C., & Harsh, J. (1988). Elements of pain and music: The aio connection. *Music Therapy, 7*(1), 15–27.

Ekblom, A., & Hansson, P. (1982). Effects of conditioning vibratory stimulation on pain threshold of the human tooth. *Acta Physiologica Scandinavia., 114*, 601–604.

Fernandez, E., & Turk, D. (1989). The utility of coping strategies for altering pain perception: A meta analysis. *Pain, 38*, 123–132.

Goodman, R. R., & Snyder. S. H. (1982). Autoradiographic localization of adenosine receptors in rat brain using [^{3}H] cyclohexyladenosine. *Journal of Neuroscience, 2*, 1230–1241.

Guieu, R., Tardy-Gervet, M. F., Blin, O., & Pouget, R. (1990). Pain relief by transcutaneous electrical nerve stimulation and/or vibratory stimulation in a case of painful legs and moving toes. *Pain, 42*, 43–48.

Hubbard, S. J. (1958). A study of rapid mechanical events in a mechanoreceptor. *Journal of Physiology, 141*, 198–218.

Lundeberg, T. (1983). Vibratory stimulation for the alleviation of chronic pain. *Acta Physiologic Scandinavia., Supplement , 523*, 1–51.

Lundeberg, T. (1984a). Long-term results of vibratory stimulation as a relieving measure for chronic pain. *Pain, 20*, 13–23.

Lundeberg, T. (1984b). The pain suppressive effect of vibratory stimulation and transcutaneous electrical nerve stimulation (TENS) as compared to aspirin. *Brain Research, 294*, 201–209.

Lundeberg, T. (1985). Naxolone does not reverse the pain-reducing effects of vibratory stimulation, *Acta Anesthesiologica Scandinavia, 29,* 212–216.

Lundeberg, T., Abrahamsson, P., Bondesson, L, & Haker, E. (1988). Effect of vibratory stimulation on experimental and clinical pain. *Scandinavian Journal of Rehabilitative Medicine, 20,* 149–159.

Lundeberg, T., Nordemar, R., & Ottoson, D. (1984). Pain alleviation by vibratory stimulation. *Pain, 20,* 25–44.

Melzack, R. (1973). *The puzzle of pain.* New York: Basic Books.

Melzack, R., & Wall, P. D. (1965). Pain mechanisms; A new theory. *Science, 150,* 971–979.

Michel, D. E. (1976, 1985). *Music therapy.* Springfield, IL: Charles C. Thomas.

Michel, D. E., & Chesky, K. S. (1990, November). *Music vibration and pain: Creative collaboration in multi-dimensional measurement.* Paper presented at the annual meeting of the National Association of Music Therapy, Washington, D.C.

Michel, D. E., & Chesky, K. S. (1993). *Music therapy in medical settings: The challenge for more rigorous research—especially in music and music vibration for pain relief.* Paper presentation at VII World Congress of Music Therapy, Vitoria, Spain.

Michel, D. E., & Chesky, K. S. (1993). *A survey of music therapists using music for pain relief.* Poster session presented at the annual meeting of the National Association of Music Therapy, Toronto.

Michel, D. E., & Chesky, K. S. (in press). A survey of music therapists using music for pain relief. *Arts in Psychotherapy.*

O'Mara, S., Rowe, M., & Tarvin, R. P. (1988). Neural mechanisms in vibrotactile adaptation. *Journal of Neurophysiology, 59,* 607–622.

Ottoson, D., Ekblom, A., & Hansson, P. (1981). Vibratory stimulation for the relief of pain of dental origin. *Pain, 10,* 37–45.

Pantaleo, T., Duranti, R., & Billini, F. (1986). Effects of vibratory stimulation on muscular pain threshold and blink response in human subjects. *Pain, 24,* 2–8.

Perl, E. R., (1971). Is pain a specific sensation? *Journal of Psychiatric Research, 8,* 273–287.

Pertovaara, A. (1979). Modification of human pain threshold by specific tactile receptors. *Acta Physiological Scandinavia, 107,* 339–341.

Quilliam, T. A., & Sato, M. (1955). The distribution of myelin on nerve fibres from Pacinian Corpuscles. *Journal of Physiology, 129,* 167–176.

Ryan, T. J. (1981). Vibration: Good or bad? *Clinical and Experimental Dermatology, 6,* 179–189.

Salter, M. W., & Henry, J. L. (1987). Evidence that adenosine mediates the depression of spinal dorsal horn neurons induced by peripheral vibration in the cat. *Neuroscience, 22*(2) 631–50.

Salter, M. W., De Koninck, Y., & Henry, J. L. (1992). ATP-sensitivity K+ channels mediate an IPSP in dorsal horn neurons elicited by sensory stimulation. *Synapse, 11*(3) 214–20.

Turk, D. C., Meichenbaum, D., & Genest, M. (1983). *Pain and Behavioral Medicine.* New York: Guilford.

Willis, W. D. (1985). *The pain system.* Basel: Krager.

III.

PERFORMING ARTS MEDICINE

PERFORMERS WITH MULTIPLE SEQUENTIAL DIFFICULTIES IN AN ARTS MEDICINE PRACTICE

William J. Dawson, M.D.

Abstract

A study was undertaken to determine why some musicians became "repeaters", with multiple hand and upper extremity difficulties, and to devise strategies to decrease these repetitive patterns. Records of instrumentalists seen in the past 10 years were reviewed, and multiple demographic and etiologic factors were evaluated. A repeater was defined as one who presented with more than one hand or upper extremity problem during this period. Repeating patients comprised 11.7% (78/667) of all arts-medicine patients and produced 24.9% (195/784) of all first visits for new problems. They averaged 2.5 new problems per patient, with a maximum of seven. Forty-two of the 78 had more than one problem type. Two-thirds (52/78) presented with more than one problem of the same type, 80% of these in the categories of overuse and trauma. One-half (38/78) presented with the same diagnosis but in a different location; overuse conditions were the cause in 22 of these 38. Music-related difficulties were seen in 25 patients, while sports participation was the cause of injury in 22. Ongoing or chronic physical difficulties, such as hypermobility, diabetes, arthritis, or other connective tissue deficiencies, were seen in only 25 patients and accounted for 66 new problems. Repeaters most often were performing professionals or active, dedicated amateurs. Most problems were produced by musculoskeletal overuse or sports-related trauma. Music-related overuse may be minimized by correct practice and performance techniques. General physical and sports conditioning may be useful for those instrumentalists having chronic connective tissue conditions, or to preserve and maintain strength, endurance, and sports-related musculoskeletal skills for all musicians.

Introduction

Performing arts medicine has become a recognized specialty only for the past 12 years, although many medical professionals throughout the world have been providing skilled care for musicians and dancers for decades. The author's personal experience in this field encompasses more than a quarter century, but practice standardization and recording of arts-medicine data have been accomplished only within the last 10 years. During this time, however, it became obvious that a large number of instrumentalists presented for treatment on more than one occasion with a new problem relating to their hands or upper extremities. The frequency of this phenomenon seemed excessive when it was compared casually to that of nonmusicians in the same practice, and yet its true cause and significance were not known.

Literature Review

A review of the pertinent English language literature of performing arts medicine was undertaken and proved to be of little assistance. Few publications addressed the concept of multiple sequential problems in musicians, and the patient populations described were not comparable to those of the author's practice. Three large orchestral surveys were reported, in which instrumentalists provided information about their own problems to the investigators. Multiple musculoskeletal complaints or problems were described by "many" musicians in a study from the Eastman School of Music by Larsson, Baum, Mudholkar, and Kollia (1993), by "a majority" of those interviewed by Caldron, Calabrese, Clough, Lederman, Williams, and Leatherman (1986), and by 62% of the orchestral musicians surveyed in the International Conference of Symphony and Opera Musicians study reported by Fishbein and Middlestadt (1988). None of these studies indicated whether the multiple problems described by each instrumentalist existed simultaneously or occurred serially, and no study dealt with precise medical diagnosis or treatment issues in these populations. The only investigators to publish data on true "repeaters" were Manchester and Flieder (1991), whose students at the Eastman School of Music were followed for a 3-year period. They found only eight students who required evaluation and treatment for sequential hand and upper extremity difficulties, out of 114 referred for care during that same time interval. The very nature of that medical practice limits the duration of time an individual will be seen for such conditions—only while remaining a student at that institution.

Why do some instrumentalists become repeaters? Several intuitive and commonsense possibilities include:

1. Presence of an underlying constitutional condition, such as benign hypermobility syndrome or arthritis.
2. Repetition of an overuse situation, musical or otherwise.
3. Repeated injury from sports participation.
4. Incomplete healing and/or rehabilitation from a prior problem.
5. Inadequate activity or behavior modifications subsequent to treatment for a specific problem.

However, confirmation or denial of these theories required precise data for support; therefore, the present study was undertaken. Three goals were set:

1. To evaluate more critically the author's own experiences and data,
2. To find reasons for, and patterns of, repeated problems in some musicians, and
3. To formulate strategies to decrease these repetitive patterns.

Method

Office medical records were reviewed for all known instrumentalist patients seen at Evanbrook Orthopaedics from the early 1980s through December 1993. These patients were seen as a usual part of the author's university-affiliated hand and orthopaedic practice and were evaluated personally by the author or by one of his five orthopaedic colleagues. Clinical information and demographic details were entered at the time of each visit.

Musicians were classified in three separate ways:

1. By their degree of musical involvement (Table 1).
2. By the class of instrument played, both primarily and secondarily (strings, keyboards, woodwinds, brasses, percussion, and miscellaneous).
3. By the type of upper extremity problem (overuse, trauma or injury, arthritis, and other conditions such as nerve compressions, masses, and developmental difficulties).

Data evaluation was performed later, with multiple demographic and etiologic factors taken into consideration; various subgroups were defined and intergroup comparisons were made. A repeater was defined as a musician who presented on more than one occasion with more than one problem involving the hand or upper extremity. This repeat visit (or visits) would be for a new or different problem/condition/injury, or for the same problem following an absence without treatment of at least 1 year, or for the same problem in a different anatomic location within an upper extremity.

Table 1. *Musician Classes*

A	Professional, performance emphasis
B	Professional, teaching emphasis
C	Conservatory or collegiate music majors
D	Skilled, active amateurs—playing regularly in organized groups
E	School musicians, grades 4–12
F	Amateur, recreational musicians—playing for themselves or family

Results

In the period under study, 784 visits were made by 667 different patients for hand and upper extremity difficulties. Seventy-eight of these patients were considered to be repeaters, and presented with 195 initial or new problems, a mean of 2.5 new problem visits per patient. The maximum number of new problems evaluated for any one patient was seven. This population of repeaters comprised 11.7% of all instrumentalist patients and accounted for 24.9% of all first visits for new problems.

Two-thirds of the repeating group (52 of 78) presented with the same problem type on more than one occasion. Eighty percent of these 52 patients were diagnosed with overuse or traumatic conditions. Eleven of the 21 patients with multiple overuse conditions described an overuse etiology for all their problems, while 15 of 20 trauma patients reported injury as the only cause of their problems. All three arthritis patients developed arthritic problems exclusively, while seven of eight musicians with other difficulties experienced their same problem type again. Simple subtraction reveals that 42 of the 78 patients presented with varied types of problems.

Same Problem

Several different patterns of problem presentation were noted. Six instrumentalists experienced exactly the same problem on a second occasion or had not achieved complete healing of their first one. One each of these performers was diagnosed with focal dystonia of the left hand, ganglion of the wrist, rheumatoid arthritis, yearly strains of hand and forearm muscles from annual music competitions, triggering digits or stenosing tenosynovitis, and fracture of the clavicle (even after the first one had healed well).

About half (38 of 78) of the repeaters later experienced the same type of problem in a different anatomic location. This group included seven musicians who were diagnosed with muscle strains, seven with trigger digits, eight with true tenosynovitis or tendinitis, nine with fractures, and four with ligament sprains. Three others noted more than one miscellaneous problem.

Problems From Music

Difficulties caused by music performance were seen in one-third of the repeater group (25 of 78 patients). All these instrumentalists were members of classes A–D, the so-called high-level musicians (regarding their skill and/or their intensity of musical activity); 15 of the 25 were performing or teaching professionals. These 25 patients presented with 39 separate diagnoses, most of which were related to musical overuse. Eleven of the 25 presented on more than one occasion with a music-related difficulty; three performers each experienced three new and separate problems. As has been reported by several investigators (Caldron et al., 1986; Dawson, 1988), keyboard and string performers comprised the majority of this group, with 19 (10 pianists, nine string players) of the 25 instrumentalists included in these two categories.

Sports Etiology

The author's practice, unlike that of many other arts-medicine health professionals, includes a significant number of performers whose difficulties were not caused directly by their music, but which had an effect on their musical performance (Dawson, 1988, 1992). Sports participation produced 38 different injuries in 22 of the 78 repeating patients; the greatest number of injuries sustained by any one person was three—and all these were fractures of the clavicle or upper humerus in a baseball umpire who was hit on three separate occasions by foul tips from a batter. Seven other performers each experienced two different injuries. These 22 patients ranged in class from symphony string players to school musicians, and the majority of the injuries produced emanated from sports involving a ball.

Nerve Compressions

Only 3 of the 78 patients presented with multiple instances of peripheral nerve compression; none of the three was diabetic. All three were diagnosed on at least one occasion with carpal tunnel syndrome, or compression of the median nerve at the wrist (two of these cases were bilateral and occurred at different times), while two also experienced ulnar nerve compression at the epicondylar groove or cubital tunnel of the elbow.

Discussion

Are repeaters as a group any different from nonrepeaters, and if so, in what ways? Data for the cohort of repeating musicians were examined for factors that might be different from those individuals who experienced only a single hand or upper extremity problem. Several differences were found and are presented in Tables 2 and 3; the statistical significance is shown when appropriate.

Table 2. *Comparison By Problem Type*
New problems of repeaters and nonrepeaters

Type	Repeaters	%	Nonrepeaters	%	Significance?
Overuse	76/195	39.0	116/589	19.7	$p > .0001$
Trauma	70/195	35.9	330/589	56.0	$p > .01$
Arthritis	9/195	4.6	41/589	7.0	
Other	40/195	20.5	102/589	17.3	

Table 3. *Comparison By Musician Class*
New problems of repeaters and nonrepeaters

Class	Repeaters	%	Nonrepeaters	%	Significance?
A	60/195	30.8	114/589	19.3	$p > .001$
B	18/195	9.2	24/589	4.1	$p > .001$
C	14/195	7.2	28/589	4.8	
D	52/195	27.2	106/589	18.0	$p > .01$
E	18/195	9.2	91/589	15.4	
F	32/195	16.4	226/589	38.4	$p > .0001$

Repeaters were much more likely to present with overuse problems and much less likely to have traumatic diagnoses than were nonrepeaters. Whether this phenomenon can be attributed to the significantly higher percentages of high-level musician classes in the repeater group is not certain; it may only indicate that a serious adult performer may be more likely to seek care for overuse problems or may be less likely to experience trauma-related conditions. By contrast, the exceptionally low percentage of class F amateur repeaters cannot be explained easily. The demographics of those musicians in class F actually may be quite similar to the data for nonmusician patients in an upper-extremity orthopaedic practice.

Characteristics of Repeaters

From the standpoint of prevention, can a repeater be identified early in his/her medical "career," and, if so, by what characteristics? Several suggestive patterns have been found, and awareness of these may help the medical professional minimize the performer's future exposure to conditions that might precipitate new difficulties.

1. Changes in a performer's musical life can lead to some of the situations that may encourage overuse problems. A new instrument, a new teacher, or a new second job frequently have been implicated as causes of repeated strains, tendinitis, or trigger digits. As the performer matures, playing increasingly difficult repertoire also can produce such problems.

2. A corollary to the above condition is change in a performer's musical class that is produced by the passage of time. Eight musicians experienced changes of this nature, caused by such life events as leaving school, returning to school or to active teaching/performing, or retirement from professional performance. The resulting increase or decrease in exposure to the effects of overuse and nonacademic job stress is easily recognized. One young percussionist and keyboard musician has been followed medically by the author for more than 15 years, from his boyhood days as a school percussionist through conservatory into the world of a professional performer; during this interval he has experienced no fewer than six different orthopaedic problems, ranging from sports trauma to performance-induced musculoskeletal overuse.

3. Continued participation in sports is a common cause of repeated injury and is seen regularly among both musicians and nonmusicians. Ball sports, most of which can be played year-round, are especially likely to produce injury to the hand and fingers (Dawson, 1990).

4. Recurrent musical stress is a recognized and accepted cause of recurrent muscle-tendon overuse conditions, especially those involving the hand and upper extremity. One teenage patient in this study was seen yearly for 3 consecutive summers because of new strain symptoms in her hands and forearms; these were caused by the marked increase in practice time and intensity needed to prepare for annual piano competitions. In each instance, her symptoms subsided completely with appropriate treatment and rest, until the next year's increased practice efforts resumed.

5. Those instrumentalists who are afflicted with ongoing or chronic constitutional or medical conditions also show some propensity for developing multiple problems. Three patients of the 78 presented with various difficulties related to an arthritic condition, two of them having been diagnosed with degenerative joint disease (osteoarthritis) and one with rheumatoid arthritis. Diabetes mellitus, especially the insulin-dependent type, often has been implicated in the production of connective tissue changes in the hand; three such diabetic patients in this series presented with a variety of these conditions, including DeQuervain's tenosynovitis, trigger digits (as many as six separate affected digits in one patient), and Dupuytren's contracture of the palmar fascia.

Hypermobility syndrome was diagnosed in 4 of the 78 repeating patients. In three of these the condition seemed to play a causal role in the development of trigger digits and of strains involving the hand and forearm muscles. However, there were an additional 25 performers without this syndrome who developed similar multiple connective tissue problems in their upper extremities. This latter group included 18 patients who were diagnosed with strains of their muscles and tendons, 16 with trigger digits, 13 with other areas affected by synovitis or tenosynovitis, eight with elbow epicondylitis and eight with rotator cuff tendinitis at the shoulder. It is postulated that this propensity for such multiple difficulties may have a genetic basis, possibly relating to the quality of an individual's connective tissue and its susceptibility to overuse or attritional conditions that may be produced by repeated physical stress. This link has not been proven, however, and future studies will be needed to confirm or deny it.

Prevention

Preventing the repetition of difficulties, whether in musicians or nonmusicians, remains an important goal of medical care. Based on the evaluation of data from the repeater group, several possible methods of prevention can be suggested. These may be useful not only for those instrumentalists who tend to repeat with the same type of problem, but also for others whose life-styles may place them at risk for several different types.

A performer may benefit from a change of practice patterns. For instance, it seems wise to increase both the time and intensity of practice for a longer period prior to a competition or audition, or before resuming music conservatory studies. The summer holiday traditionally is a period of decreased playing time for many students, and Manchester and Flieder (1991) have reported an increased incidence in students' overuse problems after they return to school in the autumn. In addition, adjusting to the artistic and technical changes in playing demanded by a new teacher or a new instrument may require a longer period of time than the performer may anticipate, especially if new overuse difficulties are to be minimized or prevented.

People, whether or not they are active performers, who have been diagnosed with various chronic or congenital connective tissue problems seem to benefit from a program of general physical conditioning, with special emphasis placed on the musculoskeletal system. Hypermobile joints are less likely to be injured when their controlling muscles are well developed and are trained to prevent excessive ranges of joint motion. For people having normal joint mobility, maintenance of muscular endurance and soft tissue flexibility also can be beneficial in prevention of overuse problems. Standard physical therapy techniques and modalities often are useful in achieving these goals; the details of prescribing and utilizing such therapy, however, are beyond the scope of this presentation.

Sports injuries can be prevented or minimized by timely training, proper conditioning, and correct use of protective equipment. Many seasonal sports are associated with a greater number of injuries to the hand in the early part of the season (Dawson & Pullos, 1981) and preseason training and practice may provide or renew the neuromuscular skills that are so necessary for safe participation. This fact is especially true for the more mature athlete, whose recreational sports performance may be hindered by slightly decreased reaction times, and who may require a longer warm-up period prior to resuming play.

Arthritis and other frequently debilitating conditions present some special considerations related to the prevention of repeated problems. As these conditions tend to progress with age, strategies designed to retard the deleterious effects of time are essential. Modifications of daily activities and the use of joint protection techniques both play a large role in decreasing stress on all joints, and they may be utilized by instrumentalists as well as others. Additional methods of modifying physical stresses may include changing one's repertoire or focus in musical life, or changing instruments or modifying their keywork when possible (the latter suggestion is especially applicable to woodwind instruments).

Study Factors

This study contains a number of factors that affect its results and that may make comparison with other study populations difficult. The patients seen in the author's practice are not a "captive audience" and do not obtain all their care for musculoskeletal problems from a single medical source; they may (and frequently did) visit other physicians during the years of this study. In addition, patients may not seek medical care for problems that they consider to be minor, thus artificially lowering the actual incidence figures for a given diagnosis. This lack of formal care may be due to a number of reasons, including financial considerations, time constraints, and skill in self-treatment. On the other hand, a goodly number of patients will self-refer to a specialist if they believe their problems to be serious enough to warrant this type of care.

In these years of increasing American emphasis on managed health care, a large number of patients now belong to health maintenance plans that have specific referral patterns and consequently do not allow their subscribers a free choice of medical specialists (including arts-medicine doctors). Many performers, including some members of large orchestras, obtain most of their musculoskeletal care from primary physicians and the remainder from a limited selection of specialists; this situation also can affect prevalence statistics because of underreporting.

The author has addressed only some demographic and etiologic factors that are pertinent to arts-medicine repeaters. No attempt has been made to discuss such other important subjects as precise diagnosis, specifics of treatment or ultimate outcome of these varied problems. These subjects properly have been the focus of many other presentations and publications in the past, and it is hoped that continued investigations along these lines will provide still more useful information to those who treat performing artists.

Conclusions

Instrumentalists who present for treatment of upper extremity problems on more than one occasion are most likely to be performers with a high level of involvement in music, such as professionals, music students and dedicated amateurs. They are more likely to sustain overuse and traumatic difficulties than to develop arthritic or other conditions. One-half of the patients in this study presented with a variety of problem types, and two-thirds suffered on more than one occasion with the same problem type.

Prevention of repeating may be facilitated by the use of correct musical practice and performance techniques, by general physical conditioning to improve flexibility, strength, and endurance, and by proper training and maintenance of sport-specific skills.

References

Caldron, P. A., Calabrese, L. H., Clough, J. D., Lederman, R. J., Williams, G., & Leatherman, J. (1986). A survey of musculoskeletal problems encountered in high-level musicians. *Medical Problems of Performing Artists, 1,* 136–139.

Dawson, W. J. (1988). Hand and upper extremity problems in musicians: Epidemiology and diagnosis. *Medical Problems of Performing Artists, 3,* 19–22.

Dawson, W. J. (1990). Upper extremity injuries in high-level instrumentalists: An end-result study. *Medical Problems of Performing Artists, 5,* 109–113.

Dawson, W. J. (1992). The role of surgery in treating musicians' upper extremity problems. *Medical Problems of Performing Artists, 7,* 59–62.

Dawson, W. J., & Pullos, N. (1981). Baseball injuries to the hand. *Annals of Emergency Medicine, 10,* 302–306.

Fishbein, M., & Middlestadt, S. E. (1988). Medical problems among ICSOM musicians: Overview of a national survey. *Medical Problems of Performing Artists, 3,* 1–8.

Larsson, L.-G., Baum, J., Mudholkar, G. S., & Kollia, G. D. (1993). Nature and impact of musculoskeletal problems in a population of musicians. *Medical Problems of Performing Artists, 8,* 73–76.

Manchester, R. A., & Flieder, D. (1991). Further observations of the epidemiology of hand injuries in music students. *Medical Problems of Performing Artists, 6,* 11–14.

CARDIAC ARRHYTHMIAS OBSERVED DURING TRUMPET PLAYING

Leigh Ann Hunsaker and Darhyl Ramsey

Introduction

In the last 20 years, awareness of the medical problems of musicians has increased greatly among physicians, performers, and teachers. This interest has expanded into the specialized field of performing arts medicine. The growth of the arts medicine field can be seen in the number of studies and informational articles in professional journals, the creation of professional journals specific to the area of arts medicine as well as the popular media of television, and newspapers. There appears to be much more attention to the effects of musical performance and playing on the body than ever before.

Much of the treatment prescribed for playing-related disorders is based on the physician's experience and insight into the demands of the musician's job (Brandfonbrener, 1989). Researchers have sought additional information from professional performers and music students about playing-related health problems. Various surveys have shown that approximately 50–75% of these musicians experience serious conditions (Lederman, 1989; Lockwood, 1989). Tendinitis and carpal tunnel syndrome were frequent complaints from players of keyboard and string instruments.

The problems experienced by wind instrument players, however, are usually of a different and less severe nature. Conditions such as protruding teeth, cold sores, and respiratory ailments have long been known to cause considerable difficulty for individual wind players. In addition to such independently existing conditions that can affect playing, the possibility of chronic health problems being caused by wind instrument playing should also be examined.

One area of investigation is the possible existence of cardiac problems in brass players. This concern has been investigated in a few studies. Tucker, Faulkner, and Horvath (1971) examined the effects of brass instrument playing upon the heart's function by examining electrocardiograms (ECGs) of brass students recorded at rest and during instrument playing. The ECGs showed evidence of altered heart response during the playing periods. The authors concluded that the physical strain caused by playing a brass instrument may result in continuing circulatory stress, with harmful results to the player.

The effects of brass instrument playing upon the heart were further investigated by Borgia, Horvath, Dunn, Von Phul, and Nizet (1975). The authors examined the ECGs of French horn players and reported irregularities in heart rhythm such as rapid heart rate changes, premature beats, T wave changes, and wandering pacemaker activity. The authors suggested that more changes in heart rhythm could be expected during the musicians' usual playing activity.

Although unsubstantiated by the data, the conclusions of these two ECG studies (Borgia et al., 1975; Tucker et al., 1971) have been presented in the more popular (as opposed to research) instrumental literature. The repetition of these conclusions by other medical researchers has led to the idea that brass instrument playing can be harmful to the heart.

Because wind instruments are widely used in school music programs, music educators must be concerned with the accuracy of such claims. Any damaging effects of playing wind instruments should be fully investigated. The alarming conclusions of Tucker et al., 1971 have not been corroborated or examined objectively. Further observation of heart response during instrument playing should be combined with a medical assessment of the findings.

Background of the Study

Information from various types of studies has been used to investigate the effects of brass instrument playing upon the heart. Research on the respiratory and circulatory responses of wind instrument players has been examined in addition to studying the action of the heart itself. The performance anxiety literature also has provided information about the cardiovascular function of musicians.

The various wind instruments have different requirements of air flow and air pressure, and thus cause a wide range of alterations in the players' respiratory and circulatory function. Bouhuys (1964) found that playing brass instruments requires more respiratory effort than playing the same pitches on woodwind instruments. Compression of the lungs and sustained high air pressures in the mouth were found to be most pronounced in people playing loud, high tones on brass instruments (Bouhuys, 1968).

Several researchers have noted that playing a wind instrument can produce a Valsalva effect on the circulatory system (Borgia et al., 1975; Faulkner & Sharpey-Schafer, 1959; Tucker et al., 1971). The Valsalva maneuver is produced by blowing against resistance, a situation inherent in all brass wind instrument playing. The high internal air pressures that trigger the Valsalva effect cause changes in the circulatory system in which venous return, cardiac output, and arterial blood pressure are altered. Additionally, there are changes in heart rate and rhythm: the heart rate slows suddenly, then gradually increases to normal or faster than normal rates (see Figure 1).

In comparative studies of various wind instruments (Bouhuys, 1964; Faulkner & Sharpey-Schafer, 1959; Tucker et al., 1971), trumpet players were found to produce higher air pressures and to exhibit greater circulatory changes than players of other instruments. The cardiopulmonary changes observed in trumpet players were more pronounced than those produced by the clinical Valsalva maneuver. Further examination of ECGs recorded during trumpet playing can provide information about the magnitude of circulatory stress encountered by the musicians.

As seen above, the entire cardiopulmonary system is affected by such demanding activities as playing a brass instrument. The use of ECG monitoring makes it possible to study the heart's response during instrument playing. An electrocardiogram of the heart's activity can indicate events in both the respiratory and circulatory systems. Borgia et al. (1975) found distinct alterations in heart rhythm (cardiac arrhythmias) in the ECGs of student and professional horn players. Tucker, Faulkner, and Horvath (1971) observed some differences in players of the various brass instruments. French horn players had many premature heart contractions, while trumpet players had the greatest and most rapid heart rate changes, as well as alterations in heart rhythm.

Several aspects of this study cast doubt upon the findings. A lack of control settings in ECG testing, questionable recording procedures, and the inappropriate application of

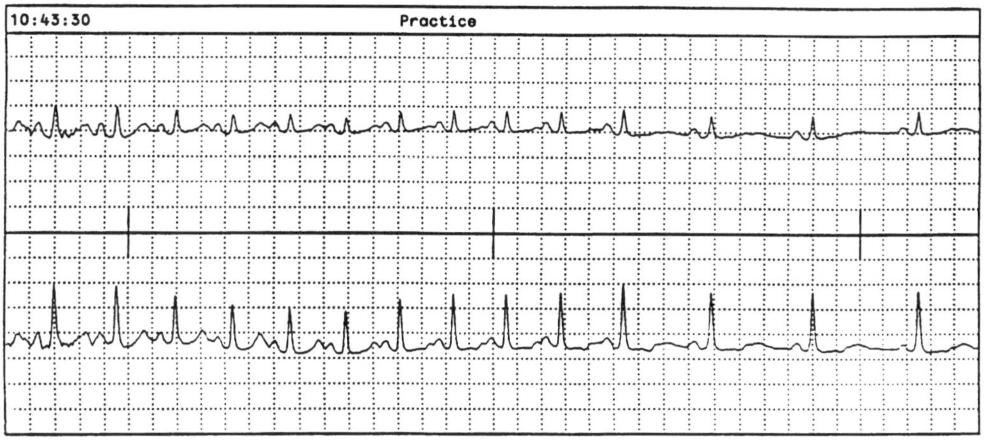

Figure 1. Valsalva Maneuver

medical data seriously undermine the conclusions of the study. The use of nonmusical playing tasks and nontypical settings to measure the heart response may have affected the outcome of the Tucker study.

Given the improvements in equipment and the knowledge that has been gained in 20 years of cardiac research, it was felt that a study that examined the heart function of trumpet players in a more natural setting would allow a more reliable medical interpretation of the findings. Therefore, the purpose of the study was to examine the effects of trumpet playing upon the heart, and to assess the clinical significance of these effects.

The research questions were as follows:

1. To determine whether there is a significant increase in heart rate during trumpet playing.

2. To compare the heart's response in two settings: Individual practice and in a performance.

3. To identify the changes in heart rhythm that occur during trumpet playing.

Methodology

Twenty-four student and professional trumpet players participated in this study. There was a wide range of abilities, as well as diverse styles of playing involved—among the subjects were members of the North Texas Lab Bands, and the Dallas Symphony Orchestra. Before beginning the ECG testing, each subject completed a medical questionnaire, providing information on personal and family medical history. Specific information on the use of beta blockers was requested; however, no one used this medication during the test. No volunteers were excluded for medical reasons.

The study included two phases: (a) a comparison of the heart rate at rest and while playing a standard etude, and (b) a comparison of heart rate and rhythm while playing selected music in both practice and performance situations. A Holter monitor was used to record electrocardiograms during the study. Subjects were given the monitor in advance in order to familiarize themselves with the process.

In the first phase of the study, playing and resting heart rates were compared in a controlled setting. Twenty-one subjects played a composite étude that included legato scale passages, rapid articulations, and lip slur patterns. After an initial rest period, the subject played the étude with a metronome. The maximum heart rate at rest and during étude playing was calculated for each subject and the results compared through a dependent t test.

The second phase of the study compared the heart's rate and rhythm responses in different playing situations. An extended ECG was recorded for eleven trumpet players during a practice session, a performance, and other activities during the day. An activity log was used to show the time of each event during the ECG.

The practice sessions consisted of each individual's usual warm up, and any other materials of his choice, including at least one complete reading of the music to be played in the subsequent performance. The subjects were instructed to practice in their normal manner; no attempt was made to indulge any additional physical responses.

The performance situations included professional and regional orchestra concerts, night club shows, chamber music concerts, and a school recital; no performances were arranged specifically for the study. Likewise, only previously programmed music selections were used in testing, in order to examine the actual demands encountered by each individual.

The two aspects of heart response that were examined in the practice and performance comparison were the mean heart rate, and the rhythm disturbance characteristic of the Valsalva maneuver. The average heart rate during performance was compared to the average rate during the practice session when the same music was played straight through. Occurrences of the Valsalva maneuver were identified on the ECGs, and classified based on the percentage of rate change between adjacent heart beats. Instances of this rhythm disturbance were classified as mild when adjacent cycle lengths varied from 10 to 24%; moderate disturbance was defined as variations of 25 to 49%; variations of 50% or more were classified as marked disturbances. The most pronounced disturbance was reported in each situation.

The third research problem was to identify additional changes in heart rhythm during trumpet playing. The Holter tapes from the controlled setting and from the live performances and practice sessions were evaluated by a cardiologist and an ECG technician.

Results

In the first phase of the study, the mean heart rate during trumpet playing was found to be significantly higher ($p < .0001$) than when resting (Table 1). Also, when compared by age groups, younger players (18–24 yrs) had a greater increase in heart rate than older musicians (25–46 yrs). This difference was significant at the $p < .02$ level (Table 2).

In the second phase of the study, nine subjects completed the comparison of practice and performance situations. Eight of the nine subjects experienced a faster heart rate during the performance; one had a slight decrease in heart rate on stage. Because different music was used by each subject, the results were not combined for statistical analysis; instead, the percentage of heart rate change between situations was calculated for each subject.

The greatest increase in heart rate occurred during a performance of the Del Borgo *Trumpet Sonata*. During practice, this player had a mean heart rate of 74 bpm; in performance, he averaged 170 bpm, an increase of 129%.

Table 1. *Comparison of Resting and Playing Heart Rates*

t Test for Dependent Measures		
Item	Resting	Playing
N	21	21
Mean	92.19	119.05
Std. Dev.	13.43	15.45
Difference in Means		26.86
t-Value		10.1397
Probability One-Tailed		.0001

Table 2. *Comparison of Heart Rate Increase in Two Age Groups*

t Test for Independent Samples		
Item	Group 1 18–24	Group 2 25–46
N	10	11
Mean	32.60	22.00
Std. Dev.	13.75	7.04
t Value		2.2554
Probability One-Tailed	0.0180	

The second aspect of heart response examined in the practice-performance comparison was the severity of the sinus arrhythmia characteristic of the Valsalva maneuver. Only 2 of the 11 subjects had more pronounced heart rate changes during performance.

For the third research problem, the ECG tapes were examined for arrhythmias occurring during any of the playing situations. All 24 subjects produced the sinus arrhythmia characteristic of the Valsalva maneuver. Eleven male trumpet players had additional arrhythmias including premature atrial and ventricular contractions, instances of atrial and ventricular tachycardia, and escape mechanisms while playing (Table 3).

Escape beats occur when the impulse causing the heart to beat is suppressed at the normal pacemaker site, allowing another area of the heart to initiate a beat. One subject produced a ventricular escape beat, while another had an escape beat originating in the atrioventricular (AV) junction. A third subject had a junctional escape rhythm, in which the AV junction temporarily assumes the pacemaking role (see Figure 2). In addition, seven

Table 3. *Subjects Producing Arrhythmias During Trumpet Playing*

$N = 24$	
Valsalva Maneuver	$n =$ 8
Premature Ventricular Contraction	8
Premature Atrial Contraction	8
Escape Mechanism	3
Right Bundle Branch Block	7
Ventricular Tachycardia	1
Atrial Tachycardia	1

subjects had a right bundle branch block, a condition in which the impulse causing the heart to beat is delayed in the conductive pathway on the right side of the heart. In one person, this delay was present throughout the ECG, but increased during trumpet playing. A second subject had an incomplete block in practice, and a normal ECG during a concert. In the other five subjects, the delay was present throughout the test and was unaffected by trumpet playing.

These arrhythmias were generally more prevalent in performances than in practice. All of the escape mechanisms occurred during performances as well as the instances of atrial

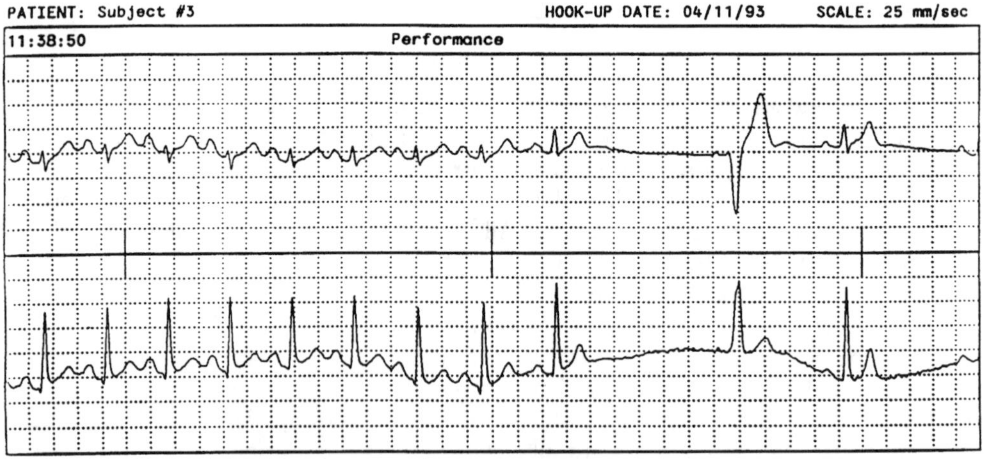

Figure 2. Valsalva Effect with AV Junctional Escape Beat

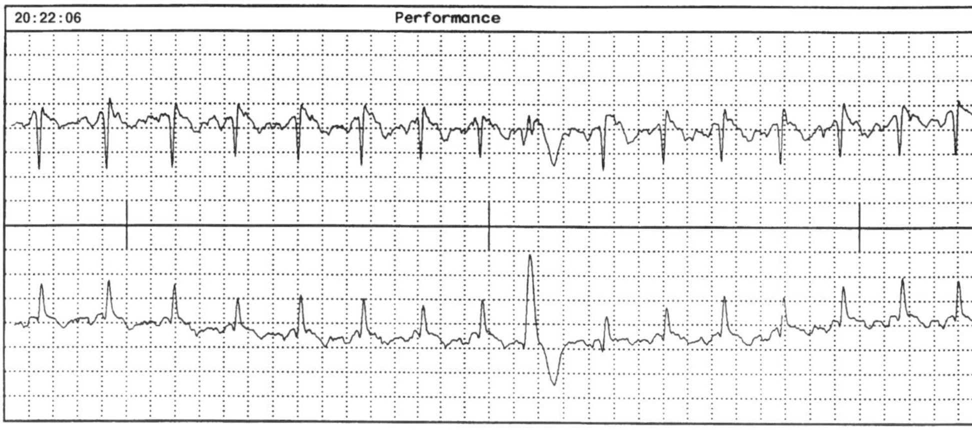

Figure 3. Premature Ventricular Contraction

and ventricular tachycardia. Likewise, the premature beats were more prevalent in performance situations. Four subjects had a total of seven premature ventricular contractions (PVCs) during practice, while 23 PVCs occurred during their performances (see Figure 3). Six subjects had a total of four premature atrial contractions (PACs) during practice, and eight PACs during performances.

In addition to these findings, the ECGs were examined for evidence of a cumulative increase in stress upon the heart during practice. In the study referred to earlier, Tucker et al., (1971) suggested this possibility after having subjects repeat an étude as many times as possible without stopping, until fatigued. The authors reported more ECG changes occurring at the end of these sessions than at the beginning.

In order to obtain a more realistic view of the requirements of trumpet playing, subjects in the present study were instructed to use their daily warm up, and to continue to practice in their normal manner. The practice sessions lasted from 20 to 90 minutes. A comparison of the first and last 5-minute segments of these ECGs showed little change in either heart rate or number of arrhythmias occurring. The ECGs of these routine practice sessions did not exhibit any type of cumulative effect in the heart response.

Conclusions

The literature suggests that musical activities such as singing and wind instrument playing cause an increase in heart rate (Gates et al., 1985; Bouhuys, 1964, 1966). Furthermore, the trumpet was found to be the most demanding in a comparison of wind instruments. The present study confirms these findings; subjects had significantly higher rates when playing the trumpet ($p < .0001$) than when resting.

The study also compared the heart's response in practice and performance situations. The subjects used for this portion of the study each chose one or more pieces of music to play while being monitored in both settings. In this type of comparison, the heart rate can indicate both the amount of work and the presence of stress in a situation. Eight of the nine trumpet players experienced an increase in heart rate during performance; the subjects experienced an average increase of 23% in heart rate on stage.

The intensity of the Valsalva maneuver produced during trumpet playing also was examined in these two settings. Of the 11 subjects involved in this comparison, only two had a more pronounced disturbance in heart rhythm during performance than during practice. All of the subjects showed some increase in rhythm change, albeit not different enough to change categories. Hence, the present study found that the heart rate usually increases during performances as a result of the body's response to the situation, while the physical effort needed to play the same music is unchanged; however, the subjects may increase their voluntary efforts unnecessarily.

The extended ECG recording made it possible to obtain additional information about heart response in a way not addressed in previous studies. There was a general pattern of more irregularities in the heart rhythm during the performance setting, although none of these changes persisted after playing. Likewise, no cumulative increase in stress upon the heart was observed during playing sessions.

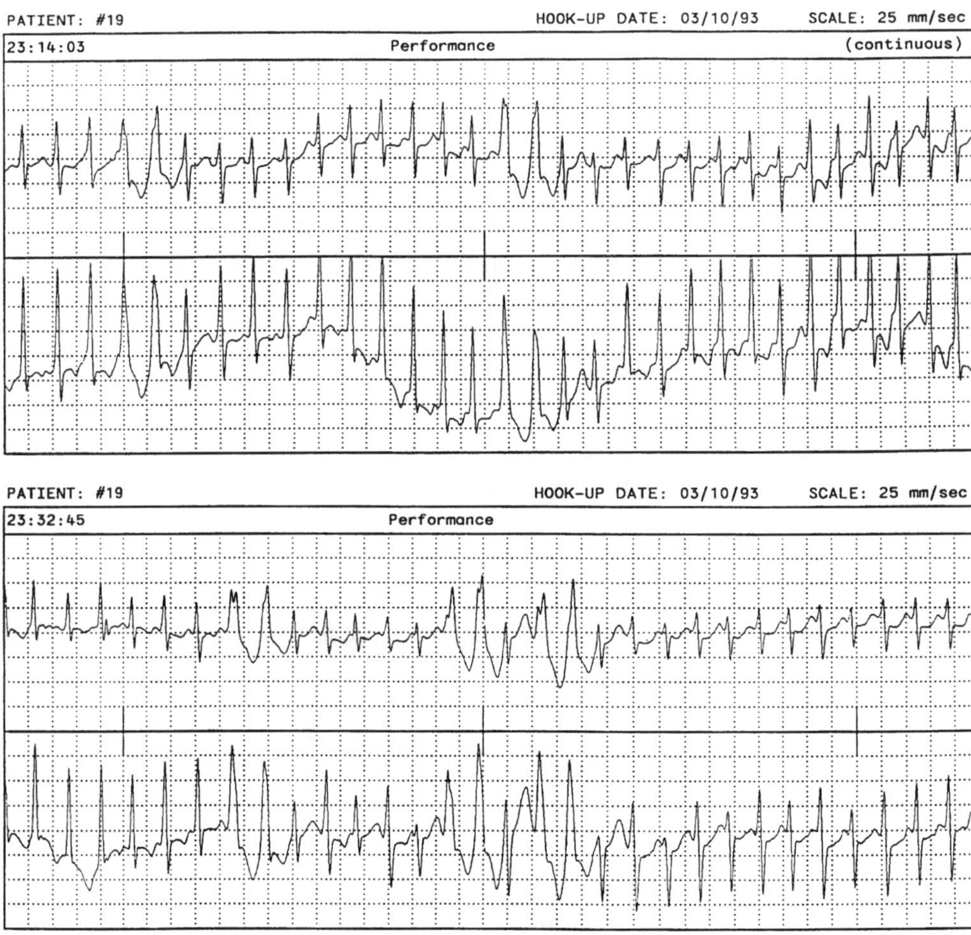

Figure 4. Complex Ventricular Arrhythmias (not induced by trumpet playing)

The third research problem identified the arrhythmias that occurred during trumpet playing. All 24 subjects produced the arrhythmia characteristic of the Valsalva maneuver during trumpet playing. Eleven subjects had additional arrhythmias similar to those reported in healthy athletes (Pantano & Oriel, 1982; Pilcher et al., 1983). Arrhythmias that were determined to be induced by trumpet playing included premature atrial and ventricular contractions, atrial tachycardia, and ventricular and junctional escape mechanisms.

Other arrhythmias observed in the study were attributed to physiological causes. One subject experienced severe rhythmic disturbances that were unrelated to trumpet playing (see Figure 4). Another had frequent premature contractions throughout the test. In addition, seven trumpet players exhibited a right bundle branch block during the monitoring period.

Although several types of arrhythmias were induced during trumpet playing, none of these ECG changes persisted after playing, and there were no signs of adaptive changes in the heart itself. Based on the data of the 24 subjects, no evidence of any adverse effect of trumpet playing on the heart was found. In the absence of other symptoms, these ECG changes can be considered normal variants that occur as a function of instrument playing.

References

Borgia, J. F., Horvath, S. M., Dunn, F. R., von Phul, P. V., & Nizet, P.M. (1975). Some physiological observations on French horn musicians. *Journal of Occupational Medicine, 17,* 696–701.

Bouhuys, A. (1964). Lung volume and breathing patterns in wind instrument players. *Journal of Applied Physiology 19,* 967–975.

Brandfonbrener, A. G. (1989). Performing arts medicine: A checkup. *Medical Problems of Performing Artists, 4,* 101–102.

Faulkner, M. E., & Sharpey-Schafer, E. P. (1959). Circulatory effects of trumpet playing. *British Medical Journal 1,* 685–686.

Gates, G. A., Saegert, J., Wilson, N., Johnson, L., Shepherd, A., & Hearne, E. (1985). Effect of beta blockade on singing performance. *Annals of Otology, Rhinology, and Laryngology 94,* 570–574.

Lederman, R. (1989). Performing arts medicine. *New England Journal of Medicine, 320,* 246–248.

Lockwood, A. (1989). Medical problems of musicians. *New England Journal of Medicine, 320,* 221–227.

Nizet, P. M., Borgia, J. F., & Horvath, S. M. (1976). Wandering atrial pacemaker: Prevalence in French hornists. *Journal of Electrocardiology, 9,* 51–52.

Pantano, J. A., & Oriel, R. J. (1982). Prevalence and nature of cardiac arrhythmias in apparently normal well-trained runners. *American Heart Journal, 104,* 762–768.

Pilcher, G. F., Cook, J., Johnston, B. L., & Fletcher, G. F. (1983). Twenty-four hour continuous electrocardiography during exercise and free activity in apparently healthy runners. *American Journal of Cardiology, 52,* 859–861.

Tucker, A., Faulkner, M. E., & Horvath, S. M. (1971) Electrocardiography and lung function in brass instrument players. *Archives of Environmental Health, 23,* 327–334.

BIOPSYCHOSOCIAL ASPECTS OF MUSIC PERFORMANCE: PERFORMING ARTS HEALTH

Cheryl Dileo Maranto

Introduction

The psychosocial and biomedical aspects of music performance have traditionally been researched as mutually exclusive phenomena, for example, musculoskeletal and other physiological problems and stress/anxiety problems have been studied independently. However, little research has addressed the interrelationships of these phenomena in musicians. My own interest in this phenomenon has evolved during the past 6 years through my offering of a course on performance anxiety for university music students.

The purpose of this paper is: (a) to provide a summary of various biopsychosocial problems in musicians; (b) to provide a new, biopsychosocial and systems theory perspective, (c) to suggest new approaches to terminology and treatment, and (d) to present new models and topics for research in this evolving field.

Terminology in Performing Arts Medicine

The general term "performing arts medicine", applied to the various performance-related problems of performers, implies to a great extent that these problems warrant medical intervention according to the medical model of treatment. Following, specific terminology in the field of performing arts medicine has typically emphasized a dichotomy of the mind and the body. For example, terms such as "musculoskeletal" vs. "nonmusculoskeletal" problems, and "medical" vs. "psychological/stress" problems have been generally used to categorize these problems. Furthermore, the journal, *Medical Problems of Performing Artists,* has included performance anxiety as a topic within the purview of medicine. Performance anxiety when treated as a medical problem by physicians often requires a drug intervention.

There are three major problems inherent in this terminology: (a) It neglects to reflect the inherent interdisciplinary nature of this field (requiring the expertise and knowledge of physicians, allied health therapists, creative arts therapists, artists, physiologists, arts educators, etc., (b) It dismisses to a large extent the interactive nature of health-related problems of artists (i.e., the mind-body relationship), and (c) The issues of prevention and healthy playing have been to a large extent undermined. Although this terminology is considered problematic at the present, it will be used to some extent in this paper to avoid confusion.

Stress, Performance Anxiety, Psychological and Physical Issues in Music Performing

Stress

How stressful is it to be a performing musician? Although there are limited data on this phenomenon, a study by Middlestadt and Fishbein (1988) reports that 69% of the 2,212 ICSOM respondents revealed that orchestral musicians experienced the same levels of stress as other professional musicians (although not specified); 23% indicated that they experienced more stress and 16% indicated experiencing less stress than other professional musicians.

There are potentially many causes of stress-related problems of musicians and student musicians.

Brandfonbrener (1988) postulated that a primary cause of stress in musicians was related to the "absolute standard of perfection" in music performance that does not allow error.

Dews and Williams (1989) identified the 10 top issues of concern for student musicians as: "(a) stress, (b) pre-performance nervousness, (c) progress impatience, (d) burnout with musical progress, (e) job insecurity, (f) feeling conflict between music and one's personal life, (g) inadequate practice facilities, (h) depression, (i) stage fright, and (j) concentration" (p. 39). Some of these issues are interrelated and may be potential sources of stress.

Theorell (in press), in a comparison of orchestral musicians to other occupational groups, found that orchestral musicians had the lowest level of job-decision latitude (control over work) and the next to lowest levels of skill discretion (learning new things and job variety), both potential sources of job stress and health problems.

In order to assess this problem, it may be helpful to categorize stressor events according to a model by Eliot and Eisdorfer (1982):

1. An acute time-limited variety, including such events as preparing for specific medical procedures (e.g., surgery, dental examinations) or for invasive medical examinations (e.g., biopsies, cardiac catheterizations) or having to confront specific evaluations (e.g., a Ph.D. defense).

2. A stressor sequence variety, whereby a specific event (e.g., death of a loved one, divorce, job loss, natural or man-made disaster) may trigger a series of stressful reactions and transitional adjustments (e.g., coping with being raped or otherwise being victimized, becoming unemployed).

3. A chronic intermittent variety, constituting repeated exposures to such stressors as student examinations, competitive performances (e.g., musical or athletic competitions), occasional medical tests or treatments, military combat or episodic physical disorders (e.g., recurrent headaches).

4. A chronic continual variety, include having to cope with a debilitating or chronic medical or psychiatric illness; prolonged marital or familial discord, often with accompanying physical or sexual abuse; and exposure to persistent occupational dangers and stressors in professions such as police work, nursing and teaching (Meichenbaum, 1993, p. 373).

Based on this categorization, stress factors of musicians and student musicians related to performing are varied and comprise all categories (see Table 1). It should be noted that this list refers only to performance- and career-related stress; most individuals also have a host of other stress factors in their lives that are not included in this paper. In addition, there have been no studies that have compared professional musicians to other occupational groups.

The most significant question that needs to be asked, which has not yet been addressed in the literature, is: What are the short- and long-term health effects of performance-related stress on the health of the musician? Will the stressors of a career as a musician ultimately impair health?

Music Performance Anxiety

In addition to stress, one must consider another problem of musicians that often, if not always, contributes to stress: performance anxiety.

Table 1. *Categories and Example Sources of Stress in Musicians*

Category	Example Sources
1) ACUTE, TIME-LIMITED	
	Auditions
	Pre-performance nervousness
	Actual Performances
2) STRESSOR SEQUENCE	
	Inadequate Practice Facilities
	Job Insecurity (Unemployment)
	Hand Problems
3) CHRONIC INTERMITTENT	
	Progress Impatience
	Conflicts with Personal vs. Professional Life
	Depression
	Stage Fright
	Concentration Difficulties
	Juries
	Difficult Performance Schedules
	High Decibel Levels
4) CHRONIC CONTINUAL	
	Perfectionism
	Burnout with Progress
	Low Job Decision Latitude
	Low Skill Discretion
	Salary Levels

Musical performance anxiety "is defined as the experience of persistent, distressing apprehension about and/or actual impairment of, performance skills in a public context, to a degree unwarranted given the individual's musical aptitude, training and level of preparation" (Salmon, 1990, p. 2).

As there is generally some anxiety present in all music performances, according to the Yerkes Dodson Law (1908), performance is optimal with moderate levels of anxiety; performance quality is diminished at both higher and lower levels of anxiety (Steptoe & Fidler, 1987).

Thus some anxiety is considered desirable in music performance. Performance anxiety is considered a problem when it significantly interferes with the music performance (Plaut, 1988). Anxiety during a performance may be either facilitating (improving performance) or debilitating (worsening performance) (Lehrer, Goldman, & Strommen, 1990; Wolfe, 1989).

Prevalence. According to the available data, music performance anxiety is ubiquitous. In a sample of 61 music students, Nagel (1987) found that 92% had problems with stage fright, and 62% felt that this adversely affected their performances.

In a study of the prevalence of performance anxiety among student and professional musicians by Wesner, Noyes and Davis (1990), 16.5% of respondents indicated that their performances were impaired by performance anxiety, and 16.1% indicated that performance anxiety had markedly affected their careers.

Fishbein and Middlestadt (1988) in a survey of 2,212 orchestral and symphony musicians, found that stage fright was the most frequently indicated severe problem that respondents experienced (of both musculoskeletal and nonmusculoskeletal types). Twenty-four percent of respondents indicated that this was a problem, and 16% indicated this was a severe problem.

Chronic performance anxiety may lead musicians to stop performing or abandon their careers. This factor is not directly assessed in the studies of performing musicians who are still active. Thus, only prevalence data as opposed to incidence data have been available to date.

Causes and Symptoms. Music performance anxiety may be multidimensional in nature. According to Brandfonbrener (1990), "as universal as it seems to be, performance anxiety has different origins, meanings and manifestations, which are as varied as the individuals in whom it occurs. Therefore, it is as meaningless to generalize about the cause of performance anxiety as it is about any psychophysiologic symptom" (p. 23).

There are of course, various theories that explain music performance anxiety according to various psychological viewpoints. According to behavioral/cognitive theory, performance anxiety is related to negative self-statements arising from distorted beliefs and expectations. Psychoanalysts may view performance anxiety as an amalgam of personality traits, fears, and conflicts that are triggered in light of the performing situation. Physiologists view performance anxiety as a heightened state of adrenergic arousal.

The symptoms of performance anxiety appear to vary according to the performer, although some common symptoms have been noted. These include: palpitations, dry mouth, shakiness, trembling voice, shortness of breath, dizziness, nausea, and bladder and rectal pressure (Plaut, 1988), and memory loss (Hiner, Brandt, Katz, French, & Beczkiewicz, 1987). There are many other emotional and cognitive symptoms of performance anxiety that are a result of the individual's personal expectations, the perceived threat of the situation, etc. For example, Lehrer (1988) has identified some core "worries" of anxious performers that include: fears of anxiety, distraction, memory lapses, receiving criticism from others, and inadequate performance.

Several studies have indicated that negative cognitive appraisal of the performing situation can be more debilitating than the state of heightened arousal (Meichenbaum, 1972; Morris & Liebert, 1970, cited in Nagel, 1990). This is illuminated in a study by Clark and Agras (1991) wherein musicians who received cognitive-behavior therapy had a greater reduction in subjective anxiety than those who received buspirone, an antianxiety drug.

Anxiety related to performing may be reflective of trait anxiety (an enduring personality characteristic) or state anxiety (anxiety that is situational in nature). It is suspected that musicians with performance anxiety may have more global anxiety problems aside from that which is related to their performances (Lehrer, Goldman & Strommen, 1990).

Steptoe (1983) presented evidence that suggested that the stresses of musical careers and stage fright were not independent phenomena.

Treatments of Performance Anxiety. In general, various interventions have been used to deal with performance anxiety with differing reports of effectiveness (Maranto, 1989; 1992). Aside from no treatment, seeing a general practitioner is often the least effective strategy in treating the problem (Fishbein & Middlestadt, 1988).

In this same survey (Fishbein & Middlestadt, 1988), it was found that 27% of the 2,212 respondents had used beta-blockers. The use of these drugs was more common among women, brass players, and among musicians under 35 years of age. The vast majority of musicians reported using these drugs without a prescription. Musicians are most likely to use these to control performance anxiety before an audition, solo recitals, challenging orchestral performances and concerto performances.

It is unfortunate that in this comprehensive study there was no attempt to correlate musculoskeletal and nonmusculoskeletal problems, as these data would have been most illuminating to the field of performing arts medicine.

Again, with regard to performance anxiety, similar and new research and treatment questions arise: What are the short- and long-term health effects of performance anxiety, particularly as they relate to immune system functioning? What are the long-term effects of beta-blockers to treat this problem? Does the presence of performance anxiety in a musician increase stress and/or health risks?

Personality and Psychological Traits/Problems of Musicians

Besides stress factors and performance anxiety, there may be various personality characteristics, traits and/or problems common or unique to musicians.

There are several estimates of the prevalence of psychological problems of musicians. Ostwald (1987) indicated that 30–50% of the artists seen at a performing arts medicine clinic had functional psychological or emotional problems. Cohen and Kupersmith (1987) revealed that although patient performers scored significantly higher on a rating scale for psychiatric symptoms when compared to a control group of nonpatients, they had lower scores than other nonperforming patients.

Ostwald (1987) postulates that "performing artist patients have developed personality patterns and coping styles that are significantly different from those of nonperforming artist patients. These differences may account for some of the special vulnerabilities as well as the special resistance to psychiatric disorders that has been observed among performers" (p. 132). Ostwald states that there are certain performers' problems for which psychotherapy appears to be relevant: critical times when the performer experiences overwhelming disturbing emotions, times when his or her career is failing, various life developments for which the performer is unprepared, times of loneliness and/or sexual frustration, and times when substance abuse is problematic.

Kanefeld (1990) has described the psychological problems of performing arts students (including musicians). Some of these problems include: loneliness and alienation, identity problems, relationship problems, trauma, career concerns, and acute stress and anxiety. The field of performing arts is replete with occupational hazards that involve job unpredictability, financial difficulties, geographic uncertainty, intense and uneven time demands, and overwhelming competition.

Bejjani and Snow (1990), in comparing psychological scores of musicians to the general population, found that musicians were similar in coping styles, except for introversion, sociability, and confidence. Furthermore, insofar as psychological stress factors are concerned, musicians exhibit more self-imposed pressure than the general population.

Marchant-Haycox and Wilson (1992) assessed personality characteristics and stress in various groups of performing artists. Among the groups of performers, musicians were the "most cynical, resigned, and world-weary group, being inactive, unsociable, submissive, unambitious and controlled, as well as low in adventurousness" (p. 1065). In addition, there was a relationship between personality variables and stress symptoms (among all types of performers). "General emotionality predicted depression, panic and migraine, and introversion was related to shoulder-ache. Adventurousness was related to liver disease, as not surprisingly was alcohol consumption" (p. 1066).

Wills and Cooper (1984, 1987) found that popular musicians suffered from above-average levels of psychological anxiety. In a similar manner, Kemp (1981) found that classical musicians also had higher than average levels of anxiety.

Treatment. According to Ostwald (1987), the psychotherapeutic process for performers should include obtaining an understanding of the specific issues relevant to performing (choice of performing modality, details of training, relationships with teachers, professional successes and failures, and career goals and aspirations). In addition, it may be useful for the therapist to share the performing experience with the patient, whether vicariously, by observing a performance, or through making music with the patient. Also, it may be useful for the therapist to assess the various aspects of the musician's relationship with his or her instrument (Ostwald, 1992) involving: physical contact, movements, sound production, public performances, care of the instrument and the cultural and historic meaning of the instrument.

Physiological Problems

Although there are numerous studies that review the physiological problems of performers, a thorough analysis of this literature is beyond the scope of this paper. These problems are also ubiquitous and are often categorized according to medical specialty, for example, neurological, orthopedic, dermatological, otolaryngologic, etc. The most common problems involve the musculature and are attributable to playing beyond muscle limits.

In the largest survey to date regarding the prevalence of physical problems of orchestral musicians (2,212 respondents), Fishbein & Middlestadt, 1988) found that 82% of respondents experienced a medical problem, and 76% indicated that this problem was severe enough to interfere with their performance. Eye strain, and neck and back problems were frequently cited problems. Severe problems that affect performance are significantly more common in women and among string players (Middlestadt & Fishbein, 1989).

Again, important research and treatment questions emerge from these data: Is there a relationship among the various factors of stress, performance anxiety and psychological traits and difficulties of musicians? What are the short and long-term health risks of psychological traits and difficulties? What are short- and long-range consequences of physiological problems? And most importantly, what is the relationship, if any, between "psychological" and "physiological" problems? Does each of these phenomena, if indeed they are separate, exert an influence on the other?

Interrelationships between Biomedical and Psychosocial Phenomena in Musicians

There are two models that may describe the relationship between biomedical and psychosocial phenomena.

The first well-accepted model described is useful in a conceptualization of performance anxiety. This model by Lang, Miller and Levin (1988) views anxiety as the result of close interactions between three loosely connected components, that is, behavioral, physiological and cognitive/verbal systems. Although highly interactive, these three systems are also to some extent independent in that they are not equally sensitive (physiological systems are the least sensitive) to stress stimuli or across individuals and may respond differentially depending on the situation. Thus Craske and Craig (1984) applied this model to music performance anxiety; the results obtained supported Lang's theory.

Concordance among these three systems may be more likely when strong emotional responses are evoked and there is extreme duress; conversely discordance is most likely in situations of moderate or low duress (a person can have an elevated heart rate, but may not feel anxious).

It is still unclear as to which of these systems activates the others and the precise sequence of these events, that is, if fearful cognitions can trigger autonomic activity and subsequently influence cognitions and behavior; or, conversely, if autonomic reactivity occurs first and subsequently influences behavioral and cognitive reactions.

A more precise, yet global perspective, the biopsychosocial model of illness (Engle, 1977) provides a most relevant way of considering the potential, if not, ever-present, interaction among biomedical and psychosocial phenomena. The biopsychosocial perspective, based on systems theory, is "a way of organizing disparate data that permits clinicians and scientists to consider various points of view and integrate them into a coherent approach to the patient" (Goldmann, 1988, p. 2). This model also stresses that "an understanding of physical or mental health is incomplete if based solely on an understanding of chemical or molecular processes.... The biopsychosocial model offers an *integrationist* vision of the traditional division between mind and body. It regards such a cleavage as a false dichotomy obscuring man's inextricable organic unity. Any monist theory that denies either the reality of our bodies and their processes or the mind and its meanings and psychologic associations is equally unhelpful in our attempt to understand health and illness" (Goldman, 1988, p. 8).

Within this model, for example, the musician with "overuse" syndrome is not viewed as a victim of incorrect playing technique and perhaps genetic predisposition to muscular problems, or as a victim of overwhelming professional tensions. Both views are accurate, illuminating and not in the least mutually exclusive.

Of particular concern within this model are the "mechanisms by which stress precipitates and exacerbates illness, lowers host resistance, and perhaps causes some diseases" (Goldmann, 1988, p. 3). In addition, the relationship between "symbolic events, thoughts and feelings influence behavior and initiate pathologic processes in humans is a challenge for future research" (Goldmann, 1988, p. 3). Furthermore, the psychosocial aspects resulting from illness are of significance as one views the progress of the illness.

Current Biopsychosocial Trends in Performing Arts Medicine

Although the biopsychosocial perspective has yet to make a significant impact on the field of performing arts medicine, several authors have realized its importance, and several studies have demonstrated its potential (at times, serendipitously).

Brandfonbrener (1988) in commenting on a national survey of ICSOM musicians (Fishbein & Middlestadt, 1988) indicated that approximately 82% of the reported problems could be viewed as stress-related. Furthermore the standard of perfection to which musicians must adhere could be the cause of eventual mental and physical health problems, including drug abuse, eating disorders and self-destructive behaviors.

She further states, "the potential for psychological stress to affect the overall health of performers is so great that all of us concerned with their well-being must be thoroughly familiar with the psychological as well as the physiological risk factors " (Brandfonbrener, 1990, p. 1).

Lippin (1992) asks: "How can one separate the physical act of playing (music) from the impact of music on health?" (p. 31). He goes on: "Music medicine physicians often request that the patient bring his instrument to the medical session. This represents a unique opportunity not only to observe the patient's technique, but also to listen to the music for its diagnostic value where one could hear the pathology in a music work. As a nonmusic patient articulates his disease through his words, perhaps the musician articulates his diseased self through his music" (p. 32).

Lippman (1991) hopes that the fast-accumulating knowledge of the role of neuropeptides in the mood-correlated vulnerability of organs and tissues will soon generate novel, more scientific methods for the musician (p. 58).

Research studies in the field of music medicine generally fall into 3 categories:

1. Those that focus on either biomedical or psychosocial phenomena alone (ignoring the other area) (Bengston & Schutt, 1992; Cohen & Kupersmith, 1986; Dawson, 1988; Fry, 1986, 1988; Harmon, 1993; Larsson, Baum, Mudholkar, & Kollia, 1993; Lockwood, 1988; Manchester, 1988; Mathews & Mathews, 1993; Newmark & Hochberg, 1987; Newmark & Salmon, 1990; Simons, 1986; Wolfe, 1990, 1989; Zaza, 1992).

2. Those that assess each of these areas independently (Caldron, Calabrese, Clough, Lederman, Williams, & Leatherman, 1986; Raeburn, 1987a, 1987b; Hiner, et al., 1987 Middlestadt & Fishbein, 1988).

3. Those that assess each of these phenomena separately with an intent to correlate (Bayer, 1982; Marchant-Haycox & Wilson, 1992; Middlestadt & Fishbein, 1988; Wills & Cooper, 1987).

4. Studies that have as their direct purpose the prospective examination of the influence each of these has on the other (Frederickson & Gunnarsson, 1992).

The results of some of these studies is summarized below.

Bayer (1982) found that the two best predictors of ill-health in musicians were the presence of performance anxiety and problems with a stand partner.

In a survey of musculoskeletal problems of high-level musicians by Caldron, Calabrese, Clough, Lederman, Williams, and Leatherman (1986), respondents indicated a link between musculoskeletal problems and performance anxiety and related autonomic symptoms.

In a follow-up study of instrumentalists with upper extremity disorders, Knishkowy and Lederman (1986), respondents revealed that stress may have been a precipitating factor in their musculoskeletal problem; three individuals acknowledge stress as a major contributing factor. These three individuals had diagnoses of thoracic outlet syndrome.

Zaza (1993) lists nonmusical activities, stress and tensions as extrinsic factors of playing-related health problems.

In an analysis of 21 instrumental musicians with occupational cramp (Lederman, 1988), factors precipitating the occurrence of occupational cramp were reported. For 2 of the subjects examined, emotional stress was reported as a predisposing factor. Raeburn (1987a, 1987b) recommends that relationships between "characteristics/coping resources, sources of stress, coping and strain/illness" be investigated in future studies of (rock) musicians (p. 81).

Ziporyn (1984) emphasized that the more tension that is involved in playing, the more likely it will be that a physical injury will occur.

Montello, Coons, and Cantor (1990) used music therapy as an intervention for performance anxiety. The goal of treatment was to help the musicians focus on "their actual process of music-making—how the body, mind and emotions interact during musical preparation and performance" (p. 49).

Wills and Cooper (1987) found six variables that significantly predicted high psychosomatic health scores in musicians: Performance-related anxiety, poor physical work conditions, performance anxiety, work over/underload related to traveling, effects on social and family life and exercise. It is noted that performance-related anxiety (accounting for 18% of the variance) played a significant part in the health of the musician.

In a study of 2,212 ICSOM musicians (Middlestadt & Fishbein, 1998), a highly significant correlation was found between the perceived occupational stress and the number of musculoskeletal problems experienced; the higher the amount of stress, the higher the number of problems that were experienced. The correlation between stress and number of problems experienced is even higher for the nonmusculoskeletal types of problems. Individuals with the highest amount of stress also tried more treatments to alleviate problems. It was also found that 67% of respondents reported experiencing some musculoskeletal problems. The musculoskeletal problems most often associated with stress involved the back and neck. Increased levels of stress were also correlated with a variety of psychological problems. No differences in perceived stress were found between men and women; however, musicians in the middle age group (30–49) reported more stress than either their younger or older counterparts.

Frederickson & Gunnarsson (1992) studied behavioral, cardiovascular, neuroendocrine and subjective fear levels of low and high-anxious student musicians during public and private performances. Significant increases in epinephrine, norepinephrine and cortisol were found for both high- and low-anxious subjects during public performance. Also, significantly higher heart rates were found particularly for high-anxious subjects during public performance. Ratings of perceived distress increased in both groups of subjects during public performance.

Implications

Although the biopsychosocial perspective has yet to be adopted as a paradigm for performing arts medicine, it is the opinion of this author that it is the most viable one to date. By its inherent reliance on systems theory, it is capable of subsuming and embracing a variety of approaches, as it provides a logical means to explain musicians and artists, in all of their complexities, in a comprehensive manner, and to provide an understanding of them as they interact with the world. "Since general systems theory originates in biology, it can embrace both mind and body, the experiential and behavioral, and the individual and the social in its overall scheme of different levels and aspects of systems operating according to the same basic principles—the need for organization, interaction of parts, control mechanisms, and maintenance of boundaries" (Goldmann, 1988, p. 31).

The implications for research and treatment follow logically:

1. The word, "medicine" in the term, "performing arts medicine" should be changed (perhaps to "performing arts health") to reflect the interdisciplinary nature of the field as necessitated by the biopsychosocial perspective. This field should involve all professionals who can contribute knowledge regarding the biomedical and psychosocial aspects of the musician and his world; elitism should be avoided.

2. Specific categories of problems in "performing arts medicine" must be changed to reflect a re-conceptualization of the musician in biopsychosocial terms. The terminology describing problems should avoid reductionistic and unilateral thinking, for example, "musculoskeletal", etc.

3. The term, "performing arts health" would also elicit more appropriate associations with prevention (as opposed to only pathology).

4. The biopsychosocial perspective can embrace a wide variety of treatment approaches that can yield to scientific scrutiny. Reductionistic approaches, for example, "medical", "psychological", etc. should become more integrative.

5. There should be a concerted effort to broaden research efforts regarding the biopsychosocial aspects of musicianship. Research methodology should similarly be broadened to include qualitative as well as quantitative procedures.

6. There should be more systematic efforts among experts to interface and integrate knowledge in this area via conferences, publications, and collaborative research.

7. Efforts at prevention of performance-related problems need to be drastically escalated. An interesting model for prevention is described by Spaulding (1988) wherein musicians are educated to various scientific fields, including biopsychosocial perspectives. Musicians are encouraged to be active participants in their own health maintenance through various biopsychosocial strategies.

A biopsychosocial paradigm of "performing arts health" may serve to unify, broaden and increase knowledge and services for musicians, a group that is indispensable to all "systems" of society.

References

Bayer, L. J. (1982). The stress process in professional musicians: An exploratory study. (Doctoral dissertation, University of Cincinnati). *Dissertation Abstracts 43*(5) #DA8223023.

Bejjani, F. J., & Snow, B. S. (1990). Use of mood scores as indices of athletic character and stress reactivity among musicians. *Medical Problems of Performing Artists, 5*(1), 45–48.

Bengston, K. A., & Schutt, A. H. (1992). Upper extremity musculoskeletal problems in musicians: A follow-up survey. *Medical Problems of Performing Artists, 7*(2), 44–47.

Brandfonbrener, A. G. (1990a). Beta blockers in the treatment of performance anxiety. *Medical Problems of Performing Artists, 5*(1), 23–26.

Brandfonbrener, A. G. (1990b). Psychological issues in performing arts medicine. *Medical Problems of Performing Artists, 5*(1), 1.

Brandfonbrener, A. G. (1988). The price of perfection (Editorial). *Medical Problems of Performing Artists, 3*(1).

Caldron, P. H., Calabrese, L. H., Clough, J. D., Lederman, R. L., Williams, G., Leatherman, J. (1986) A survey of musculoskeletal problems encountered in high-level musicians. *Medical Problems of Performing Artists, 1*(4), 136–139.

Clark, D. B., & Agras, W. S. (1991). The assessment and treatment of performance anxiety in musicians. *American Journal of Psychiatry, 148*(5), 598–605.

Cohen, B. J., & Kupersmith, J. R. (1986). A study of SCL-90 scores of 87 performing artists seeking psychotherapy. *Medical Problems of Performing Artists, 1*(4), 140–142.

Cooper, C. L., & Wills, G. I. (1989). Popular musicians under pressure. *Psychology of Music, 17,* 22–36.

Craske, M. G., & Craig, K. (1984). Musical performance anxiety: The three systems model and self-efficacy theory. *Behavior Research and Therapy, 22,* 267–280.

Dawson, W. J. (1988). Hand and upper extremity problems in musicians: Epidemiology and diagnosis. *Medical Problems of Performing Artists, 3*(1), 19–22.

Dews, C. L. B., & Williams, M. S. (1989). Student musicians' personality styles, stresses and coping patterns. *Psychology of Music, 17,* 37–47.

Eliot, G. R., & Eisdorfer, C. (1982). *Stress and human health.* New York: Springer Verlag.

Engel, G. L. (1977). The need for a new medical model: A challenge for biomedicine. *Science, 196,* 129.

Fishbein, M., & Middlestadt, S. E. (1988). Medical problems among ICSOM musicians: Overview of a national survey. *Medical Problems of Performing Artists, 3*(1), 1–8.

Frederickson, M., & Gunnarsson, R. (1992). Psychobiology of stage fright: The effect of public performance on neuroendocrine, cardiovascular and subjective reactions. *Biological Psychology, 33,* 51–61.

Fry, H. J. H. (1988). Music-related overuse in secondary schools. *Medical Problems of Performing Artists, 3*(4), 133–134.

Fry, H. J. H. (1986). Incidence of overuse syndrome in the symphony orchestra. *Medical Problems of Performing Artists, 1*(2), 51–55.

Goldmann, H. H. (1988). *Review of general psychiatry* (2nd ed.). Norwalk, CT: Appleton & Lange.

Harmon, S. (1993). Medical problems of marching musicians. *Medical Problems of Performing Artists, 8*(4), 132–135.

Hiner, S. L., Brandt, K. D., Katz, B. P., French, R. N., Jr., Beczkiewicz, T. J., (1987). Performance-related medical problems among premier violinists. *Medical Problems of Performing Artists, 2*(2), 67–71.

Kanefeld, E. L. (1990). Psychological services at the Juilliard School. *Medical Problems of Performing Artists, 5*(1), 41–44.

Kemp, A. (1981), The personality structure of a musician I: Identifying a profile of traits for the performer. *Psychology of Music, 9,* 3–14.

Knishkowy, B., & Lederman, R. J. (1986). Instrumental musicians with upper extremity disorders. *Medical Problems of Performing Artists, 1*(3), 85–89.

Lang, P. J., Miller, G. A., & Levin, D. (1988). Anxiety and fear. In R. J. Davidson, G. E. Schwartz, & D. Shapiro (Eds.), *Consciousness and self-regulation* (pp. 123–151). New York: Plenum.

Larsson, L. G., Baum, J., Mudholkar, G. S., & Kollia, G. D. (1993). Nature and impact of musculoskeletal problems in a population of musicians. *Medical Problems of Performing Artists, 8*(3), 73–76.

Lederman, R. J. (1988). Occupational cramp in instrumental musicians. *Medical Problems of Performing Artists, 3*(2), 45–51.

Lehrer, P. M. (1988). The causes and cures of performance anxiety: A review of the psychological literature. In F. L. Roehmann & F. R. Wilson (Eds.), *The biology of music making: Proceedings of the 1984 Denver conference* (pp. 32–46). St. Louis: MMB Music.

Lehrer, P., Goldman, N. S., Strommen, E. F. (1990). A principal components assessment of performance anxiety among musicians. *Medical Problems of Performing Artists, 5* (1), 12–18.

Lippin, R. (1992). MusicMedicine: The case for a holistic model. In R. Spintge & R. Droh (Eds.), *MusicMedicine* (pp. 30–38). St. Louis: MMB Music.

Lippman, H. (1991). A fresh look at the overuse syndromes in musical performers: Is "overuse" overused? *Medical Problems of Performing Artists, 6*(2) 57–60.

Lockwood, A. (1988). Medical problems in secondary school-aged musicians. *Medical Problems of Performing Artists, 3*(4), 129–132.

Manchester, R. A. (1988). The incidence of hand problems in music students. *Medical Problems of Performing Artists, 3*(1), 15–18.

Maranto, C. D. (1992). Music therapy in the treatment of performance anxiety in musicians. In R. Spintge & R. Droh (Eds.), *MusicMedicine* (pp. 273–283). St. Louis: MMB Music.

Maranto, C. D. (1989). *Performance anxiety: A meta-analysis of experimental research and clinical implications.* Paper presented at the 7th Annual Symposium on medical problems of musicians and dancers, Snowmass, Colorado, July 1989.

Marchant-Haycox, S. E., & Wilson, G. D. (1992). Personality and stress in performing artists. *Personality and Individual Differences, 13,* 1061–1068.

Mathews, J. A., & Mathews, W. (1993). A survey of rheumatic disorders in orchestral musicians. *Medical Problems of Performing Artists, 8*(1), 14–15.

Meichenbaum, D. (1972). Cognitive modification of test anxious college students. *Journal of Clinical Psychology, 39,* 370–378.

Meichenbaum, D. (1993). Stress inoculation training: A 20-year update. In P. Lehrer & R. Woolfolk (Eds.), *Principles and practice of stress management* (pp. 373–406). New York: The Guilford Press.

Middlestadt, S. E., & Fishbein, M. (1988). Health and occupational correlates of perceived occupational stress in symphony orchestra musicians. *Journal of Occupational Medicine, 30,* 687–692.

Middlestadt, S. E., & Fishbein, M. (1989). The prevalence of severe musculoskeletal problems among male and female symphony orchestra string players. *Medical Problems of Performing Artists, 4*(1), 41–48.

Montello, L., Coons, E. E., & Kantor, J. (1990). The use of group music therapy as a treatment for musical performance stress. *Medical Problems of Performing Artists, 5*(1), 49–57.

Morris, L. W., & Liebert, R. M. (1970). Relationship of cognitive and emotional components of test anxiety to physiological arousal and academic performance. *Journal of Consulting and Clinical Psychology, 35,* 332–337.

Nagel, J. J. (1990). Performance anxiety and the performing musician: A fear of failure or a fear of success? *Medical Problems of Performing Artists, 5*(1), 37–40.

Newmark, J., & Hochberg, F. H. (1987). "Doctor, it hurts when I play": Painful disorders among instrumental musicians. *Medical Problems of Performing Artists, 2*(3), 93–98.

Newmark, J., & Salmon. P. (1990). Playing-related complaints in nonclassical instrumentalists: A pilot questionnaire study. *Medical Problems of Performing Artists, 5*(3), 106–108.

Ostwald, P. F. (1992). Psychodynamics of musicians: The relationship of performers to their musical instruments. *Medical Problems of Performing Artists, 7*(4), 110–113.

Ostwald, P. F. (1987). Psychotherapeutic strategies in the treatment of performing artists, *Medical Problems of Performing Artists, 2*(4), 131–136.

Plaut, E. A. (1988). Psychotherapy of performance anxiety. *Medical Problems of Performing Artists, 3*(3), 113–118.

Raeburn, S. D. (1987a). Occupational stress and coping in a sample of professional rock musicians (Part 1). *Medical Problems of Performing Artists, 2*(2), 41–48.

Raeburn, S. D. (1987b). Occupational stress and coping in a sample of professional rock musicians (Part 2). *Medical Problems of Performing Artists, 2*(3), 77–82.

Salmon, P. G. (1990). A psychological perspective on musical performance anxiety: A review of the literature. *Medical Problems of Performing Artists, 5*(1), 2–11.

Simons, H. (1986). Health and the choral conductor. *Medical Problems of Performing Artists, 1*(2), 56–57.

Steptoe, A. (1983). The relationship between tension and the quality of musical performance. *Journal of the International Society for the Study of Tension in Performance, 1,* 12–22.

Steptoe, A., Fidler, H. (1987). Stage fright in orchestral musicians: A study of cognitive and behavioral strategies in performance anxiety. *British Journal of Psychology, 78,* 241–249.

Theorell, T. (in press). Personal control at work and health. In A. Steptoe & A. Appels (Eds.), *Stress, personal control and health.* Chichester: John Wiley.

Wesner, R. B., Noyes, R. Jr., & Davis, T. L. (1990). The occurrence of performance anxiety among musicians. *Journal of Affective Disorders, 18,* 177–185.

Wills, G. I., & Cooper, C. L. (1984). Pressures on professional musicians. *Leadership and Organization Development Journal, 5,* 17–20.

Wills, G. I., & Cooper, C. L. (1987). Stress and professional popular musicians. *Stress Medicine, 3,* 267–274.

Wolfe, M. L. (1990). Coping with musical performance anxiety: Problem-focused and emotion- focused strategies. *Medical Problems of Performing Artists, 5*(1), 33–36.

Wolfe, M. L. (1990). Relationships between dimensions of musical performance anxiety and behavioral coping strategies. *Medical Problems of Performing Artists, 5*(4), 139–145.

Wolfe, M. L. (1989). Correlates of adaptive and maladaptive musical performance anxiety. *Medical Problems of Performing Artists, 4*(1), 49–56.

Yerkes, R., & Dodson, J. (1908). The relationship of strength of stimulus to rapidity of habit forming. *Journal of Comparative Neurology and Physiology, 18,* 459–482.

Zaza, C. (1993). Prevention of musicians' playing-related health problems: Rationale and recommendations for action. *Medical Problems of Performing Artists, 8*(4), 117–121.

Zaza, C. (1992). Playing-related health problems at a Canadian music school. *Medical Problems of Performing Artists, 7*(2), 48–51.

Ziporyn, T. (1984). Pianist's cramp to stage fright: The medical side of music-making. *Journal of the American Medical Association, 252* 985–989.

A PSYCHOPHYSIOLOGICAL PROFILE RELATED TO OVERUSE INJURIES IN UNIVERSITY MUSICIANS

Revis Ann Massey

Introduction

Background and Related Literature

Overuse injuries are becoming more commonly experienced and diagnosed in performing artists just as they have been in the past among athletes and people in other occupations. Most research already conducted with overuse injuries among performing musicians has focused on the physiological or associated psychological problems. Overuse syndrome is identified by pain and loss of function in repetitively used muscles and ligaments that often involves the psychological as well as the physical well-being of the musician. Until recently, the relationships among the physiological and the psychological or emotional factors have been overlooked or ignored in treating overuse injuries.

In a survey by the International Conference of Symphony and Opera Musicians, 76% of the responding membership reported at least one medical problem they considered to be severe in terms of the effect on performance (Middlestadt & Fishbein, 1988). According to Lockwood (1989), surveys of performing musicians indicate that almost half experience playing-related medical problems, which potentially threaten or end their careers.

In a recent study at Brigham Young University (Pratt, Jessop, & Niemann, 1992), 87% of the 246 music majors surveyed reported some degree of performance-related pain. Fifty-six of these 128 students reported a reliance on themselves for treatment, after which they looked to relaxation (47%) and their teachers (43%) as the second and third treatment modes. Most reported avoidance of professional medical help.

Many of the medical and psychiatric problems of musicians are related to performance practices. Psychiatric disorders, even if not totally disabling, may have significant effects on musical performance (Clark, 1989). Performance anxiety, the most common psychological problem in musicians, has been reported to increase the incidence of overuse. It was reported to be the most common psychological problem in musicians. Amateur musicians were shown to have relatively more performance anxiety than professionals. In a survey of 48 symphony orchestras of the International Conference of Symphony and Opera Musicians (ICSOM), 39% of the 2,212 musicians who responded to the questionnaire reported some psychological problems. Ostwald and Avery (as cited in Sataloff, Brandfonbrener, and Lederman, 1991) estimated that up to 50% of the patients seen in general medical clinics are afflicted with mental, emotional, or personality problems.

Certain aspects of the musician's life-style may relate to possible risk factors for overuse. One hundred sixty-two performing musicians were surveyed by Wolfe (1990) to examine the relationships between adaptive and maladaptive musical performance anxiety and behavioral strategies used to manage this anxiety. Those with high levels of maladaptive anxiety generally reported high levels of state anxiety, shown as disruptive cognitive or autonomic responses while performing and also tended to avoid using coping strategies. There are trends seen throughout the literature:

1. Women appear to be at greater risk to develop overuse injury.

2. Players of certain instruments, such as piano, harp, violin, flute, and clarinet, have higher incidence of overuse than players of other instruments.

3. Areas of the body that seem to be injured most often are shoulders, neck area, wrists and hands, and elbows.

4. Performance anxiety plays a vital role in a musician's career as well as in the development of overuse.

5. Students have added stress of academic and financial problems.

For musicians who develop an overuse injury, therapies are effective in helping. Clark (1989) recommends a two-stage treatment:

1. control of inflammation with medication and rest, and
2. a graded return to practice.

Purpose and Rationale

The purpose of this study was to establish an overall psychophysiological profile (self-report) of student musicians in university settings as related to overuse injuries. The diagnostic and explanatory terms that follow were defined specifically for this study. The definitions for performance anxiety and overuse syndrome were taken from Ostwald and Avery (as cited in Sataloff, Brandfonbrener, & Lederman, 1991), Fry (1986), Fry (1988), Steptoe (1989), and Clark (1989). The diagnostic terms were identified in consultation with a physician who specializes in orthopedic surgery (Anderson, 1992).

Performance anxiety is defined as intense stage fright, fear, or severe apprehension on stage or in rehearsal. *Overuse syndrome* is a collective term to describe a group of disorders associated with damage to tissues, which occurs when activity exceeds the biological or anatomical limits, producing a painful condition of the hand and upper limb. *Carpal tunnel syndrome* is defined as pressure on the median nerve at the level of the carpal tunnel (wrist), the most common compression neuropathy of the upper extremity. *Cubital tunnel syndrome* is pressure on the ulnar nerve at or near the elbow joint. *Lateral epicondylitis (tennis elbow)* is pain at or near the lateral epicondyle at the elbow where the extensor muscles attach. *Dorsal wrist/hand tendinitis* is defined as pain along the course of the extensor tendons at or near the extensor retinaculum. *Muscle fatigue* is gradual increase in pain in a muscle that results from prolonged use of that muscle. *Paracervical muscle fatigue* is the gradual increase in pain in the muscles in or surrounding the shoulder and neck area. *Parascapular muscle fatigue* is the gradual increase in pain in the muscles in or surrounding the shoulder blade area.

Method

Subjects and Setting

The 278 subjects included 166 undergraduate and graduate music students from the Meadows School of the Arts at Southern Methodist University (SMU) in Dallas, Texas, and 112 undergraduate, graduate, and postgraduate music students from The University of Oklahoma (OU) in Norman, Oklahoma. They were selected randomly through music and ensemble classes at both universities. Although 278 questionnaires were returned, 77 (completed by voice students) were not used for analysis because the questionnaire was designed for problems among instrumentalists. Therefore, usable data came from a total of 201 questionnaires (111 SMU students and 90 OU students). Subjects ranged in age from 17 to 53 years.

Procedure

The preliminary test was first given to SMU students in the Fall of 1991 in a free health clinic and then later distributed at SMU and OU. To ensure confidentiality, each questionnaire was assigned a number to replace the name. The evaluation of the data was taken directly from the questionnaire. Frequency distribution and percentages were gained from analysis of each of the three profile domains:

1. A life-style/personal profile.
2. A student/musical profile.
3. The psychological symptoms in relationship to the physiological profile, as found in the diagnostic profile. The physiological profile included the symptoms from the diagnostic profile that contributed to the overall diagnosis of overuse.

For purposes of analysis, each subject was placed according to each individual diagnosis in one of two categories:

1. Subjects having overuse injuries, or
2. Subjects without overuse injuries.

Those having overuse were placed into subcategories:

1. Muscle fatigue only.
2. Tendinitis only.
3. Peripheral nerve damage only.
4. Both Tendinitis and Peripheral nerve damage.

Results and Conclusions

Twenty-six (23%) of 111 subjects diagnosed with overuse according to the diagnostic questions on the survey reported a previous diagnosis by a physician. In the Peripheral nerve damage group, 33% of those diagnosed through the survey had been diagnosed previously. In the Tendinitis group, 31% of those diagnosed through the survey had been diagnosed previously. In the Muscle fatigue group, 7% of those diagnosed through the survey had been diagnosed previously by a physician. Table 1 assigns subjects to general categories of diagnosis as determined by the diagnostic profile of the questionnaire.

Table 1. *Evidence of Overuse Syndrome*

DIAGNOSTIC GROUP	SUBJECTS	
	Number	Percent
Muscle fatigue only	55	27.36
Tendinitis only	42	20.90
Peripheral nerve damage only	7	3.48
Tendinitis and Peripheral nerve damage	7	3.48
Overuse Total	111	55.22
No overuse	90	44.78
Total	201	100.00

Results showed that 44.78% of the total subjects reported no overuse with no overlaps in reporting the diagnoses. The "Muscle fatigue only" category is derived from the diagnoses of (a) Muscle fatigue, (b) Paracervical muscle fatigue, and (c) Parascapular muscle fatigue; those subjects placed in this category presented with diagnostic symptoms for one of these three disorders. The "Tendinitis only" category is derived from the diagnoses of Dorsal wrist/hand tendinitis and Lateral epicondylitis (tennis elbow); to be placed in this category, the subjects showed diagnostic symptoms for one of these two disorders. The "Peripheral nerve damage only" category is devised from the diagnoses of Carpal tunnel syndrome and Cubital tunnel syndrome; assignment to this category required diagnostic symptoms for one of these two disorders. The category labeled "Tendinitis and Peripheral nerve damage" represents subjects who presented with symptoms of these disorders. Most subjects were in the 17–26 year-old group (82.09%). Of the total subjects, 86 were male and 115 were female with 40.30% of the females reporting overuse. Among the five ethnic groups, 20 were Asian, 11 Black, 229 Caucasian, 11 Hispanic, and 7 Other.

Subjects who exercised 20 minutes three times a week and also reported overuse constituted the largest group in the health habits category. Of the four religious preferences, most of the subjects were Protestant or Other. Most subjects did pray or meditate.

Of those who reported major life changes in the last year, the largest group also reported overuse. Of those reporting a strong support system, the largest group, 44.78% also reported overuse. Most reported being comfortable in a large group and being comfortable alone. Most reported the level of communication with a spouse or close friend as Well.

Table 2. *Academic Data Profile*

	Total	OVERUSE		NO OVERUSE	
QUESTION	Number	Number	Percent	Number	Percent
Academic Degree					
Cert. 1	4	1	25.00	3	75.00
Cert. 2	5	1	20.00	4	80.00
Cert. 3	1	1	100.00	0	00.00
UG 1	37	22	59.46	15	40.54
UG 2	40	28	70.00	12	30.00
UG 3	23	12	52.17	11	47.83
UG 4	17	9	52.94	8	47.06
UG 5	7	5	71.43	2	28.57
Grad. 1	28	14	50.00	14	50.00
Grad. 2	21	10	27.62	11	52.38
Grad. 3	5	1	20.00	4	80.00
Grad. 4	2	1	50.00	1	50.00
Postgrad	11	6	54.55	5	45.45

(table continues)

Table 2 (continued)

QUESTION	Total Number	OVERUSE Number	OVERUSE Percent	NO OVERUSE Number	NO OVERUSE Percent
Academic Major (Music)					
Composition	8	3	37.50	5	62.50
Conducting	3	1	33.33	2	66.67
Education	36	17	47.22	19	52.78
Double Major	31	19	61.29	12	38.71
History	1	1	100.00	0	00.00
Piano Pedagogy	13	8	61.54	5	38.46
Performance	90	51	56.67	39	43.33
Theory	3	3	100.00	0	00.00
Music Therapy	13	6	46.15	7	53.85
Credit hours enrolled					
0–1	2	1	.51	1	.51
2–5	17	7	3.48	10	4.97
6–9	40	20	9.95	20	9.95
10–12	27	13	6.46	14	6.96
13–15	51	27	13.44	24	11.93
16–18	61	42	20.88	19	9.45
19+	3	1	.51	2	1.00
Hours of study each week					
0–6	87	50	24.88	37	18.90
7–14	79	40	19.90	39	19.40
15–21	25	16	7.96	9	4.48
22+	9	5	2.49	4	1.99
Time of day for most study					
Morning	14	6	2.99	8	5.96
Afternoon	19	8	3.98	11	5.47
Evening	52	30	14.93	22	10.95
Late (night)	112	67	33.33	45	22.39
Listen to music while studying					
Yes	93	54	26.87	39	19.40
No	108	57	28.36	51	25.37

Table 2 shows the academic data and the incidence of overuse injuries. In reporting the results for the questions concerning academic degree and academic major, each answer has a possible total of 100%. The following academic levels had higher percentages of overuse: Undergraduate 1, 2, 3, 4, 5, and Postgraduate. The following academic majors had higher percentages of overuse: Double Major, Music History, Piano Pedagogy, Music Performance, and Music Theory. Students enrolled in 16–18 credit hours reported the greatest difference in overuse. More of those who studied late at night reported overuse.

Table 3 (below) shows the instrument history and the incidence of overuse injuries. Each answer has a possible total of 100%. The piano (n = 65) and violin (n = 21) (the largest groups) reported more overuse. Most subjects practiced late at night. The largest difference in the incidence of overuse was in the 10+ group. More subjects reported not being uncomfortable performing in a group. However the greatest difference in incidence of overuse was with those who reported discomfort performing in a group.

Each principal instrument group is described (Table 4) by the incidence of an overall diagnosis of overuse. The percentage of overuse in each group is given according to the following categories: No overuse, Muscle fatigue, Tendinitis, Peripheral nerve damage, Tendinitis and Peripheral nerve damage. Each instrument group totals 100%. In each group, the highest percentage is in the No overuse category. Woodwinds appear to have the lowest incidence of overuse, a lower percentage of Muscle fatigue and higher percentage of Tendinitis than all other groups except Brass that reported 25% in the Tendinitis diagnosis.

Table 3. *Instrument History Profile*

QUESTION	Total Number	OVERUSE Number	OVERUSE Percent	NO OVERUSE Number	NO OVERUSE Percent
Principal instrument					
Brass					
Baritone Horn	2	2	100.00	0	00.00
French Horn	11	8	72.73	3	27.27
Trombone	3	1	33.33	2	66.67
Trumpet	14	6	42.86	8	57.14
Tuba	3	1	33.33	2	66.67
Total	33	18	55	15	45
String					
Cello	8	6	75.00	2	25.00
Double Bass	3	1	33.33	2	66.67
Guitar	10	6	60.00	4	40.00
Viola	6	4	66.67	2	33.33
Violin	21	12	57.14	9	42.86
Total	48	29	60	19	40
Woodwind					
Bassoon	6	2	33.33	4	66.67
Clarinet	14	6	42.86	8	57.14
Flute	10	7	70.00	3	30.00
Oboe	4	3	75.00	1	25.00
Saxophone	3	1	33.33	2	66.67
Total	37	19	51	18	49

(table continues)

Table 3 (continued)

QUESTION	Total Number	OVERUSE Number	OVERUSE Percent	NO OVERUSE Number	NO OVERUSE Percent
Other					
Harp	1	1	100.00	0	00.00
Organ	2	0	00.00	2	100.00
Percussion	15	9	60.00	6	40.00
Piano	65	35	53.85	30	46.15
Total	83	45	54	38	46
Years playing principal instrument					
1–12	123	72	35.83	51	25.36
13–23	61	32	15.92	29	14.43
24–34	12	4	1.99	8	3.98
35–46	5	3	1.49	2	1.00
Teachers of principal instrument					
1–3	102	57	28.37	45	22.38
4–6	76	42	20.89	34	16.91
7–8	17	8	3.98	9	4.48
9–14	6	4	1.99	2	1.00

Table 4. *Principal Instrument Groups and Overall Diagnoses*

DIAGNOSTIC GROUP	BRASS n	BRASS %	STRINGS n	STRINGS %	WOODWINDS n	WOODWINDS %	OTHER n	OTHER %
No overuse	15	45	19	40	18	49	38	46
Muscle fatigue	10	30	17	35	6	16	22	26
Tendinitis	8	25	9	19	9	24	16	19
Peripheral nerve damage	0	0	2	4	2	5.5	3	4
Tendinitis and Peripheral nerve damage	0	0	1	2	2	5.5	4	5
TOTAL ($N = 201$)	33	100	48	100	37	100	83	100

For overall diagnosis of overuse, the string group reported 44% with No overuse, 35% with Muscle fatigue, and 19% with Tendinitis. The largest specific diagnosis was Parascapular muscle fatigue (40%). The next largest group was Paracervical muscle fatigue (21%). For overall diagnosis of overuse, the Woodwind group reported 49% with No overuse, 24% with Tendinitis, and 16% with Muscle fatigue. The largest specific diagnoses after No overuse were Parascapular muscle fatigue (30%) and Dorsal wrist/hand tendinitis (30%). The next largest group was Paracervical muscle fatigue (27%). For overall diagnosis of overuse, the brass group reported 45% with No overuse, 30% with Muscle fatigue, and 25% with Tendinitis. The largest specific diagnosis after No overuse was Paracervical muscle fatigue (33%). The next largest group was Parascapular muscle fatigue (24%). For overall diagnosis of overuse, the Other instrument group reported 46% with No overuse, 26% with Muscle fatigue, and 19% with Tendinitis.

String and woodwind players reported the highest stress levels according to the scale in this study. The stress level scale was devised from these five items on the questionnaire:

1. Hours of study.
2. Hours of ensemble rehearsal.
3. Hours of practice.
4. Increase in practice time.
5. Job.

Each subject had the possibility of scoring from 0–5 points. A point was given for 15+ hours of study each week, 7+ hours of ensemble rehearsal each week, 4+ hours of practice each day, if practice time had increased, and if the subject had a job along with school. The subjects were placed in their principal instrument group for analysis.

The Other Instruments group consisting of the harp, organ, piano, and percussion has the most number of subjects attributable to the large number of pianists completing the survey. This group has more Overuse than No Overuse.

Table 5. *Performance Anxiety Profile*

	Total	OVERUSE		NO OVERUSE	
QUESTION	Number	Number	Percent	Number	Percent
Uncomfortable performing (group)					
Yes	48	32	15.92	16	7.96
No	153	79	39.31	74	36.81
(alone)					
Yes	69	42	20.90	27	13.43
No	132	69	34.33	63	31.34
Performance anxiety or stage fright					
Yes	159	87	43.29	72	35.81
No	42	24	11.94	18	8.96
During recital: Cold hands					
Yes	100	60	29.85	40	19.90
No	101	51	25.38	50	24.87
Sweaty hands					
Yes	135	81	40.31	54	26.86
No	66	30	14.92	36	17.91

(table continues)

Table 5 (continued)

QUESTION	Total Number	OVERUSE		NO OVERUSE	
		Number	Percent	Number	Percent
Interfering thoughts					
Yes	127	75	37.32	52	25.86
No	74	36	17.91	38	18.91
Mind goes blank					
Yes	85	52	25.88	33	16.41
No	116	59	29.35	57	28.36

The performance anxiety scale (Table 5) was devised from the seven items on the performance anxiety profile of the questionnaire. Each subject, placed in a principal instrument group, had a possible score from 0–7 points, receiving one point for each Yes answer.

Concerning principal instrument groups and performance anxiety levels (a possible seven points), the brass players (25%) scored their highest number of points at five. The brass players seemed to have experienced greater performance anxiety, with other instrument players and woodwinds behind them. Concerning principal instrument groups and stress levels (a possible five points), the string players scored their highest number at three points. Woodwind players also scored their highest number at three points.

The Histogram below shows the number of subjects involved in each of the principal instruments groups. The following principal instruments reported a higher percentage of Overuse than No overuse: Baritone horn ($n = 2$) French horn ($n = 11$), cello ($n = 8$), guitar ($n = 10$), viola ($n = 6$), violin ($n = 21$), flute ($n = 10$), oboe ($n = 4$), harp ($n = 1$), percussion ($n = 15$), and piano ($n = 65$). Those playing 1–12 years and those with 1–3 teachers of their principal instrument had the highest percentage of overuse.

There seems to be no difference between the psychological means and modes of the two groups. Further research is needed to determine if the difference in mean averages is related to psychological factors, or if the number of subjects within groups was a determining factor. Most had not seen a doctor in the last 2 months, were not on the university health plan, and did not consider their condition to be a result of playing their instrument.

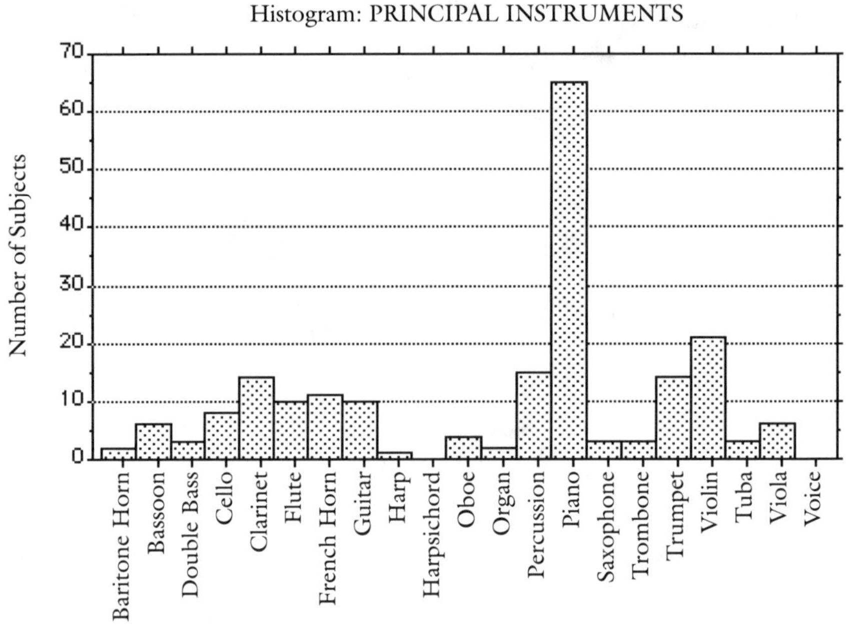

Figure 1. Number of Subjects by Instrument

Summary

The purpose of this study was to establish an overall psychophysiological profile of student musicians in university settings as related to overuse injuries that affect instrumental performance. Subjects, selected from SMU and OU, totaled 278, but only 201 subjects (111 from SMU and 90 from OU) were used for the results. A frequency distribution among categories was used to determine the profile.

Due to the specific population of student musicians involved in this study, the results cannot be reasonably generalized to include professional or amateur musicians who are not also music students. Since there were two universities represented in the study, results can be more easily generalized to other university musicians.

A summary of the life-style/personal profile found in this study of students reporting more evidence of overuse is as follows: 17–26 years old, female, Caucasian, single, raised by both parents, exercising 20 minutes three times a week, not active in a sport, consuming zero to two beers a week, reporting major life changes in the last year, working, reporting no mental illness or counseling in last 5 years, and reporting a strong support system.

Within the student/musical profile, those reporting more overuse are as follows: Undergraduate 1–5 and Postgraduate, double major, music history major, piano pedagogy major, music performance major, and music theory major, 16–18 credit hours, studying 15–21 hours a week, and studying late at night. The following instruments reported the highest degree of overuse: baritone horn, French horn, cello, guitar, viola, violin, flute, oboe, harp, piano, and percussion. Included are those who increased practice time, reported 10+ hours of ensemble rehearsal, reported performance anxiety or stage fright, sweaty hands, interfering thoughts, and mind going blank during performance. Strings reported the highest percentage with overuse and Brass was the second highest group. Brass also had the highest performance anxiety scale. Strings and woodwinds had the highest stress level scales.

Since this study was descriptive and exploratory in nature, the results do not determine cause and effect related to physiological or psychological problems of student musicians, but do show relationships and areas for further research and development. Based on the data gathered from the Performing Arts Medicine Questionnaire, there did not seem to be a relationship between the number of psychological or emotional symptoms reported in the psychological profile and the incidence of overuse injuries. However, there did seem to be a relationship between performance anxiety and overuse, which supports the related literature.

Recommendations

Further research of student musicians is recommended to more clearly define and answer the questions concerning overuse injuries. Based on the large number of responses and the high percentage of overuse among these university musicians, such continued research is recommended. Prevention and treatment of the emotional, as well as the physical, components of overuse are becoming more understood. As research in music therapy with overuse injuries is new and limited, further research using music and imagery, music-assisted breathing and relaxation, music-assisted biofeedback, and improvisational music therapy as treatment for performance-related problems is important.

Detailed intake questions, including the kind of exercise (conditioning or stretching), any sports in which the subject is involved, exactly what life changes have occurred in the last year and how significant these changes were to the subject, a detailed description of the subject's diet, and a prior and recent significant substance use and prescription medication intake are needed. A complete medical history of the subject should be taken, including major physical and mental illness within the immediate family, such as stroke, cancer, heart disease, psychosomatic disorders, epilepsy or seizures, depression, or anxiety. A psychological assessment of the subject, including an anxiety and depression test, is important for a complete diagnosis of the emotional state of the subject. Specific studies with the focus on the student's technique, posture, and education on the instrument by the private teacher would determine any relationships between these variables and the incidence of overuse. Research is recommended to determine any relationships between weight of the instrument and overuse. These more specific investigations will allow for individual attention of variables that were only studied briefly in this research.

Acknowledgment

This paper was the result of a Master's Thesis completed at Southern Methodist University under the following committee: Charles T. Eagle, Kaja Jensen, Dennis Bowers, and Bill Anderson.

References

Abel, J. L., & Larkin, K. T. (1990). Anticipation of performance among musicians: Physiological arousal, confidence, and state-anxiety. *Psychology of Music, 18,* 171–182.

Barney Dews, C., & Williams, M. (1989). Student musicians' personality styles, stresses, and coping patterns. *Psychology of Music, 17,* 37–47.

Caldron, P., Calabrese, L., Lederman, R., Clough, J. D., Stulberg, B., & Bergfield, J. (1985). A survey of musculoskeletal problems encountered in high-level musicians. *Arthritis and Rheumatism, 28 (Suppl 4)*, S97.

Clark, D. B. (1989). Performance-related medical and psychological disorders in instrumental musicians. *Annals of Behavioral Medicine, 2(1)*, 28–34.

Cohen, B., & Kupersmith, J. (1986, December). A study of SCL-90 scores of 87 performing artists seeking psychotherapy. *Medical Problems of Performing Artists*, 140–142.

Dawson, D. J. (1990, September). Upper extremity injuries in high-level instrumentalists: An end-result study. *Medical Problems of Performing Artists*, 109–112.

Dawson, W. J. (1988, March). Hand and upper extremity problems in musicians: Epidemiology and diagnosis. *Medical Problems of Performing Artists*, 19–22.

Fry, H. (1988). The Treatment of Overuse Syndrome in Musicians. Results in 175 Patients. *Journal of the Royal Society of Medicine, 81*, 572–575.

Fry, H. J., Ross, P., & Rutherford, M. (1988, December). Music-related overuse in secondary schools. *Medical Problems of Performing Artists*, 133–134.

Goodman, G., & Staz, S. (1989, March). Occupational therapy for musicians with upper extremity overuse syndrome: Patient perceptions regarding effectiveness of treatment. *Medical Problems of Performing Artists*, 9–14.

Harding, D. C., Brandy, K. D., & Hillberry, B. M. (1989, September). Minimization of finger joint forces and tendon tensions in pianists. *Medical Problems of Performing Artists*, 103–108.

Lederman, R. J. (1989). Peripheral nerve disorders in instrumentalists. *Annals of Neurology, 26 (5)*, 640–646.

Lederman, R. J., & Calabrese, L. H. (1986, March). Overuse syndromes in instrumentalists. *Medical Problems of Performing Artists*, 7–11.

Lockwood, A. H. (1989, January). Medical problems of musicians. *The New England Journal of Medicine*, 221–226.

Manchester, R. A. (1988, March). The incidence of hand problems in music students. *Medical Problems of Performing Artists*, 15–18.

Manchester, R., & Lustik, S. (1989, June). The short-term outcome of hand problems in music students. *Medical Problems of Performing Artists*, 95–96.

Middlestadt, S. E., & Fishbein, M. (1988). Health and occupational correlates of perceived occupational stress in symphony orchestra musicians. *Journal of Occupational Medicine, 30(9)*, 687–691.

Newmark, J., & Lederman, R. (1987, December). Practice doesn't necessarily make perfect: Incidence of overuse syndromes in amateur instrumentalists. *Medical Problems of Performing Artists*, 142–144.

Newmark, J., & Salmon, P. (1990, September). Playing-related complaints in nonclassical instrumentalists: A pilot questionnaire survey. *Medical Problems of Performing Artists*, 106–108.

Pratt, R., Jessop, S., & Niemann, B. (1992). Performance-related disorders among music majors at Brigham Young University. *International Journal of Arts Medicine, 1(2)*, 7–20.

Sataloff, R., Brandfonbrener, A., & Lederman, R. (Eds.). (1991). *Textbook of performing arts medicine*. New York: Raven Press.

Steptoe, A. (1989). Stress, coping and stage fright in professional musicians. *Psychology of Music, 17*, 3–11.

Steptoe, A., & Fidler, H. (1987). Stage fright in orchestral musicians: a study of cognitive and behavioural strategies in performance anxiety. *British Journal of Psychology, 78*, 241–249.

Wolfe, M. L. (1989, March). Correlates of adaptive and maladaptive musical performance anxiety. *Medical Problems of Performing Artists*, 49–56.

Wolfe, M. L. (1990, December). Relationships between dimensions of musical performance anxiety and behavioral coping strategies. *Medical Problems of Performing Artists*, 139–144.

PERFORMING ARTS MEDICINE QUESTIONNAIRE

DEMOGRAPHIC PROFILE

DATE TODAY: ____________________ ID#: ____________________________

NAME: __________________________ PHONE: ________________________

NAME OF COLLEGE OR UNIVERSITY: ________________________________

CITY: ________________________ STATE: ________ ZIP: _________________

AGE: _____ SEX: _____ DATE OF BIRTH: ______________________

COUNTRY OF BIRTH: ___________________

ETHNIC ORIGIN (Check one):

_____ ASIAN
_____ BLACK
_____ CAUCASIAN
_____ HISPANIC
_____ OTHER (Specify): ____________

MARITAL STATUS (Check one):

_____ DIVORCED
_____ MARRIED
_____ SINGLE
_____ WIDOWED
_____ (Number of children)

RELIGIOUS PREFERENCE (Check one):

_____ CATHOLIC
_____ PROTESTANT
_____ ATHEIST
_____ OTHER (Specify): ____________

Do you attend church regularly? _____ Yes _____ No

Were you raised (Check one):

_____ BY BOTH PARENTS?
_____ BY A SINGLE PARENT? (Check one): _____ FATHER
_____ MOTHER
_____ OTHER? (Specify): ____________

HABIT PROFILE

Do you exercise at least twenty minutes three times/week? ______ Yes ______ No

Do you actively participate in any kind of sports? ______ Yes ______ No

Do you pray or meditate? ______ Yes ______ No

Do you consider yourself to have a "healthy" diet? ______ Yes ______ No

How much alcohol (or the equivalent) have you consumed in the last week?

______ 0–2 beers ______ 3–6 beers ______ 1–2 six packs ______ 2+ six packs

How much caffeine (or the equivalent) have you consumed in the last week?

______ 0–2 colas ______ 3–6 colas ______ 1–2 colas/day ______ 2+ colas/day

In the past 72 hours (3 days), how many hours (average) have you slept each night?

(Check one): ______ 0–3 ______ 4–7 ______ 8+

Do you have a job other than school? ______ Yes ______ No

(If yes, check all that apply):

______ ON CAMPUS: ______ OFF CAMPUS

______ PART-TIME ______ PART-TIME

______ FULL-TIME ______ FULL-TIME

PSYCHOSOCIAL PROFILE

Have you experienced any major life changes within the past year?
(Such as change in social activities or relationships, church activities, eating or sleeping habits, pregnancy, divorce or separation, getting married, personal injury or illness, change in academic advisor or instrumental teacher)

______ Yes ______ No

Have you been treated for mental illness or consulted with a psychiatrist or other professional counselor in the past five (5) years? ______ Yes ______ No

Do you feel uncomfortable being in a large group? ______ Yes ______ No

Do you feel uncomfortable being alone? ______ Yes ______ No

How many hours did you spend last week in a social situation, such as at a party or group activity? (Check one):

______ 0 ______ 1–5 ______ 6–12 ______ 13+

Do you have a strong support system? ______ Yes ______ No

How well would you say you communicate with your spouse or close friends?
(Check one): ______ WELL
______ NEEDS SOME IMPROVEMENT (GOOD BUT AWKWARD)
______ NEEDS MUCH IMPROVEMENT
______ NO COMMUNICATION AT ALL

PERFORMANCE ANXIETY PROFILE

Do you feel uncomfortable performing in a group? ______ Yes ______ No

Do you feel uncomfortable performing alone? ______ Yes ______ No

Do you experience stage fright or performance anxiety? ______ Yes ______ No

Do your hands get cold when giving a recital? ______ Yes ______ No

Do your hands sweat when giving a recital? ______ Yes ______ No

Do thoughts of doing poorly interfere with performance? ______ Yes ______ No

Does your mind go blank during a performance? ______ Yes ______ No

INSTRUMENT HISTORY

Principal major/concentration instrument. (Check one):

______ BARITONE HORN
______ BASSOON
______ CELLO
______ CLARINET
______ DOUBLE BASS
______ FLUTE
______ FRENCH HORN
______ GUITAR
______ HARP
______ HARPSICHORD
______ OBOE
______ ORGAN
______ PERCUSSION
______ PIANO
______ SAXOPHONE
______ TROMBONE
______ TRUMPET
______ TUBA
______ VIOLA
______ VIOLIN
______ VOICE

How many years have you played this principal instrument? ______________

How many teachers of your principal instrument have you had? ______________

How long have you studied with your present teacher? ______________

Do you have a secondary instrument? ______ Yes ______ No

PRACTICE ROUTINE

At what time of day do you usually practice most? (Individually, i.e., practice room)
(Check one): ______ MORNING ______ EARLY EVENING (6–9 PM)
______ AFTERNOON ______ LATE AT NIGHT (9 PM+)

How many total hours do you usually practice every day? (Check one):
______ 0–1 ______ 2–3 ______ 4–6 ______ 7–9

Has practice time increased since last semester? ______ Yes ______ No

In how many music ensemble(s) do you now play? ______

How many total hours do you usually spend in all ensemble rehearsals in one week?
(Check one): ______ 0–2 ______ 3–6 ______ 7–10 ______ 11+

ACADEMIC PROFILE

Check one type and one year that applies to your degree:

______ CERTIFICATE	______ GRADUATE	______ UNDERGRADUATE
______ 1ST YEAR	______ 1ST YEAR	______ 1ST YEAR
______ 2ND YEAR	______ 2ND YEAR	______ 2ND YEAR
______ 3RD YEAR	______ 3RD YEAR	______ 3RD YEAR
	______ 4TH YEAR	______ 4TH YEAR
		______ 5TH YEAR

Academic major (Check one):

______ MUSIC COMPOSITION	______ MUSIC THERAPY
______ MUSIC THEORY	______ MUSIC EDUCATION
______ MUSIC PERFORMANCE	______ SACRED MUSIC
______ MUSIC HISTORY	______ ACCOMPANYING
______ PIANO PEDAGOGY	______ CONDUCTING
______ DOUBLE MAJOR	

In how many semester/credit hours are you currently enrolled? (Check one):
______ 0–1 ______ 6–9 ______ 13–15 ______ 19+
______ 2–5 ______ 10–12 ______ 16–18

How many total hours do you usually spend studying academic subjects each week?
(Check one): ______ 0–1 ______ 6–9 ______ 13–15 ______ 19+

At what time of day do you usually study the most?
(Check one): ______ MORNING ______ EARLY EVENING (6–9 PM)
______ AFTERNOON ______ LATE AT NIGHT (9 PM+)

Do you listen to music while studying? ______ Yes ______ No

TREATMENT HISTORY

How many times in the last two months have you seen a doctor for a medical problem?
(Check one): ______ 0 ______ 1–3 ______ 4+

Are you presently on the university health care plan? ______ Yes ______ No

Do you feel your physical complaints are the result of playing your instrument or some other injury such as a car accident, sports injury, etc.?
______ Yes ______ No (Please explain) ______________________________

Has a doctor ever diagnosed you as having any of the following? (Check all that apply):
______ Carpal Tunnel Syndrome ______ Cubital Tunnel Syndrome
______ Lateral Epicondylitis/Tennis Elbow ______ Muscle Fatigue
______ Dorsal Wrist/Hand Tendinitis ______ Thoracic Outlet Syndrome

If so, when were you diagnosed? ______________________________

Which of the following do you experience during stressful situations, or those in which you notice pain? (Check all that apply):
______ Numbness in the index, long, or thumb fingers
______ Pain in wrist that wakes you up
______ Recent loss of dexterity (ease in using the hands)
______ Numbness in little finger
______ Pain or soreness near "funny bone" at elbow area
______ Pain on top of wrist or hand area, especially after playing your instrument
______ Pain at the outside of elbow area
______ Muscle tension. If so, where? ______________________________
______ Tension headache
______ Neck pain
______ Muscle cramps. If so, where? ______________________________
______ Chest pain
______ Restlessness
______ Jaw clenching
______ Confusion
______ Forgetfulness
______ Crying easily
______ Speech difficulty
______ Fearful feeling
______ Concentration difficulty
______ Ragged breathing
______ Sleeping difficulty
______ Cold hands
______ Cold feet
______ Rapid heartbeat
______ Clammy hands
______ Swelling
______ Bloating
______ Fainting

IMPLEMENTING PREVENTIVE EDUCATION IN THE TRAINING OF PROFESSIONAL MUSICIANS

Crispin Spaulding

Introduction

Our purpose has been to determine criteria for the formulation and implementation of an effective prevention program at Trøndelag Music Conservatory, Trondheim, Norway. The project represents over a decade of collaborative effort between the music faculty and an on-staff interdisciplinary leader who is trained in both medicine and music. There gradually has emerged a unique curriculum based on the essential principle of developing preventive skills as an integral part of professional musical training. This highly specialized prevention model continues to evolve, being tailored by, and for, the particular needs of the institution's teachers and their students. Key elements in the prevention scheme that demonstrate a high degree of relevance and reliability will be described.

Certain conceptual subtleties accompanying the project have been discussed in an earlier article (Spaulding, 1988). We will begin with a short review of those concepts believed to have favorably disposed this program to its notable success; in short, since prevention can be validated only through active practice, making prevention work will depend at least as much on *how* an institution proceeds in evolving needed changes, as on *what* actual methods and content it chooses to employ.

Nature, in Self and Musicianship

Making ideas of prevention and avoidance meaningful to musicians means pairing a prevention paradigm with human fascination for music-making. The ideas must foster respect for our remarkable construction and function as musical organisms and cause individuals to value self-knowledge and self-authorship as a primary means to artistic aspiration. Accordingly, a robust vision of the "nature" of great musical performance has the potential to involve students directly with issues of their own biology, arouse their curiosity, and allow them to see themselves and their talent in a renewing and stimulating light.

At the heart of the nature of great playing or singing are the finest of the musical species' hallmarks: versatility and flexibility. A high-level musician is an inventive, uniquely self-expressing, daring, musical creature. We see something alive—something besides body: aliveness in imagination. Through care for, and total delight in the music, the artist relates the wonders beheld, and enables others to participate in them. It may enlighten—it may disturb; it moves, and affects. Nature sets up a live current between such an artist and audience, one imagination reaching other imaginations. This rare communication is magic, but there is no mistaking the phenomenon when it occurs: the whole world stands still for it, and breathes this kind of music in.

The degree to which prevention education will meaningfully impact technical training correspondingly depends to a great extent on how deep an anchor it sinks in the whole "nature"—including the magic—of musical performance. Interdisciplinary leaders must be able to understand musical thinking, know what is important to musicians, and be skillful in defining and executing the supportive role that music physiology is intended to play in the school. Among these skills is the needed ability to create an atmosphere of trust and confidentiality, so that people wish to share their deeper concerns and know that they will be met with a sense of immediacy and support.

Creating a forum, individually and collectively, sows the necessary seeds for formulating a prevention scheme that reflects realities of practice and performing *as they exist in that institution*. Only when prevention is tailored to the individual, and only by shaping the prevention scheme per institution in this way—by, and for, the teachers' and students' goals—can prevention succeed. Time of course will be needed to refine the implied partnership that can truly provide supportive pedagogical environment for practicing prevention. When patience, flexibility, and structural room for response characterize the collaborative effort, it will occur most naturally through two essential earmarks of any working relationship: frequent communication and quick follow-up.

Relevance as Motivation

Prevention implies taking active responsibility for self-authoring an insurance policy for the future. Educating for prevention must therefore reach beyond supplying information and enter the practical realities of daily practice and technical development. Students must be brought to seeing a direct connection between exercising preventive skills and bettering their playing skills. To achieve this it is advisable to focus instruction of selected interdisciplinary topics on a minimum of theory and a maximum of applied considerations.

When explaining to musicians' their biology, function should be emphasized; for example, the hand is an information-seeking organ, and the arm is a hanging pendulum. Attention thus drawn to the "feel" of bodily contact with instrument helps discourage unmindful use of fingers and hands. Understanding rhythmic carriage and central body support can, through self-observation and experimentation, facilitate holding and playing instruments. Discussion of basic topics like posture and breathing will also help open discussion about technique—health-focused discussion, directed toward informed choice. Understanding the biologic origins of the debilitating effects of performance nervousness, likewise encourages the student to accept and make positive use of this human aspect of his or her nature.

Working in pairs and learning from each other is a very effective way for students to explore their tension habits. This works particularly well when learning, for example, how to reduce unconscious temporal mandibular joint and neck tension. Activities such as making their own anatomical drawings using giant-sized pieces of paper and lots of color, involves musicians in their more relevant, interesting, and comprehensive nature: body *and imagination*.

Education for prevention and avoidance can provide a clearer vision of ideas—rationality, self-control, self-authorship, opportunity, responsibility, self-improvement, and critical judgement capacity. Good understanding of one's own nature can affirm for music students the great importance of biology in human and musical behavior, and can consequently show them why their biology makes them free—free to choose, and become agents, rather than spectators in their own destiny—and that when they choose health, they choose quality—in artistic development, and in life.

Individually Tailored Prevention

Structure and Content

Trøndelag Music Conservatory begins planting the seeds of preventive consciousness at the moment of audition. Through informal discussion with the candidate as he or she comes through the final audition stage, it is possible to determine the degree to which the individual has gained earlier awareness of, or experience with, physical problems related to playing. Teachers may then have the opportunity to discuss the potential students' situations, and be alert to signals deserving particular attention. In June, incoming students receive a letter about the school's prevention program, which also contains common sense advice about summer jobs notorious for overtaxing arms and hands; they are also reminded not to increase practice suddenly, and urged to plan a gradual buildup of practice pace with which to begin the school year.

In the early weeks of the fall term, students undergo an assessment process by which they may draw up a reasonably comprehensive individual health profile. Appraisal includes medical, psychological, sociological, and behavioral characteristics that may dispose the individual to difficulties. Through video filming, students have opportunity to visually study and discuss their singing or playing; each receives an early evaluation of occupational health status, along with needed advice about specific risk-factors, such as structural weaknesses in hands or lower back.

All new students take a one-semester intensive course in Music Physiology during their first term. This is a several-hour-per-week investment, devoted to instrument group and individual instruction, closely coordinated with ongoing instrument lessons and interpretation classes. There is an all-out effort to discourage single-factor thinking about health and ill-health and to replace it with a multifactorial conscious awareness of influences on the individual, such as sleep patterns, nutrition, postural and structural weaknesses, ergonomic relationship to the instrument, prior injury, being out of shape, and failing to monitor other physical activities such as lifting, carrying, and in particular, long hours of sitting and writing term papers and exams.

Understanding stress is emphasized in terms of its sources in musical life, and the difference between normal, acceptable, positive levels of stress versus constant unabated stress that makes people vulnerable to developing problems. Stress is viewed as normal and expected—even a welcome aid—when we have knowledge and skills with which to use it as stimulation, growth, and for self-expression. Understanding the principles of immune reaction to chronic stress, and learning how to actively respond, rather than react to stress, helps build needed tools for coping with performance demands. Students learn to observe and monitor their individual stress levels in conjunction with practice habits, through discussion and regular keeping of journal diaries.

Students are expected to maintain good physical condition—for example through swimming—and to incorporate in their daily routines an appropriate selection of suggested preventive strategies. During this period students are monitored for technical progress and active preventive participation. Attention is focused on providing a collective and interested support system for both students and their teachers.

Students are informed of the types and frequency of difficulties known to be associated with intensive practice, and are made aware of clinical differences between usual muscle fatigue and such conditions as tendinitis, epicondylitis, nerve compression, and focal dystonia.

Inherent in the prevention scheme is the assumption that all such disorders have a relatively long developmental process. The message to first-year students is strong and clear: these problems can be prevented; it is up to the individual to be alert to early symptoms and signs, communicate these, and alter his or her course toward health rather than toward disability.

Establishing Efficient Practice Habits

The student who practices efficiently has developed skills in practicing mentally and relies on these to minimize empty-minded hours spent (practicing mistakes) in the practice room. Efficient mental practice will mean efficient physical practice. It is especially important to reduce static neck tension characteristic of dependency on score-reading.

The efficient student of music:

1. Listens to, and compares recordings as a daily part of practice routine and values auditive rehearsal of repertoire as means of both training the mind, and expanding interpretive capacity and his own musical ideas.
2. Studies scores prior to playing them, analyzing harmony, structural landscape, and style.
3. Rehearses musical scores away from the instrument, through singing (committing instrumental music to voice), and through rhythmic rehearsal using the whole body (not just arms) for rhythmic gesture.
4. Memorizes regularly, preferring the freedom and security of being able to mentally reproduce every detail in a piece independent of actually playing or singing.
5. Knows which hours of the day in which practice will be most efficient, and sticks to them.
6. Monitors practice time, paces practice, and takes frequent pauses to rest and rebalance the work-musculature.
7. Keeps written track of practice progress.
8. Records himself often, studies his day-before tapings as part of practice routine, and employs a tape-recorder to reinforce memory by the "play-listen-play" method.
9. Enjoys improvising as part of warm-up.
10. Prepares well for lessons, and seeks criticism as a means of learning.
11. Knows how to create quiet before playing.
12. Assesses daily limits in the practice room, and knows when to quit. Sometimes the most efficient thing to do is to leave the practice room and go fishing.

When score reading is unavoidable, such as in ensemble rehearsal, the informed student can help reduce static neck tension by warming up physically before starting, taking frequent breaks, alternating seating, and taking time for a post-rehearsal rest and rebalance of the work-musculature. It goes without saying that ensemble rehearsal schedules for students ought not to exceed the expected endurance limits of nonprofessional musicians.

Quiet Time

Creating mental and physical quiet in which to make music is a skill and a necessity. Visualization of performance—mental filming of oneself playing, in all details (from relaxation, to bowings, fingerings, intonation)—is a major facilitator to both practice and prevention of injury. Students today can choose from a variety of helpful methods to deepen concentration and relaxation and tailor these according to preference and needs.

At Trøndelag Music Conservatory, autogenic training and the oriental discipline of T'ai chi chuan ("shadow boxing"), having established excellent track records, have become mainstays of the prevention program. When presented in the traditional manner, T'ai chi can offer musicians exceptional value in mental and physical integration, because it relies on non-verbal instruction, and demands acute attention to "sensing" and on ideokinetic coordination. Shadowboxing has taken over early morning practice room corridors, and increasing numbers of students employ T'ai chi to reduce concert nervousness and be assured of warm hands.

To be intelligible is as essential to the art of music as it is to human speech. Good interpreters of music must first be capable of great feeling and profound contemplation. Without great feeling—without making time for profound contemplation—something will be missing in their music. Sadly, this can be the same missing link that can make them vulnerable to developing serious injury.

Physical Responsibilities

In becoming familiar with their individual physical status, students are evaluated for structural weaknesses and disadvantageous movement and tension patterns. Structural risk factors cover a wide spectrum from mild to severe—from common lordosis for example, to a more serious condition such as scoliosis. Joint laxity, or hypermobility of joints in wrists, thumbs, fingers—or the opposite condition, as in too tight and inflexible hands—constitute risks that musicians cannot afford to ignore. These, among others, should be evaluated, and students should be carefully shown how to reduce or correct compensatory tensions so as to avoid cumulative joint trauma or a worsening situation. They may need advice about adaptive devices, such as neck straps and thumb rests; then students need support to do the preventive work necessary to avoid injury and disability.

"Exercise"

Good physical conditioning requires regular attention. Obviously there is no single prescription for exercise that is valid for all musicians. The important thing is to choose a form of exercise that is enjoyable and realistic. Even walking or biking to and from school instead of taking the bus every day, may be a good solution for some individuals.

Swimming—particularly stroking while lying on the back—is recommended for re-balancing pectorales, trapezius and upper-pole muscles involved in holding and playing instruments, and is an excellent form of physical conditioning for those who are not allergic to chlorine.

Students are warned against doing gymnastic exercises or activities that require direct weight-bearing on wrists, or a fast pace and mindless repetition that tend to put joints at risk.

Since many musicians are attracted to dance classes, they can benefit from knowing the differences in types and degrees of jeopardy to which they may be exposed in, for instance, classical ballet classes, often conducted without regard to putting stresses on hips joints and the lower back, or to already chronic static postural tension.

Physical Warm-up

Physical warm-up, prior to technical warm-up, is basic to the preventive routine. Students receive an individually tailored warm-up sequence. The sequence itself is not complicated, but its design rules are fairly strict:

1. Before doing anything else, raise body temperature.
2. Do not stretch, or push or pull on the body as a means of "warming up".
3. Begin with central-body warm-up, being sure to establish a rhythmic movement, and sing!
4. Follow your warm-up sequence carefully, and get advice before altering its pace. Use only your own sequence—no borrowing!
5. If you sleep during the day, repeat your warm-up sequence before evening practice.

Individual warm-up sequences will reflect specific needs—for example to strengthen structural weaknesses; all warm-ups are designed to prepare the central-body, iliopsoas and lower back, shoulders and trapezius first—arms and hands being last. Warm-ups may include arm and hand massage, but not as a replacement for important central-body preparation.

Rhythmic, Tonal, Gestural Unity in Playing

This theme is central to the prevention scheme and forms the basis for understanding efficient upper extremity use. By this we mean that consistent unsegmented fluidity of rhythm, movement, and tone initiated from the central body both helps to convey musical meaning and facilitates technique.

Over half of the students in an average first-year class at our institution appear to need help in this area. Through video filming and one-on-one lessons, students learn how to recognize segmented rhythm/movement/tone in themselves and in others and are shown how to connect tone with rhythmic support from the whole body. While there is no single recipe for teaching this process, students who develop the trilogy at reflex level early, demonstrate strong advantage toward avoiding static tension in playing. They report increased ease in playing, and also significantly greater efficiency in building repertoire.

Prevention Life after the Intensive Course

In their remaining years at school, students will have contact with performance physiology, in part through playing and singing at monthly departmental seminars that focus on cognitive and physiologic aspects of musical processes. Other participation in ongoing body classes or individual consultation is elective. Three types of consultation are most frequently sought:

1. Request from instrument teacher and student, to check for unnecessary tension-holding.
2. Special problem-solving at instrument lessons.
3. Cooperative teaching during weekly interpretation classes.

Highest elective attendance occurs in T'ai Chi chuan classes, and in sessions devoted to ideokinesis, visualization, and relaxation skills.

The school offers a graduate year seminar in Concert Preparation for extending and deepening cognitive and physiological process, which involves extensive reading and presenting of material from various fields, and leads to writing a thesis in the student's chosen area of interest. The allowed interdisciplinary scope is broad and may be directed toward either teaching or solo careers. During this several hours per week commitment, participants take a refresher intensive course, and can choose to gain teaching experience in music physiology. In addition to the thesis, the course has two exams, carries half a year's credit load, and is graded, with outside examiners.

Concluding Remarks

It is important to note that both content and structure of prevention programs will necessarily differ substantially from institution to institution, and that the value of a model will only be as useful to other institutions as is their subsequent dedication to doing the required serious work of appropriately "remodeling" it from the ground up. This is of course because prevention, unlike medication, and because it does not lend itself well to prescription, can only be approached through conscious awareness of individuals who live and work in the institution.

The currently employed prevention scheme in Trondheim combines risk-education, individual appraisal, self-knowledge and self-monitoring, as well as highly specialized applications to technique in playing and singing, as means to securing and supporting musicians' active participation in maintaining health in relation to high-level performance goals. We make no claim that science is going to "save us"—but conscious awareness has a fair chance.

By choosing tactics that more closely resemble those in musical art, musicians can benefit from taking elements of hard-and soft-sciences seriously—to know themselves, so that they can self-forget, and do the magical thinking in performance that rivets imaginations. Such music pedagogy is innovative, inspired, and full of moral and musical integrity. Education for responsibility is versatile and powerful education.

References

Brandfonbrener, A. G. (1990). Joint laxity in instrumental musicians. *Medical Problems of Performing Artists, 5*, 117–119.

Dennett, D. C. (1984). *Elbow room: The varieties of free will worth wanting.* Cambridge: MIT Press. Bradford Book.

Gould, S. J. (1987, June). Bushes all the way down. *Natural History, 96*, 12–19.

Gould, S. J. (1987) *Urchin in the storm.* New York: W. W. Norton.

Spaulding, C. (1988). Before pathology: Prevention for performing artists. *Medical Problems of Performing Artists 3*, 135–139.

Wilson, F. R., Wagner, C., & Homberg, V. (1993, October–December). Biomechanical abnormalities in musicians with occupational cramp/focal dystonia. *Journal of Hand Therapy*, 298–307.

Woolfolk R. L., & Lehrer P. M. (1984). *Principles and practice of stress management.* New York: Guilford Press.

IV.

PROFESSIONAL ISSUES AND THEORETICAL PERSPECTIVES IN MUSICMEDICINE

PROFESSIONALISM IN MUSIC THERAPY AND MUSICMEDICINE: ISSUES OF THE PAST AND FUTURE

Rosalie Rebollo Pratt

Abstract

The issue of professionalism has permeated the history of music therapy since the time of the 1940s and is now a topic of great interest to leaders in the field of MusicMedicine. The history of Music Therapy in the 1950s shows a clear relationship between that profession and medicine. The growth of Music Therapy and the development of MusicMedicine have focused attention on the need for a doctoral-level program that will be disposed toward interdisciplinary training and research and the establishment of MusicMedicine in one of several directions: as a specialty of medicine, an independent approach in healthcare, or an adjunct modality. Questions of appropriate curriculum, courses of study, accreditation, research paradigms, team teaching among disciplines, and the relationship of MusicMedicine to fields such as Music Therapy, Special Music Education, and hospital arts programs have been raised and must be discussed thoroughly by leaders in all these fields. As we do so, it behooves us to consider the past events in the development of these fields and to consider the wisdom and experience of all those who have guided these other professions and, in so doing, have created and directed the guidelines and training programs we currently follow. A Ph.D. degree program proposal will be defended on the basis of relevance to present needs in the field, and the research and theory needed to establish MusicMedicine as a peer rather than an adjunct medical specialty.

The Fundamental Question

The issue of professionalism has permeated the history of Music Therapy, particularly from the time of the 1940s. Since that period, both Music Therapy and the other creative arts therapies have expanded throughout the world, and the field of MusicMedicine has come into being. The networking of music therapists and physicians is not a new idea, and the early history of the profession clearly shows the relationship between the two fields from the very beginning. Throughout the histories of Music Therapy and MusicMedicine, there has always been the underlying concept of growth, development of programs, and response to research and clinical needs. The growing focus on what is now called Arts Medicine has prompted today's healthcare professionals to show interest in the influence of the creative arts on human behavior, including music as it affects the human life process. This trend is evidenced in such developments as the Alternative Medicine Institute at the National Institutes of Health in Maryland and the recent creation of the Rosenthal Alternative Medicine Research Center at Columbia University that is based on the Stanford University model. The movement toward serious investigation of alternative healing approaches has produced new research paradigms created by joint efforts of MusicMedicine and Music Therapy professionals working with experts from the medical field. It is clear that carefully controlled and meticulously reported data are needed to convince the broader international scientific community of the specific effects of music on the healing process. It is also clear that we must begin to bring some agreement to our common understanding of MusicMedicine, Music Therapy, Special Music Education, and how these fields relate. The questions that arise from this inquiry are: How do we define these fields in terms of professional development, accreditation, and contribution to healthcare? How do we address the needs of the young people in all three fields?

Charles Eagle has reminded us of the need to confront basic issues. Michael Thaut has shown us the wisdom of asking fundamental questions in the research lab. Examples of therapies that are based in eastern medical traditions have helped us realize the privilege we have as a new field to discuss and investigate research questions that have not been addressed thoroughly by western and more traditional systems of healthcare. The stunning, state of the art equipment in the Health Science Center here at the University of Texas/San Antonio has shown us the opportunity we now have to test our hypotheses in ways we never before dreamed.

The question that intrigues me the most is that of developing a MusicMedicine curriculum at the doctoral level, because I see this as the only way in which we will finally discover the body of theory we need as a field. Perhaps the most crucial question we face at this crossroads is that of our training programs. It is time to look squarely at the issue of bringing MusicMedicine, Special Music Education, and Music Therapy to a level where in-depth research can be pursued with a direct focus on the relationship between music and human well-being. Our students are as frustrated as we by degree programs that stop at the master's level and beg for continuation so that basic issues may be thoroughly investigated. Students in existing Music Therapy and Special Music Education and MusicMedicine programs continually inquire about a doctoral program that will focus primarily on music and well-being, and we must now address their requests. In so doing, we must face some fundamental questions that have been and continue to be asked by interested students, a group that also includes those from disciplines such as premedicine, medicine, psychology, nursing, and family science. Should we consider a curriculum that will lead us toward becoming a medical specialty? Should we develop distinct programs, in MusicMedicine, Music Therapy, and Special Music Education? Should we review current research paradigms and revise them in order to accommodate the interdisciplinary studies that are needed? Which courses should be involved in training doctoral-level students who seek a closer dialogue with health scientists? And how can we seek accreditation of such a program and direct its graduates toward a productive future in health care? Today, we meet as international colleagues who are discussing a future that must now address these issues. As we move ahead, let us emulate two great minds of the past. Plato's intuition and vision have inspired all of us who followed him; Aristotle's meticulous eye for scientific detail taught us the value of rigor and intellectual discipline. Above all, however, let us look to our past and learn from the ideas of those who were the leaders before us. This collective wisdom and the lessons of history will guide us as we move together toward a new era of music in medicine.

The Historical Legacy

It was largely the overcrowded conditions of military hospitals during World War II that served as an impetus to the development of adjunctive therapies in those facilities. Ainlay (1948), a physician of the time, claimed that music was considered unimportant by the military until the numbers of wounded men were such that alternative strategies were needed in the hospitals. At first, there were random organizations for instrumental and vocal ensembles, and it soon became clear that patient choice of music was important. Ainlay was responsible, in large part, for the song books and instrumental texts that were developed and published by the U.S. Army and War Department.

Schneider, Unkefer, and Gaston (1968) describe the influx of volunteers during World War II into the hospitals. The expansion of these music programs increased quickly in mental hospitals and the idea of activities for these patients caught on rapidly. It was soon apparent that continued use of music for hospitalized and institutionalized people would have to become more organized. Thus it was that in 1944 the institution that has since been renamed Michigan State University established the first curriculum designed specifically to train music therapists. The first academic course (didactic and laboratory) was taught in 1946 at the University of Kansas. Soon other colleges and universities established degree courses. In 1950, the National Association for Music Therapy (NAMT) was organized, making possible greater unity and standardization through its constitution and various committees on education, clinical practice, research, and certification and registration (Schneider, Unkefer, & Gaston, 1968, pp. 2–4). In 1968, Schneider, Unkefer, and Gaston noted that, since World War II, activity therapists had been contributing directly to the specific treatment goals of patients. Music was used by volunteers, therapists, and specialists. When specialized training of music therapists developed, these new professionals became recognized members of the activity therapists' team.

Between 1951 and 1962, 12 *Yearbooks of NAMT* were published concurrently with the NAMT *Bulletin*. Immediately prior to the *Bulletin*, the *Hospital Music Newsletter* was in circulation. The January 1953 issue of the NAMT *Bulletin* is historically significant because it contains the NAMT "Minimum Music Therapy Requirements" for the undergraduate training leading the B.A. or the B.M. degrees in music therapy, or the B.M.T. (Bachelor of Music Therapy). The specific core courses were three: Psychology of Music (4 semester hours); Influence of Music on Behavior (3–5 semester hours); and Hospital Orientation (2 semester hours). The following note accompanied the listing of these courses:

> It is assumed that these courses will include the role of Music in therapy, and will be taught by people with experience in that field. These core courses are the actual professional courses of the Music Therapy curriculum. In order to meet the desired high standards of the content, the first two courses should follow other required courses in Psychology. It is essential, therefore, that these be taught only by highly competent people from the field of Psychology (*Bulletin of the NAMT,* Jan. 1953, *3*[1]:3).

Since these courses were taught by psychologists, a concern arose concerning the proper application of psychology to music. Dr. Abraham Pepinsky commented on this point in 1954, when he noted that musicians needed to "make proper application of the theorems offered or implied in them" (p. 8).

In 1954, both the New England Conservatory of Music and Florida State University were offering the B.M. in music therapy. Music therapy degrees were also offered at the time at the New England Conservatory (Arthur Flagler Fultz) and The Florida State University (Don Michel). Weigl (1954) reported music therapy activity in England, France, Switzerland, Austria, Denmark, Norway, and Sweden. He mentioned that England was the only one of these countries with government support of its program (p. 12). On January 1955, NAMT was incorporated under the laws of the State of Michigan as a nonprofit organization, and Ray Green served as the first president. Initially, the new music therapy organization established a working relationship with the psychiatric profession. The standards for the baccalaureate degree in music therapy as they appeared in the Jan. 1953 *Bulletin of the NAMT, 2*(1), clearly required "a minimum of 6 months residence internship in an approved neuropsychiatric hospital with an established music program" (p. 3).

In September 1958, the criteria for registration of music therapists were stated by NAMT. After 31 December 1960, all those seeking registration would have to complete a 4-year course from an institution that had received full approval from NAMT *(Bulletin of the NAMT,* Sept. 1958, *7*(3), 3). The American Medical Association acknowledged the position of music therapy by inviting NAMT in May 1959 to send a representative to a meeting of the AMA *Joint Committee to Study Paramedical Areas in Relation to Medicine.* The meeting was held in Chicago, Illinois, and E. Thayer Gaston was the representative of NAMT.

One of the most striking features of the first *Bulletins* is information showing the close association of NAMT with the medical profession. Both medical doctors and psychologists contributed regularly to the *Bulletin.* For example, in 1961 Karl Blanke contributed an article on music therapy and internal medicine. Blanke claimed that music works as therapy when it bypasses the intellectual function and goes immediately to the unconscious level. He described the deep-rooted, psychological connection within the sick person to the healing power of music. Through this connection, the sick person can be restored to health and harmonious well-being (pp. 17–23). This philosophy is remarkably reminiscent of the ancient Greeks' position on the topic of health. By 1962, NAMT had members in Canada, England, Germany, Austria, Italy, New Zealand, Hawaii, the Philippines, Argentina, Brazil, and Japan. The profession had gained universal stature in the eyes of musicians and physicians alike. Professional music therapy organizations and societies sprang up throughout the world.

The first issue of the *Journal of Music Therapy* was published in March 1964. Editor Bill Sears stated that the new journal would publish "original investigations and theoretical papers pertaining to music therapy or any of the other related fields (inside cover). The June 1964 issue of the journal cited 170 current studies of the effects of music on human mood, behavior, and physical function. At the same time, Erwin Schneider (1965) published an extensive list of references in the *Journal of Music Therapy.* The bond between music therapy and psychiatry was stronger than ever. Charles Eagle was the administrative assistant to E. Thayer Gaston on a 5-year grant from the National Institute of Mental Health (NIMH) awarded to Gaston at Kansas University. The program had emphasized research activity and direct clinical application.

President Muskatevc reported that the NAMT had been invited in the Spring of 1965 to present a program on man and music to a conference of the American Psychiatric Association. In 1965, the state mental hospitals in the U.S. were employing the largest number of music therapists ever. By 1966, music therapists were practicing privately and in the therapeutic community. Toward the end of 1966, music therapy programs had been established in U.S. schools; clinical training centers for music therapists had been organized; music therapists were now certified and registered; and literature in the field was developing (Muskatevc, 1996, 117–119). In 1961, 500 people were certified as music therapists, and a central office in Lawrence, Kansas was opened.

Behaviorism became an important tool in music therapy research and clinical practice after 1968. Clifford Madsen (1968) stated that music therapy is a method of behavioral manipulation and therefore can automatically be considered as falling within the purview of the behavioral modification movement (p. 70). In the same article, Madsen suggested that music might be used for desensitization, hypnosis, specific conditioning, or a reward for appropriate behaviors (p. 71).

Another thrust in the direction of research was made by George Duerksen (1968), when he commented that "the most reliable way to increase knowledge in music therapy is through scientific research. Treatment of patients usually improves as health sciences are able to abandon 'intuitive' approaches and base their activities on scientifically derived and validated knowledge" (p. 95).

E. Thayer Gaston (1968) was among the strongest supporters of music therapy from its inception as a profession. His was the guiding voice in the organization of NAMT, the formulation of policies, certification and registration requirements, and the general direction of the field. He warned against taking music therapy methods from one country or another without regard for anthropological or cultural differences. He urged music therapists to pay more attention to the needs of individual cultures and societies. In 1969, Gaston was appointed Liaison Officer to The American Medical Association during the 19th annual NAMT conference. An AMA representative had met with officers of NAMT and directors of training and clinical programs in music therapy in order to discuss music therapy as one of the allied health professions. Gaston maintained a strong relationship with the medical profession until his death on 3 June 1970.

In 1971, Donald Michel reported to the NAMT about music therapy programs throughout the world. He described strong programs in Brazil and developing programs in Argentina, Uruguay, and Peru. Michel saw considerable activity in England, where professional training had existed since 1968. He noted the work of Juliette Alvin at the Guildhall School of Music. The improvisational approach was favored in England over the behavioral modification strategy. Michel also reported that the British training program included a 1-year, post graduate course for persons with a bachelor of music degree (or the equivalent) at the Guildhall School. The Nordoff and Robbins approach was very much favored by British therapists. Michel also noted a strong developing program in Holland, the first book about music therapy in German by Teirich, a Viennese training center for music therapists, and music therapy practitioners in Switzerland. Michel reported strong Orff and Freudian influences in these programs. He found that French psychologists and psychiatrists had expressed great interest in music therapy. He also said that there was a strong program in Oslo supported by conservatories and the University of Oslo. Michel also discussed the effect of live music performance and improvisation as therapy techniques (pp. 94–95). His final comments stressed the need for open-mindedness as a prerequisite to world leadership in the field.

The 1970s saw legislation that brought about mainstreaming of special education children into public school classrooms. Special music educators joined hands with music therapists to meet the needs of these children. In 1979, Music Education for the Handicapped was organized two American music educators, Meg Peterson and Rosalie Rebollo Pratt, and two French psychiatrists, Pierre Rabischong and Régis Pouget. A symposium at the University of Montpellier convened therapists, educators, physicians and psychologists from nearly every continent and the interdisciplinary dialogue began in earnest. A second symposium sponsored by MEH at Brigham Young University in Utah convened several hundred therapists, physicians, and educators from as far away as Africa. The American Association of Music Therapy (AAMT) began as the Urban Federation of Music Therapy (UFMT) at New York University in 1966. It later became AAMT in 1971 and offered a certification in music therapy from approved institutions.

Meanwhile, The International Society for Music Education, an organization under the aegis of UNESCO, created a variety of commissions to address issues important to music educators throughout the world. In 1974, at the 11th congress in Australia, ISME created the Commission on Music Therapy and Music in Special Education, which, in 1988, officially changed its name to the Commission on Music in Special Education, Music Therapy, and MusicMedicine. At a conference in 1987, the Commission held a special meeting at Brigham Young University in Utah, where world leaders in music therapy, special music education, and physicians interested in both fields met to discuss current training programs. The proceedings of that conference, *Music therapy and music in special education: The international state of the art,* contain program descriptions from Brazil, Canada, England, Argentina, Portugal, Australia, the Peoples' Republic of China, France, Germany, Poland, Israel, and the United States. Among the 31 issues identified by the conference participants were those related to professionalism. These included concern about duplication of research efforts, identification of basic competencies for music therapists and special music educators, more formal interaction among therapists, educators, and physicians, communication among countries concerning program requirements, additional professional training, special training in new technology, regular review of certification requirements, and effective collaboration with other health professionals. The research contributions of special music educators and music therapists reported in the literature are now joined by an emerging group of MusicMedicine specialists who are conducting research in areas that pertain to educational as well as clinical and institutional issues.

The International Arts Medicine Association (IAMA), under the leadership of Richard Lippin, has sought to promote interdisciplinary as well as international dialogue. Recent cosponsorship of an arts medicine leadership conference in Tokyo, with Dr. Yoshihito Tokuda, produced excellent research papers from both east and west and forged a new bond among arts medicine practitioners. Participants met at Hasegawa Psychiatric Hospital and Tokyo Medical College, where arts medicine flourishes. The proceedings of this milestone event will be published in 1996 by MMB Music.

The International Society for Music in Medicine (ISMM) has distinguished itself by the five major conferences it has cosponsored, the experimental research it has fostered, and the publications it has produced. *The International Journal of Arts Medicine (IJAM),* published by MMB Music, and edited by Rosalie Rebollo Pratt, is the official journal of both ISMM and IAMA.

A conference sponsored by the Miller Clinic in New York City 2 years ago presented a panel discussion about a doctoral curriculum in arts medicine. This idea is discussed frequently at other international forums. A proposal that outlines a specific curriculum and list of courses for a doctoral degree in MusicMedicine is presented in this volume for discussion. The proposal has already been seen by department representatives from all disciplines at Brigham Young University. It has also been reviewed by members of ISMM, and copies have been sent to faculty at the University of Texas/San Antonio, as well as other arts medicine leaders interested in this concept. It is hoped that the proposal will spawn fruitful discussion among us all and that together we will develop ideas for bringing a doctoral-level program into being.

The Future

As I researched the history of Music Therapy, Special Music Education, and MusicMedicine, and reflected on the many conferences, publications, my own research and that of many others, it seems to me that our destiny is to collaborate yet to maintain the distinctions of our field specialties, because it is both in collaboration and distinct expertise that we will gain the answers for our role in the future of healthcare. The most difficult part of this collaboration will be dissolving those boundaries that are territorial in nature rather than discipline-generated. Our habits—since Descartes encouraged us to dichotomize mind and body—have discouraged us from interdisciplinary dialogue, an adventure we should now seek out eagerly. The most satisfying research I have been a part of has always been as an equal partner with a colleague from Medicine or Music Therapy. My message to all of you is to seek similar professional liaisons that will help us all gather more truth about human health, education, ad well-being.

The pioneering efforts and daily contributions of the leaders in MusicMedicine and Music Therapy are noted with deep gratitude and appreciation. Their contributions to research and clinical practice, training programs, publications, and research as well as efforts to foster relationships among the fields represented in MusicMedicine have brought us to this place in the history of the field. To those who have done so much in MusicMedicine, Special Education, and Music Therapy, tribute is paid for the work from which future generations will all benefit. Let us begin now in earnest to face new challenges and move together toward a new and exciting chapter in MusicMedicine, Special Music Education, Music Therapy, but, transcending all of these, human well-being.

References

Ainlay, G. W. (1948). The place of music in military hospitals. In D. M. Schullian & M. Schoen (Eds.), *Music and medicine* (pp. 322–351). New York: Henry Schuman.

Arrington, G. E., Jr. (1953, June). Music in medicine. *West Virginia Journal, 49,* 152–165.

Barger, D. A. (1979). The effects of music and verbal suggestion on heart rate and self-reports. *Journal of Music Therapy, 14,* 158–171.

Beardley, G. L. (1882–1883). The medical uses of music. *New England Medical Monthly, 26,* 214–216.

Bernaerts, A. (1946, Jan.) La danse, la musique, et la médecine. *Bruxelles médical, 26,* 40–43.

Blanke, K. F. (1961, Sept.). Music therapy experiences in the practice of internal medicine. *Bulletin of the National Association for Music Therapy, 10*(3), 17–23.

Boxberger, R. (1963). *A historical study of the National Association for Music Therapy.* Unpublished doctoral dissertation, University of Kansas, Lawrence.

Brocklesby, R. (1749). *Reflections on ancient and modern music with the application to the cure of diseases.* London: M. Cooper.

Browne, H. E. (1952, Jan.). The use of music as a therapy. *Mental Hygiene, 36,* 90–103.

Bulletin of the NAMT (1953, Jan.). *2*(1), 3.

Bulletin of the NAMT (1954, Jan.). *3*(1), 8.

Bulletin of the NAMT (1958, Sept.). *7*(3), 3.

Carpenter, N. C. (1958). *Music in the medieval and renaissance universities.* Norman, OK: University of Oklahoma Press.

Cawston, F. G. (1932, Feb.). Music and medicine. *South African Medical Journal, 6,* 119.

Duerksen, G. (1968). Comment. *Journal of Music Therapy, 5,* 95.

Eagle, C. T., & Dubler, G. (1971). Recent findings in psychology of music research. *Journal of Music Therapy, 8,* 152–167.

Garrison, F. H. (1948). Medical men who have loved music. In D. M. Schullian & M. Schoen (Eds.), *Music and medicine* (pp. 190–217). New York: Henry Schuman.

Gaston, E. T. (Ed.). (1968). *Music in therapy.* New York: Macmillan.

Gaston, E. T., & Schneider, E. H. ((1965). *An analysis, evaluation, and selection of clinical uses of music in therapy.* Lawrence, Kansas: The University of Kansas.

Gilbert, J. P. (1979). Published research in music therapy 1973–1978. Content, focus, and implications for future research. *Journal of Music Therapy, 16,* 102–110.

Iverson, L. F. (1967). The necessity for a multidisciplinary approach to music therapy. *Journal of Music Therapy, 4,* 106–107.

Larson, B. H. (1928). Music in medicine. *Journal of the Michigan State Medical Society, 27,* 203–206.

Licht, S. (1946). *Music in medicine.* Boston: New England Conservatory of Music.

Madsen, C. K. (1968, Sept.). A behavioral approach to music therapy. *Journal of Music Therapy, 5,* 69–71.

Masserman, J. H. (1955). *The practice of dynamic psychiatry.* Philadelphia, Pennsylvania: W. B. Saunders.

Michel, D. E. (1971). Music therapy: An idea whose time has arrived around the world. *Journal of Music Therapy, 8,* 90–95.

Muskatevc, L. C. (1966, Dec.). Blueprint for growth. *Journal of Music Therapy, 3,* 117–119.

NAMT minimum music therapy requirements. (1953, Jan.). *Bulletin of the NAMT, 2*(1), 3.

Pepinsky, A. (1954, Jan.). Comments. *Bulletin of the NAMT, 3*(1), 6.

Pratt, R. R. (Ed.). (1985). *The third international symposium on music in medicine, education, and therapy for the handicapped.* Lanham, Maryland: University Press of America.

Pratt, R. R. (1985). The historical relationship between music and medicine. In R. R. Pratt (pp. 237–269).

Schneider, E. H. (1965). The status of music therapy. *Journal of Music Therapy, 2,* 105–106.

Schullian, D. M., & Schoen, M. (Eds.), (1948). *Music and medicine.* New York: Henry Schuman.

Teirich, H. R. (Ed.). *Musik in der Medizin: Beiträge zur Musiktherapie.* Stuttgart: G. Fischer Verlag.

Van de Wall, W. (1923). *Music in correctional institutions.* New York: J. B. Lyon.

PROPOSAL FOR A DOCTORAL DEGREE IN HEALTH SCIENCES: EMPHASIS IN MUSICMEDICINE

Rosalie Rebollo Pratt

Introduction and Rationale

The fields of Arts Medicine, in general, and MusicMedicine, in particular, have developed dramatically in the 1990s. Medical science is reaching out to arts medicine professionals by inviting research studies through new institutions such as the National Institutes of Health Institute for Alternative Medicine, and the new Rosenthal Alternative Medicine Research Center at Columbia University. MusicMedicine, special music education, and music therapy students usually pursue study in their fields up to the master's level. After that, they are usually left with the option of adapting their specialty to doctoral degree programs belonging to other disciplines such as counseling, clinical psychology, and family sciences.

This proposal has been created to respond to two needs:

1. A degree program that can support in-depth research in MusicMedicine, and
2. A venue to the general scientific community.

Since the 1950s, when music therapy developed its first curricula and standards; the 1970s, when Special Music Education emerged as an area for dealing with problems of special learners; and the 1980s, when MusicMedicine began to take shape, the need for a theory base underlying all three fields has become more pressing. These fields had in practice already crossed disciplinary boundaries and established the need for communication among scientists, artists, educators, and therapists. The task was then, and is now, clearly one of developing a theoretical position that supports and even demands interdisciplinary cooperation and investigation. It is equally clear that any theory base will emerge only from consistent, rigorous, and pertinent research studies, which will develop only within the setting of a doctoral program. The direction of MusicMedicine, and perhaps, Music Therapy and Special Music Education, moves most naturally toward an academic residence that can encompass broad philosophical questions concerning human well-being; a residence that welcomes both the arts and sciences in a free but rigorous inquiry.

Health Science in the broadest sense involves human well-being in every aspect of the term. Therefore, this 74-credit-hour degree is proposed for inclusion in either a Department of Health Sciences or, perhaps, within a College of Human Sciences, because these seem the most logical places to house a program of this kind. In either of these environments, there is an emphasis on prevention, which is both the present and future focus of healthcare and education, and a primary goal of Arts Medicine in general. Health Sciences can logically house interdisciplinary courses such as psychoneuroimmunology and biofeedback, both significant components in health programs of the 90s. These two courses also lend themselves to team teaching among music and health sciences faculty. In addition, the proposed program offers the three formal didactic courses necessary for U.S. biofeedback certification (through the Biofeedback Certification Institute of America). This liaison between music and biofeedback has strengthened considerably as current research studies using the combined tools prove to be effective strategies in general stress reduction and, more specifically, increased heart rate variability and decreased heart rate. Biofeedback practitioners are also experimenting in the specialized area of neurofeedback with the use of background music during neurofeedback sessions with children whose primary diagnosis is Attention Deficit/Hyperactive Disorder (AD/HD).

Entry Evaluation of Students

At Brigham Young University, our experience with applicants to the M.A. degree program in music education, emphasis in music as it affects the human life process, has been that these students come from a wide variety of backgrounds and disciplines. Those coming from premedicine, psychology, nursing, or family science, for example, range from experienced musicians with advanced skill on an instrument to those with little theoretical or practical background. One common factor, however, is an intense interest in and fascination with music. It seemed to the area faculty that this student did not necessarily require the same theoretical, historical, and practical training as students in the traditional specialties. We have worked out a system of independent readings with appropriate area faculty to establish a basic literacy in theory and history. Studio lessons are included on a study list only if they will contribute to the goals of the student's program. It is for this reason that we have 8–10 electives in music courses. The other electives, which number 7–9, allow the student, with his or her committee endorsement, to pursue those out-of-department courses that will educate best in the knowledge needed to support the thesis inquiry. For example, a student with a baccalaureate in piano performance who is interested in a thesis about anxiolytic music for women in childbirth, applied most of her 7–9 out-of-department hours to midwifery and birthing courses in the College of Nursing; her 8–10 hours in music were devoted largely to expanding her knowledge of MusicMedicine, Music Therapy, and issues of psychology, musical affect, and the like. Another example is a registered nurse in the program who is interested in the effects of music on children with learning disorders. Her out-of-department hours are spent largely in Educational Psychology and Special Education. Her in-department hours are largely devoted to independent readings in theory and history. What is most amazing to our faculty is the efficiency and interest shown in theory and history by these special students, who acquire a great deal of knowledge within a relatively short period of time.

On the doctoral level, a similar approach could be applied by carefully assessing on an individual basis the strengths and weaknesses of applicants to the program. This course of action encourages interdisciplinary dialogue and promotes the Renaissance student needed in a degree of this kind. Advisory committees must include faculty from the sciences and arts and this alchemy fosters greater understanding among colleagues as well as clarification and growth in MusicMedicine.

Future Employment

Although the proposed degree program includes the coursework required for biofeedback certification—an increasingly sought after stress reduction intervention—the original intent in creating the program is to work toward a recognized specialty (MusicMedicine) within the field of medicine. A model such as this would logically follow a master's program such as the M.A. in music education, emphasis in music as it affects the human life process, Brigham Young University. During the past 3 years in which the M.A. program has been in place, a biofeedback research lab has been created in the BYU Music Department, experimental research is conducted by all students in the program, and several research grants have been obtained, including a recent one from the EJLB Foundation in Canada. In addition, a Hospital Arts program, funded by Very Special Arts through Arts Access/Utah, has put several hundred music majors and community members into the local hospital wards, retirement homes, the State Hospital, and Family Support Center, where these volunteers play and sing for patients. A close relationship has been established between the BYU Music Department and Utah Valley Regional Medical Center, which has allowed faculty and students to pursue experimental research studies in the cardiology, stroke rehabilitation, oncology, and premature baby intensive care units. Medical doctors from this hospital have worked as co-investigators in these studies and have given the researchers complete support. During the last year, the certified nurse/midwives of Utah Valley have worked closely with Drs. Spintge and Abel and faculty and students from the BYU Department of Music to develop a research project concerning chronotropic cardiac control of women in childbirth. The results have encouraged the researchers to continue for another year to increase the sample size.

Graduates of the BYU Master of Arts degree program have found employment as biofeedback specialists, neurofeedback specialists, and stress reduction specialists. They can gain certification as specialists in biofeedback and neurofeedback and, as such, may be employed in existing medical practices, medical groups, or as part of workshop teams organized by physicians to enhance patient health. This last is a growing phenomenon in family practice as well as some specialties. The author has been invited to present lecture/workshops in the incorporation of MusicMedicine in private practices, hospitals, institutions, and medical centers. A manual about the steps involved in this procedure is being prepared for publication in 1995.

All of these efforts have resulted in a strong, vital, and developing training program. The greatest drawback is that a master's level program usually lasts for only 2 years and simply does not give the student or faculty member enough time to develop significant data. It is also difficult to gain enough financial support for master's level programs to develop sufficient data to bring evidence up to the level of significance. All of these reasons gave impetus to the current proposal, which is now presented.

Curriculum for a PhD in Health Sciences, emphasis in MusicMedicine

	Credits	Title	Faculty
	3	Review and Process of Health Information	HS
	2	Behavioral Health	HS
	2	Graduate Seminar in Health Sciences	HS
	1	Relaxation & Stress Management	HS
*	5	Psychoneuroimmunology	HS
**	5	Biofeedback: Prin. & Techniques	HS & Music
**	9	Dissertation	HS & Music
Subtotal	27		
Music Dept.			
	5	Influence of Music on Behavior	Mus.
	5	Psychology of Music	Mus.
	5	Music Research Techniques	Mus.
Subtotal	15		
Psych. Dept.			
	3	Human Neuropsychology	Psych
	3	Hormones & Behavior	Psych
Subtotal	6		
Zoology Dept.			
	4	Principles of Physiology	Zool
	3	Neurophysiology	Zool
	3	Endocrinology	Zool
Subtotal	10		
Ed Psych Dept.			
	3	Counseling Theory	EdPsych
	3	Effective Counseling	EdPsych
Subtotal	6		
Statistics Dept.			
	5	Stats for Research Workers 1	Stats
	5	Stats for Res. Workers 2	Stats
Subtotal	10		

TOTAL CREDIT HOURS – 74.
* = new course. ** = team teach

Biofeedback Certification-60 supervised internship hours. Other internships considered.

Figure 1. Curriculum for Doctoral Program in MusicMedicine

Explanation of Courses

Six departments contribute to the coursework in this degree proposal. The role each plays in the program provides a particular strength that makes the model unique.

Health Sciences core

Health Sciences contributes:

1. general health sciences information and background,
2. strong psychoneuroimmunology and biofeedback* coursework that allows for team teaching, and
3. the Dissertation.

Music Department core

The Music Department provides three discrete courses, 5 credit hours each:

1. Psychology,
2. Influence of Music on Behavior, and
3. Research techniques.

In addition, the Music Department faculty share the responsibility for training in biofeedback, and the Dissertation.

Psychology Department

The Psychology Department offers strong neuropsychology and behavioral components.

Zoology Department

The Zoology Department contributes the emphasis on physiology* and endocrinology.

Educational Psychology Department

This area gives the model a strong counseling* component.

Statistics Department

The 10 hours of coursework in statistics gives the student strong background in statistical theory and application.

Health Sciences, the department that is proposed as the degree-grantor, offers the following in course content: "The Review and Processing of Health Information" provides source information and evaluation plus content review of contemporary research in health sciences. This course gives the student an overall picture of current developments and trends. "Behavioral Health" provides an analysis of current research and theory concerning health behaviors and psychological factors in the cause, prevention, development, and treatment of physical and behavioral illness and disorders. This course ties in well with the "Psychoneuroimmunology" offering, a 5-credit hour course that will cover the theoretical foundations and literature of the field, including the research that is currently being done with

---

*Course needed to meet requirements for Biofeedback certification

music. The "Biofeedback" course will be team taught by faculty from Health Sciences and Music. This course covers basic theory and techniques in the use of basic equipment, including electromyogram (EMG), electrodermogram (EDG), electrocardiogram (EKG), and temperature modules. In addition, an Electroencephalogram (EEG) unit will be used to instruct students in the use of neurofeedback as it applies to operant training of persons with a primary diagnosis of Attention Deficit Hyperactive Disorder (AD/HD). A "Graduate Seminar in Health Sciences" covers seminal readings and discussion, while the "Relaxation and Stress Management" includes basic general strategies that are useful in working with persons needing tools to facilitate stress reduction. The 9-hour "Dissertation" is jointly supervised by faculty from Health Sciences and Music. The credit hours in the Health Sciences area total 27, with 14 of those hours team taught or team supervised by faculty in both Health Sciences and Music.

"Influence of Music on Behavior" is a 5-credit hour course in which students will have the opportunity to explore and examine the effects of music on trained and untrained listeners, composers, performers, and persons with special needs. Seminal works, journal articles, and the basic literature covering all periods of human life will be included. In addition to physiological and emotional effects, students will also look at anthropological and cultural issues and how these are different in all societies. "Psychology of Music" is also a 5-credit hour course that will cover foundations of music, acoustics, basic information about the brain and its function, musical behaviors, testing and evaluation. The "Influence" and "Psychology" courses are conceived as distinct but complementary. "Research Techniques" is a 5-credit hour course that begins with an overview of all music research approaches, but focuses mainly on experimental and descriptive research techniques. Students will cover studies in both techniques and be introduced to statistical theory and research design strategies. All students construct experimental and descriptive research designs, both of which are part of the course requirements. The credit hours in music come to 15, plus the shared 14 hours with Health Sciences.

Six credit hours are completed in the Psychology Department. "Human Neuropsychology" is a 3-hour course that provides a critical study of brain-behavior relationships. "Hormones and Behavior" is a 3-credit course that studies that neural and endocrine mechanisms underlying behavior. Ten credit hours are taken in Zoology. "Principles of Physiology" is a 4-hour course covering general principles of physiology and control of organ systems. "Neurophysiology" is a 3-credit hour course that addresses that physiology of nerve cells and neuronal interactions. "Endocrinology" is a 3-hour course that includes the study of mammalian hormones.

Six credit hours in Educational Psychology provide coursework in counseling. "Counseling Theory" is a 3-hour course that includes various theories of counseling, current research, and accepted practices. "Effective Counseling" is a 3-credit hour course that includes a lab and covers basic interviewing and helping skills for students in professional, paraprofessional, peer, or lay counseling.

Finally, these students will take 10 credit hours in Statistics. "Statistics for Research Workers 1" is a 5-credit hour course that gives the student a background in probability, estimation, tests of hypotheses, regression, analysis of variance, and nonparametric methods. "Statistics for Research Workers 2" is a 5-credit hour course that covers analysis of covariance, multiple regression, linear models, designs of experiments, and sampling.

This brings the grand total of credit hours to 74. Since each student applicant to the program will have a different background in both music and sciences, a certain amount of flexibility is in order. It is important that students are thoroughly assessed in terms of skills and knowledge and that, in cases where the student already has completed a course, electives be substituted for those hours that are waived and that these electives be chosen either in or outside the field of music according to the student's needs in background coursework and skills level. Above all, each student is an individual with varying skills and knowledge and with different research interests. Advisory committees must work with the student to design a course study list that will provide the best possible experience and direct the student's efforts most effectively toward a successful dissertation completion.

In addition, it is equally important for the faculty involved in the program to constantly monitor the progress of students so that revisions and alterations may be made to the basic program model as well as to the individual student's coursework list. Although the basic core of knowledge is required for all students in the program, individual needs and dissertation thrusts make it mandatory to monitor program and student progress at all times. The interdisciplinary nature of the program will mean that collegial cooperation and dialogue are essential to success. Although the earliest European universities of the Renaissance were accustomed to such interchange, the present systems of higher education do not lend themselves geographically and socially to this kind of dialogue.

The creation of this proposed program has meant many hours of contact with colleagues across the campus. It has also pointed out the need for university administrators to address the subject of interdisciplinary studies and thus to open up lines of communication among professors from all disciplines. In addition to this interdepartmental dialogue and cooperation, we need to address the need for intercampus exchange. Our students will greatly benefit from the knowledge and research of colleagues in other institutions. A consortium of campuses would allow a student to complete some of the coursework with a colleague whose research specialty is focused on a particular area of interest. Those involved in the consortium could decide how many credit hours could be completed on another campus with such an expert and then transferred to the degree-granting institution. Such a policy would give all of these students the benefits of contact with leading scholars and resources within the consortium, not unlike the earliest students of the Middle ages who traveled from city to city to study from the masters in their field of interest. It would also be a fine example of intellectual humility, even largesse that gives students a clear message: Knowledge and truth are discovered through respectful and collegial, but rigorous dialogue, investigation, and assessment.

The issue of an appropriate practicum and/or internship must also be addressed. If the student wishes to certify in biofeedback, for example, 60 hours of supervised internship with a certified specialist must be completed. It is important to address other types of practica or internships that might be useful to the student. Dialogue with organizations such as The National Association for Music Therapy, The American Association for Music Therapy, The American Medical Association, and The International Society for Music Education, to name just a few, will be useful in addressing this issue. Other organizations that do not grant certification, but are involved in the furtherance of arts medicine, such as The International Society for Music in Medicine, and The International Arts Medicine Association, should also be integrally involved in discussions of program development and accreditation.

Matters of accreditation, ethics, professionalism, and the like will require much thoughtful discussion among colleagues of all disciplines involved in this program. Our music departments and schools are currently under accreditation from agencies such as the National Association of Schools of Music. We must now tackle the issue of a degree that primarily involves health sciences as well as music, plus four other departments. How can we achieve recognition within the health sciences as well as the general medical and healthcare community? This brings us to the topic of MusicMedicine as a specialty in field of medicine. The proposal offers coursework for subsequent certification in biofeedback and neurofeedback. The coursework outside of music lays an important foundation in the behavioral sciences and also provides the student with important research and counseling skills.

This proposal is but a first step. It is made for one reason only: to bring this issue to the table for discussion. We can no longer delay the implementation of a doctoral program in MusicMedicine. The literature shows us that, without a doubt, we lack a body of theoretical knowledge on which we can build a strong and viable program. Our research must be thorough, in depth, and worthy of consideration by our colleagues in the sciences, who must also be ready to help us design research paradigms that fit nature and characteristics of music.

Our early history shows the close liaison, for which E. Thayer Gaston was largely responsible, between music therapy and the medical field. It seems logical that it is once again time to take up this dialogue and expand it to the Health Sciences, which figure so importantly in current healthcare reform programs. As we take up these challenges, let us pause to remember the incredible devotion and hard work of those pioneers who led us so truly in the past and emulate their courage and efforts. Let us also catch sight of the vision that will lift us into a new era of healthcare that embraces the art we all love so well.

ACCESS TO THE LITERATURE OF MUSICMEDICINE THROUGH CAIRSS™ (COMPUTER-ASSISTED INFORMATION RETRIEVAL SERVICE SYSTEM™)

Charles T. Eagle and Donald A. Hodges

INTRODUCTION

Research—Practice—Theory.

1. *What* is being done in each of these three aspects?
2. *How* is it being done?
3. *Who* is doing it?
4. *Where* in the world is it being done?
5. *When* was it done?
6. *Why*?

These are the six essential questions in any discipline or profession, including MusicMedicine. Without resolution of the what, how, who, where, when, and why of MusicMedicine, it shall not be taken as seriously by collegial observers of the art/science, nor will we researchers, practitioners, and theorizers of it be fully confident of ourselves. As a consequence and, most importantly, the patients, clients, and students whom we serve through the knowledge and skills of MusicMedicine will not be nurtured to the fullest extent possible. Nor will they or we be served if an interconnecting paradigm is not envisioned among the three aspects of research, practice, and theory.

Wisely and succinctly, Gaston (1968) has said that "without practice and research, theory is impotent and unproven; without theory and research, practice is blind; and without theory and practice, research is inapplicable" (p. 408). To fail to have evidence of any one of the necessary three legs of the tripod of research, practice, and theory in MusicMedicine is to court failure in all three. The *success* of our discipline depends, therefore, on knowing the composition of the tripod and the relationships among its three legs. Only then can we rise to a higher level of confident attainment in MusicMedicine, metaphorically standing on the tripod and accessing a felt world view of who we are in the discipline—confident but not arrogant, philosophical and also practical, caring, and providing meaning in life. This is the foundational intent of the CAIRSS™ for Music Project, both as process and product.

The Computer-Assisted Information Retrieval Service System™ (CAIRSS) has been developed to meet the need for a single comprehensive source of literature pertaining to the function of music in nature...in its art and science...its art/science. More specifically, *CAIRSS for Music*™ (Hodges & Eagle, 1992) is a bibliographic database of music research, its clinical and educational practice and theory. CAIRSS has been developed to meet the evidential requirements of practitioners who need to know the latest and best clinical music procedures described in the literature, of researchers who need to know about the published music studies relevant to their own, and of theoreticians who need to know why something has happened in the findings reported in music research literature. As has become readily apparent, this literature (hereinafter called by the inclusive term "research") is reported in many publications throughout the world, making identification of and access to the research sometimes nearly impossible, but certainly time-consuming and frustrating.

Recent advancements in technology have aided in the search for relevant music literature with several electronic strategies. For example, some music research literature can be identified in such many-topical electronic databases as EMBASE, ERIC, and MEDLINE. However, there is only one database that is devoted solely to the music research literature: *CAIRSS for Music*. Researchers from any location in the world now have immediate and easy electronic on-line access to computerized searches of thousands of relevant periodical articles in music research, from hundreds of journals published worldwide. The purpose of this chapter, then, is (a) to describe the historical development of CAIRSS and the current operational status of the resulting database, (b) to present a description of the contents of CAIRSS, and (c) to provide speculations of the envisioned future directions for CAIRSS.

HISTORICAL DEVELOPMENT OF CAIRSS

CAIRSS was established in 1969. A thorough investigation of finding published music research literature was instigated in an attempt to bring it together into a single, comprehensive source. Over the ensuing years, a global search has been made to identify and collate published music research, relevant particularly to medicine but also to psychology, education, therapy, and other related areas. Support for this process has been provided by several institutions, including the National Association for Music Therapy (1970–1977), Southern Methodist University (1975–1994), Texas Woman's University (1972–1975), University of Miami (1969–1972), and University of Texas at San Antonio (1988–1994).

As the CAIRSS Project has continued, no less than 21 formal presentations have been made about its progress and results, to such international audiences as dance therapists, drama therapists, music educators, music performers, music therapists, neurophysiologists, physicians (various), psychoacousticians, and psychologists (Eagle 1976b, 1978b, 1978c, 1979b, 1979c, 1980d, 1986, 1989, 1990, 1993a, 1993b; Eagle & Dubler 1970; Eagle & Hodges 1978, 1994; Eagle & Lathom 1972; Eagle, Miniter, & Drennan 1977; Eagle & Prewitt 1973; Hodges & Eagle 1993a, 1993b, 1994a, 1994b). Among these, the first formal results of the CAIRSS Project were presented to a meeting of the Music Teachers National Association (Eagle & Dubler, 1970), and subsequently published (Eagle & Dubler, 1971). In all, 11 publications have carried informational details about *CAIRSS for Music* (Eagle 1976c, 1979a, 1980a, 1980b, 1980c, 1992, 1994; Eagle and Dubler 1971; Eagle & Hodges 1992; Eagle & Miniter 1985; Eagle & Prewitt 1974).

The initial, first generational efforts of *CAIRSS for Music* eventuated in a printed series of three indexes. The three index volumes were computer-generated (mainframe) from a series of evolving software programs: KWOC (Keywords Out Of Context),[1] KWIC (KeyWords In Context), WADEX (Word And Author Index) (Ripperger, Wooster, Juhasz, Falconer, Roach, & Stanton 1966), and, finally, the nine subroutines of COWAX.[2] The last subroutine of it provided the final format for the printing of the three indexes.

The first index publication was *Music therapy index, Volume 1* (Eagle, 1976a). This volume contained bibliographical citations of music research—with music therapy as the central focus—published between 1960 and 1975. The second was *Music psychology index, Volume 2* (Eagle, 1978a). The change of title reflected an evolving philosophy due to the expanding relevance of literature in music research, especially to medicine and psychology as well as music therapy. This can be seen especially in its subtitle: *The international interdisciplinary index of the influence of music on behavior: References to the literature from the natural and behavioral sciences, and the fine and therapeutic arts for the years 1976–77.* The third and final printed volume was *Music psychology index, Volume 3* (Eagle & Miniter, 1984); it contained relevant citations published 1978–1980. Summary data of the three index volumes indicate over 6,000 bibliographic entries covering music research literature from 1960–1980. These citations are listed under more than 16,000 keyword descriptors and names of authors found in those references.

With the publication of *Volume 3* in 1984, work on *CAIRSS for Music* ceased. The enormity of the subject had become overwhelming, due to the following reasons: First, new professional organizations in MusicMedicine, such as the International Arts Medicine Association, International Society for Music in Medicine, and Performing Arts Medicine Association, were being established during the 1980s. Second, there was an increasing number of national and international conferences specifically oriented to the function and use of music in various medical specialties and settings. Third, there was an increasing number of related refereed journals that began publication, including *International Journal of Arts Medicine, Music Perception,* and *Music Therapy Perspectives.* Fourth, a holistic art/science philosophy had led literally to hundreds of sources of thousands of relevant articles. Fifth, a "revolution" in computer hardware and software was under way by the early 1980s, and consequently, a change in technology for operating CAIRSS became obvious. Sixth, it became clear that an index of citations built only from a listing of keyword descriptors in the titles and authors of articles (i.e., through KWOC, KWIC, WADEX, and COWAX mainframe computer programs) was inadequate in providing users the essential information from within the published articles. Seventh, more immediate access to published literature via online computer services, rather than through time-delayed printing and distribution became apparent (i.e., printed indexes had become passé). The convergence of these seven major factors led to the conclusion that a complete overhaul of the CAIRSS Project was necessary if it were to continue in operation effectively and efficiently.

Taking into account these developments, plans were made to secure the second generation of CAIRSS toward the end of the 1980s.

1. Searches were made of several electronic databases of medical literature (including MEDLINE and EMBASE) using the keywords "music" and "music therapy." Searches also were made "by hand" of other appropriate publications and bibliographies.

2. Thirty-nine relevant fields of information were determined. These fields not only included the most pertinent ones of other bibliographic retrieval systems, but also ones that the developers considered worthy of inclusion for users of CAIRSS.

3. Desktop computers were purchased.

4. Several software programs were reviewed for relevancy; these included *Bookends, Double Helix, Pro-Cite, Filemaker,* and finally, *Filemaker Pro.* The combination of these four factors resulted in the renewed input of bibliographic materials into CAIRSS.[3]

5. At the same time, however, work began toward the development of a technique to determine keyword descriptors from *each article*—not just the titles—of each bibliographic entry in the database. This effort has resulted in a thesaurus of search terminology compatible to languages used by medical *and* music professionals. Thus, not only has a modern, more sophisticated, and user-friendly CAIRSS database been built, but a more complete

and compatible language base for music researchers has been devised. (See Eagle, 1994: *CAIRSS thesaurus, Volume 1.*)

Parallel with these activities taking place at Southern Methodist University in its Department of Music Therapy: Medicine & Health (DMT) during the late 1980s, the Institute for Music Research (IMR) was established at the University of Texas at San Antonio. IMR was created to promote research primarily in the areas of music psychophysiology and music technology, the activities of IMR being organized into three main categories: computer services,[4] conferences,[5] and dedicated research.[6] Part of these activities at IMR included the development of an extensive database, primarily of research in music education. Subsequent consultation between the directors of DMT and IMR led to the merger of the two databases, resulting in an appropriately expanded version and institutionalization of *CAIRSS for Music.* In turn, NOTIS[7] was selected as the delivery system for CAIRSS. NOTIS is a comprehensive system for libraries, allowing for a wide range of management and processing functions and also to offer on-line catalogs. It is this cataloging capability that is now being used for CAIRSS. Because NOTIS automatically runs on the INTERNET, a worldwide computer network, CAIRSS is now accessible as a free bibliographic service to all users anywhere in the world.[8]

DESCRIPTIVE CONTENTS OF CAIRSS[9]

Citation Holdings

Currently, there are over 11,000 citations in CAIRSS. Eighteen "primary journals" form the nucleus of the database; these are so identified because more than 50% of the articles in the periodicals pertain to music research. This means that every article (including perhaps, those on art, dance, drama, etc.) that has ever been published in these journals over the years is cited in CAIRSS. This means, too, that citations of articles from these journals are added to the database as they are received on an ongoing basis. These primary journals are: *Arts in Psychotherapy, Bulletin of the Council for Research in Music Education, Bulletin of the National Association for Music Therapy, Contributions to Music Education, Hospital Music Newsletter, IJAM: International Journal of Arts Medicine, Journal of the Association for Music and Imagery, Journal of Music Teacher Education, Journal of Music Therapy, Journal of Research in Music Education, Medical Problems of Performing Artists, Music Perception, Music Therapy, Music Therapy Perspectives, Psychology of Music, Psychomusicology, The Quarterly: Research in Music Teaching and Learning*, and *Update: Applications of Research in Music Education.* Besides the primary journals, there are 969 additional different journals (mostly medical and psychological) published worldwide, from which pertinent articles have been selected and are currently cited in CAIRSS. There is a variety of these secondary sources that have been identified, including reference listings from 'hand searches' and from other databases such as MEDLINE and EMBASE. In addition, another 551 journals have been identified that contain relevant articles. Thus, there currently is a total of 1,538 journals identified as having pertinent references that are published in 42 different countries in 20 languages.

Citation Contents

The information for each citation in the CAIRSS database, taken from a copy of the original article, contains the following:

1. Names of all authors.
2. Complete title and subtitle of the article, and, if in a non-English language, the title appears in [brackets].
3. The number of authored references and/or bibliography cited in the article.
4. Classification from among 12 types of documents (e.g., case study, empirical study, literature review).
5. The name of the journal.
6. The country of publication.
7. ISSN designators.
8. CODEN designators. ISSN and CODEN allow reference librarians to order more easily the article desired.
9. The language of the article is stated.
10. Information concerning the existence of an English abstract.
11. Date of publication.
12. Volume number.
13. Issue number.
14. Inclusive page numbers.
15. A list of keyword descriptors.

The keywords have been determined from an analysis of 5,000 articles, the citations of which were randomly selected from CAIRSS. The resulting 2,500+ keyword and keyword-phrase descriptors have been taken directly from the title, subtitle (if any), author(s), abstract (if any), and the body of the article. Word form conventions were determined and term relationships devised. From this process, an additional 24 broad categories of terms—that appear in uppercase letters in the list of keywords for any particular article—were developed to aid the user in making a more broad and more inclusive search of the database. These categories include those such as BRAIN, DENTISTRY, PERCEPTION, SURGERY, UPPER LIMB, and WOODWINDS. The resulting purpose of these unique search features has been to increase the probability of the user making more accurate and quick "hits" of relevant citations.

Citation Summaries

Articles. Based on further analysis of the 5,000 selected articles in CAIRSS relevant to their 12 *types*, findings indicate that 42% of the articles in the database are empirical studies, 21% program reviews, 11% theoretical studies, and 6% case studies. Among the 20 different *languages* of the articles, 90% have been published in English, 4% German, 2% French, and 1% Polish. Regarding the *year of publication*, the most significant datum is the rate of publication. Since 1960 and over a period of 33 years, music research has been published an average of 48% more each year than the immediate preceding year

The summary data concerning the *broad categories* of keyword descriptors reveal that 24% of the 5,000 articles pertain to THERAPY; 13% each to EDUCATION, MUSIC TYPES, and PSYCHOLOGY; and 12% to PERCEPTION. Although not designated broad categories as such, a frequency count reveals that 20% of the 5,000 articles have the term "performing arts medicine" as a keyword phrase, and 13% "music therapy."

Journals. An analysis made of the 1,538 journals identified as having published music research literature indicates that the *countries of publication* are as follows: 51% USA, 12% England, 8% Germany, and 4% France.

In an attempt to determine the types or kinds of journals represented in the database, *categories of journals* were determined from the 987 primary and secondary journals currently appearing among the citations of the approximately 11,000 articles in CAIRSS. Findings from this categorical analysis reveal the following: In the category of "Medicine: Specialty Boards": 48% of all journals, the highest number being those in psychiatry, neurology, dentistry, and surgery. (Significant is the fact that every medical specialty, as listed by the National Library of Medicine, has published music research literature.) In the category of "Medicine: Other Specialties": 5% of all journals, the largest number being those in behavioral medicine, sports medicine, geriatrics, and occupational medicine. In the category of "Medicine: General": 14% of all journals. In the category of "Therapeutic Arts & Sciences," 16% of all journals were found, the highest number of these published in psychology, 'general' therapy, music therapy, and physical therapy. In the category of "Arts, Humanities & Sciences": 17% of all journals, the largest number being those in education, music, 'general' science, and biology. Overall then, two-thirds, or 67%, of all journals cited in CAIRSS are those in the categories of medicine. One-third, or 33%, are those journals in the categories of the arts, sciences, and humanities.

FUTURE DIRECTIONS OF CAIRSS

Although the initial experience has been positive, there are several additions and improvements envisioned for CAIRSS.[10]

Inter-Library Loan Service. To provide an inter-library loan service that will allow users to order and obtain copies of selected and desired articles not readily available.

Scanned-In Abstracts. To develop a process that will allow for scanning-in abstracts, summaries, and/or opening and closing paragraphs of articles. In turn, these items will become available on-line to users.

Scanned-Full Text. To place the full text of articles in the database that will allow users to read the complete article—including figures, tables, and illustrations—on-line. As a result, the user will be able to print out the text of the desired article at remote locations.

CONCLUDING STATEMENT ABOUT CAIRSS[11]

CAIRSS for Music has been in preparation for 25 years. Initial efforts resulted in the publication of three hard-copy volumes: *Music Therapy Index, Volume 1* and *Music Psychology Index, Volume 2* and *Volume 3.* Although the printing of CAIRSS has ceased, efforts have been, are currently, and will remain dedicated to producing a continually updated and current on-line, computerized database of music research literature, available worldwide. Through collegial collaboration, the goals of *CAIRSS for Music* remain:

1. To continue to develop a state-of-the-art computerized information retrieval service system for recording information of scientific and artistic value in music research.

2. To serve as a clearinghouse for all information relevant to music research, both published and unpublished.

3. To promote scientific inquiry into all aspects of the function of music, principally among those in the disciplines of music psychophysiology, music therapy, MusicMedicine, and music education.

4. To facilitate networking among music researchers, clinicians, and theorists.

Endnotes

[1]Joseph Youngblood of the University of Miami formulated the KWOC program specifically for CAIRSS.

[2]E. A. Ripperger of the University of Texas at Austin generously provided the COWAX program.

[3]Staff members at Southern Methodist University, who have contributed most significantly to this aspect of CAIRSS have included Dennis Bowers, David Luce, Thomas Mogyordy, Kathryn Riddle, Susan Plyler Scott, Cathy Weldin, and especially Kobie Temmingh. Thomas Eagle of Texas Instruments, Inc. also contributed significantly.

[4]MRIS (Music Research Information Services) is a gopher server that serves as a gateway to CAIRSS, TIME (Technology In Music Education)—a database of music-related hardware and software products, a bulletin board for sharing music research information, and a number of related services, including connections to remote sites. All are offered as free services, available worldwide via the INTERNET.

[5]The first conference sponsored by IMR was "Setting an Agenda for Neuromusical Research," held January 21–23, 1993. The second conference was "Technological Directions in Music Education," December 2–4, 1993, and the third: "Vth International Symposium on MusicMedicine," a conference of the International Society for Music in Medicine (ISMM), jointly sponsored by ISMM, IMR, the University of Texas Health Science Center at San Antonio, and the International Arts Medicine Association. The Second "Technological Directions in Music Education" was held January 26–28, 1994.

[6]Research projects include a variety of studies in neuromusicology and music technology.

[7]David Sebald of the University of Texas at San Antonio made the final selection of NOTIS, after investigating various options for a delivery system for CAIRSS.

[8]Staff and faculty members at the University of Texas at San Antonio, who have contributed most significantly to CAIRSS, include John Conyers, Jack Frost, Debra Harris, Sandra Rickett, David Sebald, Joe Stuessy, Sue Tyner, Kim Walls, and Fred Zapata.

[9]This section is has been abridged and edited from the materials found in: Eagle 1994: *CAIRSS Thesaurus, Volume 1.*

[10]The intent is to maintain CAIRSS as a free service; however, there is a modest cost for the *CAIRSS Thesaurus.* When the inter-library loan service and the full-text system become available, there will be a small nonprofit fee attached. In both of these circumstances, full compliance will be made with prevailing copyright restrictions.

[11]For information about CAIRSS, to become a registered user, or to acquire a copy of the *CAIRSS Thesaurus,* please send your name, address, phone, fax, e-mail address, and professional affiliation (clinic, hospital, university, etc.) to:

Dr. Donald A. Hodges, Director
Institute for Music Research; Division of Music
University of Texas at San Antonio; San Antonio, TX 78249-0645
phone: (210) 691-5317; fax: (210) 691-4381; e-mail: dhodges@lonestar.utsa.edu

In the meantime, you may log on via the following:

1. Access your local network and enter: **telnet runner.utsa.edu**
2. at login, enter: **imr**
3. at password, just press return.

References

Eagle, C. T. (Ed.) (1976a). *Music therapy index: Volume 1: An international interdisciplinary index to the literature of the psychology, psychophysiology, psychophysics and sociology of music.* Lawrence, KS: National Association for Music Therapy.

Eagle, C. T. (1976b, October 23). *How to use the music therapy index.* Paper presented at the 27th annual conference of the National Association for Music Therapy, Milwaukee, Wisconsin.

Eagle, C. T. (Ed.) (1978a). *Music psychology index: Volume 2: The international interdisciplinary index of the influence of music on behavior: References to the literature from the natural and behavioral sciences, and the fine and therapeutic arts for the years 1976–77.* (Formerly, *Music Therapy Index.*) Denton, TX: Institute for Therapeutics Research.

Eagle, C. T. (1978b, October 21). *The computer-assisted information retrieval service system (CAIRSS) for music therapy.* Paper presented at the 1st International Symposium for Music Therapy Training, Herdecke-Ruhr, West Germany.

Eagle, C. T. (1978c, November 14). *CAIRSS for music therapy.* Paper presented at the 29th annual conference of the National Association for Music Therapy, Atlanta, Georgia.

Eagle, C. T. (1979a). The computer-assisted information retrieval service system (CAIRSS) for music and music education. In S. D. Miller (Ed.), *Research Reports: Texas Music Educators Association.* (pp. ix, 1–23). Houston: TMEA.

Eagle, C. T. (1979b, February 10). *The computer-assisted information retrieval service system (CAIRSS) for music and music education.* Paper presented at the annual conference of the Texas Music Educators Association, Ft. Worth, Texas.

Eagle, C. T. (1979c, June 29). *An overview of the CAIRSS System for music therapy: Implications for creative arts therapies.* Paper presented at the conference on creative arts therapies, sponsored by the American Psychiatric Association, Washington, D.C.

Eagle, C. T. (1980a). The computer-assisted information retrieval service system (CAIRSS) for music. *Proceedings of the Loyola music symposium* (n.e.). New Orleans: Loyola University College of Music.

Eagle, C. T. (1980b). Bibliographical research in music therapy. In R. Gibson (Ed.), *The Use of the Creative Arts in Therapy* (pp. 42–44). Washington: American Psychiatric Association.

Eagle, C. T. (1980c, February 15). *CAIRSS (Computer-assisted information retrieval service system) for music.* Paper presented at the 3rd annual Loyola music symposium, New Orleans, Louisiana.

Eagle, C. T. (1986, December 11). *Exploring research in music and medicine.* Paper presented at the music and health conference, Eastern Kentucky University, Richmond, Kentucky.

Eagle, C. T. (1989, October 29). *Retrieving the literature of MusicMedicine.* Paper presented at the 4th international symposium of the International Society for Music in Medicine, Annenberg Center for Health Sciences at Eisenhower, Rancho Mirage, California.

Eagle, C. T. (1990, March 2–3). (Consultant and participant), Symposium on information retrieval in arts medicine, Philadelphia, Pennsylvania.

Eagle, C. T. (1992). Retrieving the literature of MusicMedicine. In R. Spintge and R. Droh (Eds.) *Music in medicine: Proceedings of the 4th international symposium of the International Society for Music in Medicine* (pp. 391–404). St. Louis: MMB Music.

Eagle, C. T. (1993a, November 3). *The research literature in MusicMedicine.* Paper presented at an "Evening of presentations," Institute for Music Research, University of Texas at San Antonio, San Antonio, Texas.

Eagle, C. T. (1993b, November 4). *The research literature in MusicMedicine.* Paper presented at the University of Texas Health Sciences Center at San Antonio; San Antonio, Texas.

Eagle, C. T. (1994). *CAIRSS thesaurus: The cross-indexed reference of keywords in bibliographical citations of art-science.* San Antonio: Institute for Music Research, University of Texas at San Antonio.

Eagle, C. T., & Dubler, G. D. (1970, April 15). *Recent findings in psychology of music research.* Paper presented at the annual convention of the Music Teachers National Association, Miami Beach, Florida.

Eagle, C. T., & Dubler, G. D. (1971). Recent findings in psychology of music research. *Journal of Music Therapy, 8*(4), 152–167.

Eagle, C. T., & Hodges, D. A. (1978, February 3). *The CAIRSS system for music.* Paper presented at the research symposium on the psychology and acoustics of music, University of Kansas, Lawrence, Kansas.

Eagle, C. T., & Hodges, D. A. (1992). CAIRSS for music in arts medicine. *International Journal of Arts Medicine, 1*(2), 21–25.

Eagle, C. T., & Hodges, D. A. (1994, March 18). *Access to the literature of MusicMedicine through CAIRSS (Part 2).* Paper presented at the 5th international symposium of the International Society for Music in Medicine, San Antonio, Texas.

Eagle, C. T., & Lathom, W. B. (1972, August 17). *A computer-assisted information retrieval system in music therapy: Implications for the physical and neuropsychological foundations of music.* Paper presented at the workshop on physical and neuropsychological foundations of music, Ossiach, Austria.

Eagle, C. T., & Miniter, J. J. (Eds.). (1984). *Music psychology index: Volume 3: The international interdisciplinary index of the influence of music on behavior: References to the literature from the natural and behavioral sciences, and the fine and therapeutic arts for the years 1978–80.* Phoenix: Oryx Press and Denton, TX: Institute for Therapeutics Research.

Eagle, C. T., Miniter, J. J., & Drennan, C. (1977, October 27). *The CAIRSS project: Past, present, and future.* Paper presented at the 28th annual conference of the National Association for Music Therapy, Anaheim, California.

Eagle, C. T., & Prewitt, S. A. (1973, November 2). *A computer-assisted information retrieval system in music therapy: A word-and-author index of published studies.* Paper presented at the 24th annual conference of the National Association for Music Therapy, Athens, Georgia.

Eagle, C. T., & Prewitt, S. A. (1974). A computerized bibliographical index in music psychology and music therapy. *Journal of Music Therapy, 11*(4), 181–201.

Gaston, E. T. (1968). Planning and understanding research. In E. T. Gaston (Ed.) *Music in therapy* (p. 408). New York: Macmillan.

Glassman, L. R. (1985). Review of Eagle, C. T. & Miniter, J. J. (Eds.) Music psychology index, Volume 3. *Arts in Psychotherapy, 12*(2), 120.

Hodges, D. A., & Eagle, C. T. (1992). *CAIRSS for music.* The INTERNET.

Hodges, D. A., & Eagle, C. T. (1993a, February 11). *Long distance access to music research literature.* Paper presented at the annual conference of the Texas Music Educators Association, San Antonio, Texas.

Hodges, D. A., & Eagle, C. T. (1993b, October 28). *CAIRSS for music: Long-distance access to music research literature.* Paper presented to the Joint North American Music Therapy Conference, Toronto, Canada.

Hodges, D. A., & Eagle, C. T. (1994a, February 12). *Long distance access to music education research.* Paper presented at the annual conference of the Texas Music Educators Association, San Antonio, Texas.

Hodges, D. A., & Eagle, C. T. (1994b, March 18). *Access to the literature of MusicMedicine through CAIRSS (Part 1).* Paper presented at the 5th International Symposium of the International Society for Music in Medicine, San Antonio, Texas.

Regelski, T. A. (1980). Review of Eagle, C. T. (Ed.) Music psychology index (Vol. 2). *Journal of Music Therapy, 17*(4), 223–227.

Ripperger, E. A., Wooster, H., Juhasz, S., Falconer, D., Roach, F. A., & Stanton, P. L. (1966). WADEX: Word and author index: Description and program documentation. Unpublished monograph, *Applied Mechanics Reviews*, San Antonio, Texas.

Sharpe, A. T. (1976). Review of C. T. Eagle: Music therapy index: An international interdisciplinary index to the literature of the psychology, psychophysiology, psychophysics and sociology of music, Volume 1. *Journal of Music Therapy, 13*(4), 184–185.

A COGNITIVE MODEL OF MUSIC IN MEDICINE

Cheryl Dileo Maranto

MIND-BODY COMMUNICATION

There is increasing evidence to support the fact that communication occurs between the mind and body. Although the review presented in this paper is not intended to be comprehensive, the work of several significant researchers will be mentioned. According to Goleman & Gurin (1993), "scientific evidence for the mind's influence on the body now comes from three converging areas of research: (a) physiological research, which investigates the biological and biochemical connections between the brain and the body's systems; (b) epidemiological research, which shows correlations between certain psychological factors and certain illnesses in the population at large; and (c) clinical research, which tests the effectiveness of mind/body approaches in preventing, alleviating, or treating specific diseases" (p. 8).

Physiological Research

Recent research (Pert, 1987; Pert & Snyder, 1973) has identified the role of neuropeptides and specific neuropeptide receptors in facilitating biochemical messages within the brain, from the body to the brain and from the brain to the body. Pert (in Goleman & Gurin, 1993) indicates that this network comprises a biochemical correlate of emotions, and, indeed, emotions may provide the basis for mind-body communication. Pert speculates that emotions (and in particular, the suppression of emotions) may directly influence health in a negative manner.

A recent landmark study supports this speculation (Spiegel, Bloom, Kraemer, & Gottheil, 1989). In this research, women with metastatic cancer met together in a support group while also receiving medical treatment for their conditions. It was found that the women who received psychosocial support lived on the average twice as long as women who received medical treatment only.

Felten (in Goleman & Gurin, 1993) has found evidence that nerve fibers are contained in virtually every organ of the immune system directly, thus providing direct biological connections between these nervous and immune systems; in addition, neuroendocrine mechanisms are triggered by this innervation. It is therefore possible that there is a direct link between a person's thoughts, attitudes, perceptions, emotions, etc., and functioning of the immune system. If this is the case, the individual may assume an active role in his or her health.

Several authors (Ader, 1988; Ader & Cohen, 1975) demonstrated rather vividly that learning processes could influence immune responses and that the placebo response could be learned. Therefore, it is very likely that the brain exerts influence over immune functioning.

Physicist David Bohm (1987, 1989) suggests that the connection between the mind and body is through a third phenomenon: meaning. These three entities cannot be separated as they form a whole. Meanings *are* the body and they *are* the mind; they are similar ontologically.

Furthering these theories, Dossey (1991) indicates that meaning is inseparable from a person's thinking and affect. He provides a number of medical situations wherein a person's medical condition is directly attributable to the meaning he or she ascribes to the situation.

Epidemiological Research

Although there is still controversy in the literature about specific personality variables and the propensity for specific diseases (e.g., cancer, arthritis), a generic "disease-prone" personality has been identified (Friedman & Booth-Kewley, 1987). This is characterized by depression, anger/hostility, anxiety and perhaps other factors. These factors appear to increase the general risk for disease.

In addition, there is a suspected relationship among anger and hostility and heart disease. Without a doubt, an individual's coping strategies, particularly with regard to stress and anxiety may exert an important influence on health. "Individual differences in the way people cope may be at least as important as the stressors themselves in determining health or illness. A variety of psychological factors—including mood, personality characteristics, coping style, suppression of anger, hopelessness, psychological vulnerability, and defensiveness—can all affect the way a person deals with stress and thus can potentially modulate the impact that stress will have on the immune system" (Pelletier, 1993, p. 29).

Factors that appear to be related to positive coping include: reframing the issues of life into challenges rather than threats, commitment to something meaningful, perceiving a sense of control over decisions, and having a supportive social environment (Pelletier, 1993).

Clinical Research

Although the mind/body approaches are varied, and research examining the effectiveness of specific techniques is in progress, there is support for various stress management and psychotherapeutic strategies such as: meditation, biofeedback, cognitive therapy, exercise, hypnosis, as well as various clinical uses of imagery. Current research in this area is studying: the effects of relaxation on various medical problems, such as hypertension and migraine headaches; the effect of anger and anger control on heart disease; immunological changes associated with group therapy in cancer patients; and the effects of group therapy and coping strategies on health problems of AIDS patients (Goleman & Gurin, 1993).

There has already been a significant amount of research that has studied the influence of music on health (Maranto, in press; 1993a; 1993b).

COGNITIONS AND HEALTH

From the previous sections, an argument (although not necessarily exhaustive) has been presented wherein the connection of the mind, body (and meaning) have been described. Furthermore, characteristics of a "disease-prone" personality have been identified, and psychosocial factors related to health and disease have been mentioned.

If a person's perceptions, thoughts, and feelings are related to immune system activity and health in general, many medical diseases can be considered "thinking and feeling" disorders. If this is the case, cognitive therapy may provide at least one viable way to change or modify what the mind tells the body, and subsequently facilitate health. In addition, cognitive therapy provides one way to examine the meaning of life events and health/illness for the individual.

COGNITIVE PSYCHOTHERAPY

A thorough description of cognitive therapy would be above and beyond the limits of this paper. However, several points regarding cognitive therapy and health are essential.

Beck (1993) discusses specific "stress syndromes" such as anxiety, depression and hostility (all of which have been directly related to health risk). He states that each of these syndromes "comprises a specific controlling cognitive constellation and the resultant behavioral inclinations and affect" (p. 348). A characteristic of these is that they tend to selectively identify and process stimuli consistent with them and ignore stimuli that are incongruent. Problems in these areas (i.e., idiosyncratic cognitive patterns) "become hyperactive and lead to overmobilization of the voluntary nervous system and autonomic nervous system. Concurrently, the system of buffers and adaptive functions (objectivity, perspective, reality testing) becomes strained and is progressively less effective in counteracting the dominance of the controlling cognitive constellation" (p. 357). The general aim of treatment is to reduce the hyperactivity of the relevant cognitive constellation and to facilitate more adaptive functioning.

COGNITIVE MUSIC PSYCHOTHERAPY

One approach to cognitive therapy is described in this paper, that is, cognitive music psychotherapy (CMP). In CMP, techniques of cognitive therapy are integrated with music therapy processes. This is not to imply that cognitive therapy is ineffective without music, as this is certainly not the case. There is indeed a wealth of scientific evidence that supports its clinical effectiveness. This is also not meant to imply that music therapy alone or based on other theoretical models is not an important treatment for health-related problems, as the literature in this area is rapidly expanding (Maranto, in press; 1993a; 1993b).

Music therapy as a nonverbal type of treatment, as opposed to forms of verbal therapy, may provide (among other benefits) the following: (a) more direct access to thinking and feeling states; (b) an opportunity to "contain" feelings for periods of time so that these can be explored, examined and worked through for the individual; (c) nonverbal expression of thinking and feeling states that are not yet within the verbal domain for the individual; (d) the elicitation of imagery and associations that are not accessible through verbal means; (e) more direct physiological benefits for the individual than verbal methods and (f) the freedom to explore and "try-out" various solutions to his thinking and feeling problems through music exploration and creativity.

Cognitive Music Psychotherapy Techniques

Various techniques are used in cognitive music psychotherapy for assessment and/or treatment. All experiences within music may be used (listening, improvisatory, performing or composing) according to various goals and needs of the person. The following is a partial list and brief description of some techniques (although not comprehensive) that are relevant to individuals with health problems.

Spontaneous Individual Improvisation within the group (instrumental or vocal)

This is used to assess thinking patterns associated with fears, anxieties, and self-concept related to the person's health. Individuals write down or verbally report their automatic thoughts (concerning themselves and others) as they occur before, during and after their individual improvisations.

Song Analysis

This may be used to examine individuals' rational and irrational thinking and belief systems regarding their health through their identification with and interpretation of various song lyrics. In addition, specially selected songs may be selected that can elicit feelings regarding particular meanings of their illness.

Music and Imagery

The individual listens to music in a relaxed state following a specific imagery suggestion related to health and/or mind-body communication. In addition, this procedure is used to facilitate rehearsing of goals and coping strategies.

Music and Time-Projection

In a relaxed state, individuals are asked to imagine themselves in a situation in the future. This provides some perspective to the individual's current situation and often provides a clear picture of his expectations regarding his health.

Music-Based Relaxation with Autogenic Suggestion

Individuals become progressively more relaxed as they listen to music while also receiving autogenic suggestions. These suggestions are thought to counter distracting and anxiety-provoking automatic thoughts. This technique is used to facilitate both relaxation and pain management.

Theme or Issue-Centered Group, Dyadic, or Individual Improvisation

This can be most varied, and can precede or follow any of the other experiences. It allows individuals opportunities to experiment with new thinking and beliefs, express feelings and beliefs, practice new coping patterns, achieve perspective on their illness, receive direct feedback from others musically and verbally, can provide insight to behavior patterns, etc.

Free Improvisation (Instrumental or Vocal) Dyadic, Individual or Group

This can facilitate the expression of feelings, bring insight into ways of thinking and behaving relative to health, provide opportunities for practicing coping skills, provide a source of feedback and facilitate the development of group cohesiveness and support. In dyadic treatment, these methods provide a way to nonverbally challenge absolutist or dichotomous thinking regarding the illness.

Song-Writing

Individuals are given opportunities to create their own music, and/or lyrics that reinforce new ways of thinking about health. Individuals can use these materials as prompts for rational thinking in challenging situations.

Systematic Desensitization with Music

Music is used to entrain relaxed physiological responses as the individual is verbally exposed to progressively greater anxiety-provoking situations imaginally.

Song Histories

A technique wherein patients bring in songs to describe their "life histories" so that they can get a better perspective about the events of their lives, and their thinking, feelings and belief systems relevant to these events and their health.

Process of Cognitive Music Psychotherapy

The following outline describes a process of cognitive music psychotherapy with specific goals at each stage. It is deliberately general to provide a general overview of a treatment approach. Specific music therapy techniques are included according to the goals of each stage.

Stage 1. Self-Awareness and Conceptualization

1. During this stage, the individuals use music to achieve greater self-awareness of their lives in general (song history), their health (specifically) and identify a specific health-related problem area (with specific goals). Also, a therapeutic relationship is established based on "client-therapist resonance."
2. Thinking, beliefs and feelings with regard to this problem are identified and expressed (song-analysis, spontaneous solo improvisation)
3. Dyadic improvisation between the client and therapist is used to identify aspects of irrational internal dialogue regarding health (with the client and therapist switching roles).
4. Identification of individual meanings of the problem and health (music and imagery)
5. Consistent monitoring of irrational thoughts and beliefs regarding health.

Stage 2. Learning New Thinking

1. Identification of strengths and resources (free group improvisation).
2. Learning new coping skills with regard to life situations. (Music-based relaxation and/or systematic desensitization, theme centered group improvisation.)
3. Putting health problem into perspective (Music time projection)
4. Practicing new thinking skills regarding health. (Music and imagery with coping strategy rehearsal; song-writing)

Stage 3: Applying and Evaluating New Skills

1. Testing and modifying new skills (theme-centered group music improvisation)
2. Practicing goals with regard to health (music and goal rehearsal)
3. Practice skills in vivo; learning strategies for possible relapse
4. Evaluating success according to medical, psychological, social criteria, etc.

CONCLUSIONS

Cognitive music psychotherapy can provide one strategy to deal with health risks associated with those factors that may make an individual prone to disease. Also, this strategy is focused on the development of coping skills, which appear to be instrumental in health maintenance. Because the literature supporting the various linkages between the mind and the body is burgeoning, the mind's role in health, that is, its thoughts, feelings, beliefs and meanings will undoubtedly receive increasing attention. Cognitive therapy provides an approach to understand and modify what we say to ourselves and ultimately to our bodies. Music may permit a rapid nonverbal access to these thoughts and feelings, may allow full expression of feelings and provide opportunities for enhancing the cognitive therapy process. As there is virtually no research yet in cognitive music psychotherapy, it is essential that this process be tested both clinically and empirically.

References

Ader, R., & Cohen, N. (1975). The influence of the psyche and the brain on immunity and disease of susceptibility: A critical review. *Psychosomatic Medicine, 41,* 159.

Ader, R. (1988). The placebo effect as a conditioned response. In R. Ader, H. Weiner, & A. Baum (Eds.), *Experimental foundations of behavioral medicine: Conditioning approaches.* Hillsdale, NJ: Erlbaum.

Beck, A. (1993). Cognitive approaches to stress. In P. Lehrer and R. Woolfolk (Eds.), *Principles and practice of stress management* (pp. 333–372) New York: Guilford Press.

Bohm, D. (1989). Meaning and information. In P. Pylkkänen (Ed.), *The search for meaning.* Wellingborough, Northamptonshire, England: Crucible.

Bohm, D. (1987). Soma-significance: A new notion of the relationship between the physical and the mental. In D. Factor (Ed.), *Unfolding meaning* (pp. 72–120). London: Routledge & Kegan Paul.

Dossey, L. (1991). *Meaning and medicine.* New York: Bantam Books.

Friedman, H. S., & Booth-Kewley, S. (1987). The disease-prone personality. *American Psychologist, 42,* 539–555.

Goleman, D., & Gurin, J. (1993). *Mind body medicine.* Yonkers, NY: Consumer Reports Books.

Maranto, C. D. (in press). Research in music and medicine: The state of the art. In M. A. Froelich (Ed.), *Music therapy for hospitalized children: A child-life approach.*

Maranto, C. D. (1993a). Music therapy and stress management. In P. Lehrer & R. Woolfolk (Eds.), *Principles and practice of stress management* (pp. 407–442) New York: Guilford Press.

Maranto, C. D. (1993b). Applications of music in medicine. In M. Heal & T. Wigram (Eds.), *Music therapy in health and education* (pp. 153–174). London: Jessica Kingsley.

Meichenbaum, D. (1993). Stress inoculation training: A 20-year update. In P. Lehrer & R. Woolfolk (Eds.), *Principles and practice of stress management* (pp. 373–406). New York: Guilford Press.

Pelletier, K. (1993). Between mind and body, stress emotions and health. In D. Goleman & J. Gurin (Eds.), *Mind body medicine* (pp. 19–38). Yonkers, NY: Consumer Reports Books.

Pert, C. (1987. The wisdom of the receptors: Neuropeptides, the emotions and body-mind. *Advances, 3*(3) 8–16.

Spiegel, D., Bloom, J. R., Kraemer, H. C., & Gottheil, E. (1989). Effect of psychosocial treatment on survival of patients with metastatic breast cancer. *Lancet, 21,* 888–891.

Spiegel, D. (1990). Facilitating emotional coping during treatment. *Cancer, 66,* 1422–1426.

MUSICAL MYTHOLOGY AND THE ETHICS OF ENCHANTMENT

Cynthia Snodgrass

Every professional field has its own peculiar ethical dilemmas and special frameworks. The doctor serves within the bounds of the Hippocratic oath, and the attorney must function within "the scope of the law". The priest moves within the realm of a binding oath to God and the watchful eyes of superiors. The politician must uphold the public trust, while staying afloat (especially today) in a sea of journalistic inquiry into his or her personal affairs.

Of course, in each of these cases, we know that simply expecting our professionals to conduct themselves in an ethical manner does not make it happen, and it does seem sometimes that the ethical fabric of society itself is becoming increasingly frayed. Polls tell us that we no longer trust our elected representatives, and that there exists, across the board, an erosion of trust in the traditional professions. We used to take for granted a certain distrust for used car salespeople—now we extend little more to our professionals.

The subject of ethics may not be currently in vogue; however, it is for this very reason, then, that the subject of musical ethics is of special importance. Furthermore, there is at present a veritable explosion of people who are using music and sound as therapeutic tools, both inside and outside the traditional settings of medicine and music therapy. Because of the nature of this renaissance, and due to the nature of music itself, the field of musical healing or MusicMedicine holds, like the other professions, its own peculiar ethical dilemmas. Music is a very powerful entity. As Plato has written in *The Republic,* "...rhythm and harmony penetrate deeply into the mind and take a most powerful hold on it..." (Lee, D [translated], *The Republic*, 1987, p. 163). Music speaks directly to the soul, and it has an emotional (even physical) effect on people that can be so subtle, and yet so strong, that the ancient sages often spoke of music's power to enchant the listener in terms of ethics. It is especially important, therefore, that, as the current renaissance of musical healing unfolds, the ethical considerations raised by music's power also be acknowledged and given careful consideration.

I would like to approach this subject from a somewhat unlikely vantage point, in the hopes that through this more circuitous route we will come eventually not only to the significant issues of ethical concern, but to a deeper understanding of those considerations, as well. Rather than beginning from the traditional casuistic approach of case studies written for the individual practitioner, I would like to begin from the arts themselves—from the realms of music, myth, and literature. David Fideler (1993) has written recently that:

> The life of each civilization—and every individual—is influenced by underlying [beliefs systems and] mythologies... In our century, psychology has shown that those who do not believe that their lives are shaped by an underlying mythology are always those who are the most captivated by its spell. (p. 3)

So, rather than approach the power of music (or sound) through the use of technology that measures, or biology that is monitored, I would like to begin from the vantage point of deeply embedded cultural attitudes and perceptions—for our folk tales and mythologies often lie hidden so deeply within the bedrock of our everyday lives that we can easily miss the fact that we are actually standing on top of them or living out of them.

This kind of investigation began during the current year in Hungary when I heard a simple, unassuming children's folk-song; it is a song that most Hungarians learn during childhood. It concerns music's ability to heal, and it is inextricably bound up with Hungary's cultural and political history. The song goes like this:

Gólya, gólya, gilice.	Stork, stork, little bird,
Mitöl véres a lábad?	Why is your leg bleeding?
Török gyerek megráta,	A Turkish child hurt it.
Magyar gyerek gyógyitja	A Hungarian child will heal it,
Sippal, dobbal, nádihegedüvel.	With pipes, drums and reed violins.

The song speaks of a time when Hungary was invaded by the Ottoman Turks. The Hungarians lost the Battle of Mohács in 1526, and for 150 years the Turks ruled much of what is now modern-day Hungary. So it is that, in this song, a Turkish child is responsible for harming the stork, and it is a Hungarian child who is responsible for healing it—"with pipes, drums, and reed-violins".

The bird in the song—a stork—is significant, as Hungarians (like many others) teach their small children that it is the stork who brings new babies. The stork is a symbol of new life—so the song describes, symbolically, how, during the Turkish invasion of Hungary, the country's lifeblood was poured out and the possibility for new life was in peril. It is, therefore, all the more poignant, that the healing of the stork's leg (and by inference, the return of new life) comes through the medium of music—"with pipes, drums, and reed violins". In this deceptively simple children's song we find a rich depth of cultural meaning, and the truth that music does heal.

Additionally, László Dobszay, in *A History of Hungarian Music,* has noted that Hungary's musical history is traceable back to the 9th century, but that echoes of even earlier practices can be identified. These earlier practices include simple, repetitive songs of two or three notes that once were the religious ritual songs, the incantations and chants of the ancient shamans. They are today, he says, still found "in certain children's songs and folk customs" (Dobszay, 1993, p. 9).

We may never know with certainty which particular shaman's melodies and rituals lie hidden within this little song about the stork, but we do know it to be a children's folk song, simple and repetitive in its rhythms, likely to have ancient connections with shamanic practice, and to be a song which Hungarian children learn as part of their early cultural shaping that unquestionably expresses the certain belief that music is able to heal. In a very real way, the melodies and rhythms of the ancient Magyar shamans can still be heard to echo in this little song that speaks positively about music's healing powers.

In the midst of Hungary, where the folk traditions are still strong and accessible, and where the western classical traditions are so vibrant, I began to wonder what other cultural attitudes towards musical healing are found in the folk tales and mythologies of western culture. What do our myths and our fairy tales teach us about musical healing and ethical behavior? How are musical healers portrayed? What do our myths and legends tell us we *should* feel about musical healers? And finally, I wondered, what lessons, if any, might those deeply-embedded attitudes impart to those of us who wish to see music continue to blossom as a healing art?

While researching this question of musical ethics, I found that the relationship between music and medicine is as ancient as human memory itself. The history of western music is founded on positive accounts of music's enchantment over nature and humanity. Music has been portrayed as being able to heal the body physically, to uplift the spirits emotionally, to inspire a work crew, to cause people to dance, or to lull peacefully to sleep. Our western folk-tales, as well, are full of such positive stories. Another Hungarian example comes to mind—that of the tale of Palko the Piper—in which Palko used the charms of music to make the tale's characters dance, as well as to lull an insomniac princess to sleep. In doing so, he won both the princess and his fortune.

But what of the negative accounts? I discovered an equal number of stories in which music's enchantment played a negative role. Some tales told of music that would not stop. For instance, the Brothers Grimm tell the story of a boy who obtains a bow that will shoot anything he aims at, along with a fiddle that will make anyone who hears it dance (Baring-Gould, 1906, p. 430). Using the bow, the boy first shoots down a bird, which falls into a bush full of thorns, and then, when a man goes into the bush after the bird, the boy begins to play the magic fiddle. The boy makes the man dance among the thorns until he finally promises the boy a huge sum of money in order to be set free from the music, the thorns, and the dancing. Interestingly, it seemed that many of the most detailed accounts (and perhaps the best-known accounts) about musical healers left the reader with a certain ambiguity regarding their ethical behavior! Perhaps it is simply the nature of myth or fairy-tale (or those from certain regions), but it seemed that for every uplifting tale of enchanting music sung by sweetly-voiced angels who guided listeners softly into beautiful, heavenly surroundings, I found tales of an equally-enchanting music that enticed listeners into strange or foreboding places, such as those inhabited by elves or fairies—or worse!

From classical mythology come stories of the Sirens, mythical beings—part bird, (often) part woman—who with their enchanting voices lure sailors to destruction and death. Only by first filling his men's ears with wax so that they could not hear, and then having himself tied fast to the ship's mast, could Ulysses take the risk of opening his ears to the magical sounds of the Sirens and not rush, seduced by the sound, to his death. "The Sirens [were] ...winged beings, rushing over the earth, seeking everywhere the lost Persephone" (Baring-Gould, p. 429). The word "siren" itself comes from a Greek word meaning "to pipe or whistle" (Baring-Gould, p. 429), and this rushing, whistling sound has been associated in folk tales with the wind, as well as with Elves, creatures who have the power to sing you into the netherworld of death's kingdom. In Scandinavian ballads, we are told of youths who were allured away by the sweet strains of Elfen maidens (Baring-Gould, p. 427); in German tales, the elves' singing is called *Alpleich* or *Elfenreigen,* and children are cautioned not to listen to it (Baring-Gould, p. 426). Goethe has set this well-known folk belief in the haunting words of his poem, "The Erlking, " which reads:

> Who rides by night in the wind so wild?
> It is the father, with his child.
> The boy is safe in his father's arm,
> He holds him tight, he keeps him warm
> (Goethe, 1983, p. 87).

The child, however, begins to hear the Elfking singing in his ear. His father tells him, no, you are only hearing the wind. As the Elfking continues to lure the child into the other world with promises of meeting his elfin daughters who will cradle him, dance with him, and sing him beautiful lullabies, the father tells the child that he is only hearing the wind among the willows. Then, being gripped tightly by the Elfking, the child screams out:

> Now struck with horror the father rides fast,
> His gasping child in his arm to the last,
> Home through thick and thin he sped;
> Locked in his arm, the child was dead
> (Goethe, translated by C. Middleton, 1983, p. 87).

This haunting tale may also be equally well-known to many through the driving rhythms of Franz Schubert's musical setting, *Erlkönig.*

In several of these proceedings' *clinical* tales, we have heard documentation that music's influence can be either positive or negative. Likewise, the belief that music (or sound) can be connected to either good or evil is solidly embedded within our *cultural* and *mythological* tales, as well. If you will indulge me, I would like to take a look at two better-known figures of musical healing—one from the world of folk-tale, and the other from the realm of classical mythology.

The figure from the world of folk-tale, who represents music's charms, for better *and* for worse, is the famous Pied Piper of Hamelin. Most people raised in western-European culture have grown up with the story of the Pied Piper and know the tale, but may not recall all the details of the story—especially those concerning the Piper's "darker side." This tale can be traced through several sources, but here, I will use the poem setting by Robert Browning.

We are told that the problem began some time in the 14th century, when the town of Hamelin, Germany was overrun by a plague of rats. Says Browning (1898):

> Rats! They fought the dogs and killed the cats,
> And bit the babies in the cradles,
> And ate the cheeses out of the vats,
> And licked the soup from the cooks' own ladles,
> And even spoiled the women's chats
> By drowning their speaking
> With shrieking and squeaking
> In fifty different sharps and flats (p. 209).

The people were more than upset, and they threatened the Mayor of Hamelin with expulsion if he did not do something immediately. Desperate, the Mayor was ready to resign himself, when there came a knock at the door:

> "Come in!"—the Mayor cried, looking bigger:
> And in did come the strangest figure!
> His queer long coat from heel to head
> Was half of yellow and half of red
> And nobody could enough admire

The tall man and his quaint attire
[The Piper] advanced to the council-table:
And, "Please you[r] honours," said he, "I'm able,
By means of a secret charm, to draw
All creatures living beneath the sun,
That creep to swim or fly or run,
After me so as you never saw!
And I chiefly use my charm
On creatures that do people harm,
The mole and toad and newt and viper;
And people call me the Pied Piper."
And his fingers, they noticed, were ever straying
As if impatient to be playing
(Browning, 1898, pp. 210–11).

The Mayor and the townspeople were ecstatic, and, when the Piper asked for the sum of 1,000 guilders as his fee, they flourishingly begged and insisted that he take not *one* but *50* thousand guilders. So,

Into the street the Piper stept,
Smiling first a little smile,
As if he knew what magic slept
In his quiet pipe the while
And ere three shrill notes the pipe uttered,
You heard as if an army muttered;
And the muttering grew to a grumbling;
And the grumbling grew to a mighty rumbling;
And out of the houses the rats came tumbling
From street to street he piped advancing,
And step for step they followed dancing.
Until they came to the river Weser,
Wherein all plunged and perished!
(Browning, 1898, p. 212).

The people were overcome with joy and danced about, but now that the rats were gone, they thought better of their grand generosity. When the Piper asked, fairly enough for his 1,000 guilders, the Mayor offered him not 50 *thousand,* but 50 *only,* as his pay. The piper grew angry and threatened the people with a different kind of music; but now that the cure had been effected, the townspeople had changed their tune. So,

Once more he stept into the street
And to his lips again
Lain his long pipe of smooth straight cane;
And ere he blew three notes [so sweet]
There was a rustling that seemed like a bustling
Of merry crowds justling at pitching and hustling,
Small feet were pattering, wooden shoes clattering,
Little hands clapping and little tongues chattering

Out came the children running
Tripping and skipping, ran merrily after
The wonderful music with shouting and laughter
(Browning, 1898, p. 215).

The children, like the rats before them, followed the piper, in their case, out of town towards Koppenberg Mountain:

When lo, they reached the mountain-side,
A wonderous portal opened wide,
As if a cavern was suddenly hollowed;
And the Piper advanced and the children followed,
And when all were in to the very last,
The door in the mountain-side shut fast
(Browning, 1898, p. 216).

In Browning's tale, only one lame boy was left to tell of the children's enchantment. He had seen into the mountainside, in which there was a fantastic land, which the Piper, in his music, had promised to all who followed him. The cave in this story is common to many German fairy tales, which speak of an enchanted land beneath a mountain, from which music often emanates, and from which people sometimes never return. In Browning's words, the boy describes what he saw:

waters gushed and fruit-trees grew
And flowers put forth a fairer hue,
And everything was strange and new;
The sparrows were brighter than peacocks here,
And their dogs outran our fallow deer,
And honey-bees had lost their stings,
And horses were born with eagles' wings...
(Browning, 1898, p. 216).

Then the boy says:

And just as I became assured
My lame foot would be speedily cured,
The music stopped and I stood still,
And found myself outside the hill,
Left alone against my will,...
(Browning, 1898, p. 216).

In a cruel twist of fate, as though the Piper had decided to return one broken promise with another, and just as the boy was certain that by listening to the Piper's music he would be healed, the musical spell was broken; the boy was left to question why the magical healing had not worked for him, and to mourn the loss of his friends. The magic was over, and 130 children were lost.

The moral of this story is meant to be that one should always keep a promise. Truly, much of the story deals with broken promises: the town did not pay the Piper the promised amount; the Piper, in return, took the town's children, leaving behind one small, lame boy disillusioned and, literally, disenchanted, having been promised music's miracles. But, there is more here than meets the eye (or ear). The fairy-tale offers some important lessons for the healer/healee relationship, and lying below the surface of this simple story are profound questions concerning the healer's ethical conduct. The Piper had a valid point to make about his need for payment, but in choosing to misuse his healer's powers, he acted in a manner morally reprehensible. The tale makes its simpler moral point—however, it *also* leaves the reader with certain feelings of ambiguity and distrust, as well as the subliminal message to exercise caution when dealing with musical healers—or fear of what one might lose!

Let us look now at another ambiguous figure from the realm of ancient mythology—the mythical figure of Orpheus. The legends tell us that Orpheus was "presented with a lyre by Apollo [himself] and instructed by the Muses in its use; he enchanted with its music not only the wild beasts" (Peck, 1962, p. 1145), but he transplanted trees and rocks as well (Apollonius Rhodius, translated by R. C. Seaton, 1980, p. 5). Orpheus' powers were described in the *Argonautica,* as he was said to be among those who accompanied Jason and the Argonauts on their search for the golden fleece. When the great ship Argo would not be hauled into the water, Orpheus' lyre coaxed the ship into being launched (Guthrie, 1952, p. 28); he was able to calm storms, and he set the rhythms by which the oarsmen rowed (Guthrie, 1952, p. 28); once, when the Argo came too close to where the Sirens called, his lyre drowned out the Sirens' song and saved the men from destruction (Apollonius Rhodius, translated by R. C. Seaton, 1980, pp. 355–56); and, the pure strains of Orpheus' lyre lulled to sleep the dragon who guarded the golden fleece (Guthrie, 1952, p. 28).

The figure of Orpheus, however, is probably best remembered for the tragic loss of his wife, Eurydice. Orpheus is completely devastated and overcome with grief; he can do nothing but sing of the sorrow of his lost love. He finally comes to Hades, the Underworld ruled by Pluto and Persephone, who hold only hearts of stone in regard to the fates of mere human beings. Virgil (translated by MacKail, 1950), in the fourth book of the *Georgics,* tells us that with the magic of his doleful melodies, Orpheus is able to soften the hearts of Hades' rulers.

> Startled by his song from the deep sunken realm of Erebus thin shadows rose and phantoms of the lost to light, millionfold as birds shelter in the leaves when evenfall or wintry rain drives them from the hill; ...Nay, the very halls of death and Hell's recesses were amazed, and the Furies with livid serpents twined in their tresses; Cerberus held his triple jaws agape, and Ixion's whirling wheel hung motionless in the wind. (p. 350)

Reversing the very course of nature, Pluto and Persephone allow Eurydice to return with Orpheus to the upper world, on the condition that she follow directly behind him and that he not look back at her, until they have reached the realms of light.

Some versions say that Orpheus panicked—that he was anxious to know if Eurydice were really still behind him—so he turned, and she was lost. But Virgil (1950) paints a picture of an Orpheus so sure of his own powers that he thinks he can do anything, for he turns "...when a sudden madness seized the unwary lover, surely to be forgiven, if Death knew forgiveness" (p. 350). Here, Orpheus is certain that his musical powers had reversed the course of nature once, and that the gods would surely forgive him again. Omnipotent in his self-assurance, Orpheus abuses his power, and loses everything. Unlike the Piper, who purposefully chose to abuse his charms, Virgil's myth of Orpheus leaves the reader with a picture of a musical healer, much less in control, vulnerable himself to the charms of his own enchantment.

Now one might argue that we rationalistic moderns are no longer affected by ancient myths or folk-tales. But, I imagine that most everyone has heard the story of the Pied Piper at some point, and one does not have to be a scholar of the Classics to be influenced by the stories of the ancient world in the form of grade-B movies—witness, for example, *Hercules, The Ten Commandments,* or *Jason and the Argonauts.* Let us also recall the words of David Fideler (1993) "that those who do not believe that their lives are shaped by an underlying mythology are always those who are the most captivated by its spell" (p. 3).

So, assuming that some distrust of music healers may exist on the part of a public who has been raised on these myths and tales, and who currently are wary of the professions in general, what can professional music healers do to counteract what might be called the "Pied Piper Syndrome"?

Public perception of musical healers may well vary, depending upon whether one practices inside or outside the traditional arenas of music therapy and MusicMedicine. Within the field of MusicMedicine these issues of public distrust and professional ethical conduct are being addressed in a number of ways. The NAMT now has a Code of Ethics, and, within the last 10 years, there has been an attempt to monitor and to set appropriate standards for educational curricula within the field (see, for example, Maranto (1981), Maranto (1989), Edwards, Eagle, Pennebaker, and Tunks (1991), and Taylor (1989). Music and medicine are being brought together in some new and exciting ways, and if, as Plato taught, music is a moral entity, then, musical ethics is a very important part of medical ethics.

Questions of language and its usage are being raised. What do we mean by the word "healing"? Are we using it in the same context that the general public hears it? Do we mean "physical cure" or "restoration and wholeness"? In the realm of morality, which the Piper's tale originally addressed, what are we promising people? And, what can we actually deliver?

Musical practitioners are calling for consistent, well-documented evidence concerning music's ability to heal. For example, Spintge (1992) has written that "the reputation of music therapy/MusicMedicine and its acknowledgment by the medical community depends on how it meets the scientific and therapeutic standards of state-of-the-art health care and science" (p. 347). Maranto (1991) has suggested that a systematic approach be taken by isolating the different kinds of musical events to be tested for, and then cataloguing them in a standardized list to be used in all future research (pp. 43 and 53–54), providing a means for consistent monitoring across the field.

Brunner (1992) has pointed out that precisely because music can be such a powerful therapeutic modality, the music healer should not be practicing as a lone ranger, but rather be functioning as part of a team where support and knowledge can be shared. He writes that "as we continue to expand our use of music for healing and transformation, ...we need to proceed responsibly, fully aware that what we do may have powerful and unexpected effects on individuals". Musicians will need to work along with trained psychologists or other professionals to address situations that may arise as a result of a patient's interactions with music" (Brunner, 1992, p. 84). Likewise, Rosalie R. Pratt has called for better communication between international scholars, including a computer base that would hold translated abstracts that would allow international and equal access to current research (Pratt, 1992, p. 9).

Precisely, perhaps because of the Pied Piper syndrome, the onus of honesty and integrity falls squarely onto the shoulders of the musical healer. Honesty and integrity are key to any good healer/healee relationship and in order to develop trust, a practitioner must not only be honest with his/her clients, but must also be honest with him/herself. Howard Brody, in *The Healer's Power,* suggests that the word "power" be introduced into the biomedical-ethics vocabulary for ongoing discussion and examination. While he speaks from a physician's perspective, his advice is applicable to all who take on the healer's role. He cautions his readers against the abuse of power when in the healer's position, requiring an inner honesty and analysis of motivation that will signal to the practitioner when the darker forces of his or her healing power might be present. He quotes John Ladd:

> suggesting three components of the responsible exercise of power: [1] Realism: being aware of the true consequences of one's acts or omissions; [2] Accountability: being ready and able to give an explanation of one's use of power [3] Purposiveness: having a specific end toward which the power is directed. (Brody, 1992, p. 42).

The ongoing endeavor to include discussion of ethical issues in both classroom and clinical settings must continue. Teaching students a core of ethical thinking and ethical principles that can be applied in a number of different settings will help to insure good, ethical practice, and, at the same time, counterbalance the Pied Piper syndrome.

If, however, the onus for honesty and integrity falls to the musical healer who serves within a traditional medical setting, then it is no doubt doubled for those who work outside that sphere. Outside the traditional sphere, the questions of power may be even more important, as the sound traditions that are being used often spring from a specific religious context, and/or they are part of spiritual or religious training and practice. As such, they may encompass or encounter the world of the spirits. There are currently some new and exciting ways in which music and healing practices are being recovered and combined; however, the questions of standardized training, documentation, and ethical conduct are much more unclear outside the traditional medical sphere, and the means for monitoring, as well as the rules for regulation, simply do not exist. Unfortunately, (or fortunately, depending upon how you look at it) the definitions, the expectations, and the boundaries in nonmedical settings are somewhat fuzzier. For instance, as sacred musical rituals are recovered, many of which involve the use of magic, is the music healer, then, also using the magic? And, if so, is she or he trained sufficiently well to be using that magic? Furthermore, how does one define the ethics of magic?

In his article on sonic entrainment, Jonathan Goldman raises questions about the ethical uses of hemi-sync techniques. With such powerful technology, he says, there must be some restraints upon its usage, or "we may be unleashing a Pandora's box to an unsuspecting public" (Goldman, 1992, p. 207). Many of the current sound and vocal techniques are subtly invasive and questions concerning invasion and the client's autonomy need to be asked and respected. When might entrainment stop and a kind of mind control begin?

Or, when a music healer has developed a computerized healing system that generates sound-tones into the body and claims to heal physically, however that system has never truly been submitted to the scrutiny of objective inquiry and verification, where does high technology stop and possible deception begin?

Or, when a musician, working in a medical setting, claims authority based on the authenticity of a musico-historical tradition, but the field of modern musicology tells us that the specific music and the solid historical foundations for that practice simply do not exist, when does informed recovery of musical tradition stop and the world of make-believe begin?

Or, when music from the healing rituals of other cultures is transposed and shared in a variety of settings for Western clients, wherein the music and its healing intent are taken out of their original cultural context, when does respect and responsibility for sacred tradition stop and our love of experimentation and entertainment begin?

These are all ethical questions. They may not be comfortable ones, but they are important ones, as musical healers from both inside and outside the "medical establishment", can have a deleterious effect on the public's perception of the entire field, and they address some of those ethical dilemmas that are peculiar to the field of professional music healing.

Having served as a hospice chaplain for 5 years and as a geriatrics chaplain for 2½ years, I have used music in many settings and know how powerfully it speaks to people's souls. I also know how confused people can become when faced with their own or others' illnesses. The confusion of illness can bring desperation and vulnerability—it can, at the same time, be a powerful catalyst for deeper understanding of self and self-care. Likewise, musical healers who use music's charms may have a powerful effect on people during those especially sensitive times. In *The Third Ear,* Joachim-Ernst Berendt (1985) encourages his readers to drop the ancient prejudice against listening to the Sirens' song, to release their distrust and immerse themselves in the fullness of sound's enchantments (p. 34). Plato, on the other hand, many years ago, cautioned his listeners, saying that anything that enchants, by its very nature, also deceives. So, here we stand, along with many 20th-century clients, caught not between Scylla and Charybdis, but somewhere between Plato's caution and Berendt's abandon—wanting to find the shaman who lives within music's milieu, but wanting *not* to run into the Pied Piper. One answer, as to whether we meet the shaman or the infamous Piper, lies within those simple folk-tales and ancient mythologies, which remind us to be ever mindful, and to hold ourselves and others accountable to a high standard of ethical conduct.

References

Apollonius Rhodius. (1980). In R. C. Seaton (Translator) *Argonautica.* Cambridge, MA: Harvard University Press.

Baring-Gould, S. (1906). *Curious myths of the middle ages.* London: Longmans, Green.

Berendt, J.-E. (1985). T*he third ear.* New York: H. Holt.

Brody, H. (1992). *The healer's power.* New Haven, CT: Yale University Press.

Browning, R. (1898). *Complete works,* Vol. 4). New York: Fred DeFau.

Brunner, L. W. (1992). Theme and variations. In D. Campbell (Ed.), *Music and miracles* (pp. 74–88). Wheaton, IL: Theosophical Publishing House.

Dobszay, L. (1993) *A history of Hungarian music.* Budapest: Corvina.

Edwards, M. C., Eagle, C., Pennebaker, J., & Tunks, T. (1991). Relationships among elements of music and physiological responses of listeners. In C. D. Maranto (Ed.), *Applications of music in medicine* (pp. 41–57). Washington, D.C.: National Association of Music Therapy.

Fideler, D. (1993) *Jesus Christ: Sun of God.* Wheaton, IL: Quest Books.

Goethe, J. W. von. (1983), In C. Middleton (Editor & translator), *Selected Poems.* Boston: Suhrkamp/Insel Publishers.

Goldman, J. S. (1992). Sonic entrainment. In R. Spintge & R. Droh, *MusicMedicine* (pp. 194–208). St. Louis, MO: MMB Music.

Guthrie, W. K. C. (1952). *Orpheus and Greek religion*. London: Methuen.

Maranto, C. D. (1981). Ethics in music therapy: A programmed text. Dissertation Abstracts International, vol. 42/03/A, p. 1043 (University Microfilm No. AAD 81–17637).

Maranto, C. D. (1989). The educational standards of the National Association for Music Therapy, Inc. and the Temple University research studies on music therapy education and training. In R. R. Pratt (Ed.), *Music therapy and music in special education*, vol. 2 (pp. 78–80). St. Louis: MO: MMB Music.

Peck, H. T. (Ed.). (1962). *Harper's dictionary of classical literature and antiquities*. New York: Cooper Square.

Plato. In D. Lee (Translator) (1987) *The republic*. New York: Penguin.

Pratt, R. R. (1992). The new interface between music and medicine. In R. Spintge & R. Droh (Eds.), *MusicMedicine* (pp. 6–29). St. Louis, MO: MMB Music.

Spintge, R. (1992). Toward a research standard in musicmedicine, music therapy. In R. Spintge & R. Droh (Eds.). *MusicMedicine* (pp. 345–349). St. Louis, MO: MMB Music.

Taylor, D. (1989). A professional music therapist's opinion concerning competencies needed by the entry-level practitioner. In R. R. Pratt, *Music therapy and music in special education*, vol. 2 (pp. 115–48). St. Louis, MO: MMB Music.

Virgil. In J. W. MacKail (Translator) (1950) *The Georgics*. New York: The Modern Library.

THE EFFECTS OF MUSICAL RHYTHM ON BODY AND MIND: THE INTERACTION FIELD OF THE TA KE TI NA RHYTHM PROCESS

Reinhard Flatischler

TA KE TI NA—four sounds from a rhythm language used by various indigenous cultures as a tool for healing mind and body through rhythm. TA KE TI NA is also the name of a rhythm process I have developed over the last 25 years in which participants experience the healing power of rhythm in a special *interaction field.* In this field, musical rhythms gradually build up rhythm consciousness while strengthening and relaxing body rhythms such as breathing and the heartbeat. In the process of exploring the parameters of rhythmic influence on body and mind, I will describe the dynamics of the TA KE TI NA rhythm process. I am encouraging others to research this phenomenon because I believe the healing power of rhythm is an important remedy for many of the psychological, physiological, and spiritual problems we face today. Now that rhythm and drumming are regaining worldwide interest, many people are responding to a strong inner call to reclaim their knowledge of the effects and power of rhythm.

Traditional Views of Healing with Rhythm

Can musical rhythm improve physical and mental well-being? Can it promote healing? Our answers lie in the knowledge of ancient cultures, kept alive by small groups and tribes in such places as India, Korea, Indonesia, Africa and Brazil, to name a few. I have studied drumming rituals at length in these places and have learned about the central role musical rhythm plays in healing. Although we cannot simply imitate exotic rituals in order to revive this ancient knowledge, the underlying principles of how rhythm affects our mind and body are the same in all cultures. Today, as we listen to the rhythms of these indigenous cultures, we find that each one has focused on a particular rhythmic phenomenon (e.g., polyrhythm in Africa, extended cycles in India) and developed it to a very high form along with specific types of drums well suited to express these rhythms. The great variety of sounds from different cultures might lead us to assume that they are following different laws. It can be shown, however, that the ancient knowledge of healing with rhythm follows the same laws throughout the entire world.

The people of these cultures view body, mind, and soul as one entity, and they show us that the influence of rhythm must be directed to all these realms of our being. After studying these rhythms and the effects of the interaction fields between drum sounds and the listener, I asked myself if a rhythmic interaction field could be developed that would enhance the rhythmic knowledge and power of a Westerner in today's world.

Musical Rhythm, Body Rhythms, and Mind Rhythms: The Connection

I was encouraged in my search by the late great German physiologist Dr. Hans-Peter Koepchen, who made this remarkable statement in his lecture "Primary Internal Neurovegetative Rhythmicity" at the Fourth International MusicMedicine Symposium, Annenberg Center for Health Sciences, Eisenhower, Rancho Mirage, California, 28 October 1989: "Every disease is caused by a dysfunctioning of rhythm." Therefore disease means that certain organs, cellular systems, and the more subtle organizations of our nervous system are undergoing a rhythmic disturbance. As indigenous cultures have always known—and as we are just now rediscovering—body rhythms and mind rhythms are interconnected and sometimes, as in the case of brain waves, identical. A subtle (but measurable) change of brain wave rhythm will cause dramatic changes in our perception. Maxfield (1994) has reported that brain waves can easily be tuned to certain frequencies through drumming.

Study of the connection among our body, nervous system and consciousness leads us to believe that a highly developed and active rhythmic consciousness will have an effect on our natural body rhythms. Two questions arise:

1. Do we all have the ability to achieve synchronicity with more or less complex musical rhythms?

2. Can we all receive healing through the power of rhythm?

The Primal Rhythmic Imprint

My 20 years of practical rhythm study in many different cultures has revealed that every human has a ***primal rhythmic imprint***, or ***primal rhythmic knowledge***. This imprint—the most subtle form of mind rhythm—is an energy field containing knowledge of the laws of nature and rhythmic archetypes. It exists in the embryonic stage before external influence begins. However, the primal rhythmic imprint is only empowered by stimulation from the outside—our mother's heartbeat, her rocking movements, and the rhythm of her speech as we grow in the dark and quite loud environment of her womb. It seems that a foundation of trust or anxiety, love or hate, "yes" or "no" to life is transferred from mother to embryo through sound and rhythm. If there is no, or little, rhythmic stimulation at this stage, the primal rhythmic imprint is forgotten. But it remains in us as a potential, a seed that can be brought to life in later years. As we connect with it, we awaken the rhythmic power that lives within.

I began my work on the interaction of musical rhythms and body/mind rhythms because I saw that rhythmic dysfunction in the body disappears when we access our primal rhythmic knowledge. By expanding their rhythmic consciousness in the TA KE TI NA process, many people have improved their health. In a research group with participants suffering from asthma, arrhythmia and high blood pressure, 80% of them reported a perceptible improvement of their well-being and a decrease of their symptoms after three successive 4-day TA KE TI NA sessions.

The Dynamics and the Possibilities of Rhythmic Interaction Fields

TA KE TI NA is an interaction field that allows musical rhythms to awaken our primal rhythmic imprint. The effect of a given rhythm depends largely on the field that exists between that rhythm and the listener. Whether we create this field intentionally or it forms by itself through a certain situation, a certain effect is produced. For example, if you lie down and, without moving, listen to a recorded rhythm, you will experience a different effect than if you were to move in synchronization with the same rhythm played by a drummer. To stimulate your thinking about the conditions and qualities of existing interaction fields, the following are some possibilities:

1. Listener lies motionlessly with recorded rhythm, then with rhythm played live.

2. Listener sits, or stands motionlessly with recorded rhythm, then with rhythm played live.

3. Listener moves freely in or out of synchronization with the rhythm (same pattern as in #1). The drummer plays without changing the pattern to fit the movement; or the drummer responds to the movement but keeps a basic rhythm.

4. Listener moves only one part of the body (finger, arm, foot, etc.) either in or out of synchronization with recorded or live drumming.

5. Listener is guided to move in synchronization with recorded or live drumming.

6. Listener moves with given steps in synchronization with a simple, steady beat, while a second drummer plays different but related rhythms. Listener gradually attempts to coordinate clapping or arm movements with second drummer's accents, and thus *two* different rhythmic layers simultaneously sound.

7. Same as #6, but now part of a group in circle formation, all moving to the same rhythm, thereby providing mutual support for each other's steps.

The Two Realms of a Rhythmic Interaction Field

Before going deeper into how the TA KE TI NA field works, let us first look at the two realms that connect in an interaction field:

External musical rhythms
Seven different layers of rhythmic phenomena existing in all forms of music:

- Pulsation
- Cycle
- Pulsations in the Interval
- Offbeats
- Rhythmic figures
- Sounds of rhythmic figures
- Tempo

Body and mind rhythms
Rhythms of our daily life:

- Rhythms of the sleep and awake states
- Rhythm of walking
- Rhythm of breathing
- Rhythm of heartbeat
- Rhythm of brain waves
- Glandular rhythm
- Primal rhythmic imprint

The body rhythms in the right column proceed downwards from the visibly physical to the subtle—the primal imprint encoded with all the information of our mind and body rhythms. I have found that an expanded rhythmic consciousness can have a permanent effect on body rhythms like breathing and the heartbeat, moving them toward a relaxed and harmonious stability.

Basic Rhythmic Phenomena and Their Effects

The column on the left shows eight rhythmic phenomena found in all forms of music, each representing a different rhythmic quality. A fully developed musical rhythm includes all eight layers. Each one contributes it own rhythmic dynamic and has its own effect on the listener. The following briefly summarizes these effects:

Pulsation: Connects us with the feeling of being carried, allowing something to happen on its own accord, induces deep grounding and an energy flow towards the earth; connects with self-confidence and relates to our life force, our heart pulse.

Cycle: Connects us with timelessness and inner silence. In traditional Indian music each cycle has its own effect, for example, two- and four-beat cycles—earth feeling, extroversion, grounding; three- and six-beat cycles—rocking, trance inducing, leading into regressive states; connected with subconscious states (in deep sleep we breathe in a three-beat cycle: inhale exhale—rest); five-beat cycle—vitalizing, but with a centering effect; nine-beat cycle—dissolves body sensations, leads into mind (should be balanced with two- or four-beat cycles); twelve-beat cycles—perfect rhythm, deep, balanced trance, more awake than a three-beat cycle with less regression inducing effect. With these few examples, I offer this reminder: The influence any rhythm has on mind and body depends mainly on the field in which it appears.

Pulsation in the interval: Empty spaces (intervals) between pulses react like air columns or vibrating strings—they divide into two, three, and four equal parts, thus creating sensitive points in that space. A simple pulsation subdivided into two equal parts creates an extroverted movement and a downward, "into the earth" feeling. The same pulsation subdivided into three equal parts creates a trancelike state and introversion.

Offbeats: They are the sensitive points in the empty space between the basic pulses. Some have a strong tendency to induce deep relaxation; others induce great tension.

So far we have been talking about rhythmic archetypes—found in the music of all genres, all cultures. With the next layer (rhythmic figures and their sounds), we enter the world of creation, the world of complex musical forms. The archetypal realm certainly holds the greatest power to heal and at the same time contains all the building blocks for the creation of rhythm and music. The effect of a given rhythmic figure depends on its factors or ingredients, namely, Pulsation, Cycle, and Beat. There are also Offbeat combinations, on one side, and, on the other, sound itself. If, for example, we play a rhythm with a rattle instead of a bass drum, the effect is dramatically altered. Or we could play a different drum with different combinations of open and muffled sounds to change the effect of a given rhythm.

Pulsation is the most elementary form of musical rhythm. Sometimes we hear it in its pure form, such as the sound of a *Moktak* (large woodblock) used to accompany Zen chanting, the many forms of Native-American drumming, and the clapping that accompanies tribal chants the world over. Pulsation, as the purest form of audible rhythm, is a highly effective means for influencing our rhythmic system. Shamanic cultures throughout the world have found that a simple drumbeat of four and a half beats per second will soon induce deep trance. The research done by Melinda Mo Maxfield, mentioned previously, illustrates how this beat simply synchronizes the rhythm of the brain waves with the drumming frequency of four and a half cycles per second. These particular waves, called Theta waves, appear in sleep, daydreaming states and trance states.

Synchronization: The Central Power of an Interaction Field

The dynamic of the synchronization process that occurs between the drumbeat and the brain waves is a very important force in such an interaction field. To fully understand rhythm-fields, it is important to know about the power of synchronization. Here are three examples of this phenomenon:

1. Christiaan Huygens, the inventor of the pendulum clock, discovered by chance that two clocks in close proximity will eventually begin to swing their pendulums in synchronization. When he stopped them and moved them into different rhythms it only took about half an hour for them to swing back into synchronization. However, if the clocks were placed in different rooms, they lost their synchroneity.

2. A similar phenomenon exists among fireflies. Thousands of fireflies flash in synchroneity in a time exposure of a nocturnal mating display. Each insect has its own rhythm, but the sight of its neighbor's light brings the flashing rhythm into synchronization.

3. Perhaps you have experienced the phenomenon that occurs when several people are walking in the same room in different, apparently unrelated tempos. When each connects his steps to his own vocal sound, an interaction field is created. The people will gradually begin to synchronize their steps in various ways; some will join in the same pulsation, others will meet with their steps in half time or double time. I have performed this experiment throughout the world and have found that there is usually someone who voluntarily resists this process by clearly stepping differently than the others. Whatever reason a person may have, a very important fact is demonstrated: We can resist the power of synchronization voluntarily. Synchronization only happens if we allow it to happen. However, it also happens when we go into a trance state and when we are connected to the subconscious or the unconscious.

Opening the Channel between Different Realms of Our Consciousness

In music and in daily life, these two realms are always interacting with each other. On one side, the realm of letting go and allowing something to happen on its own accord—just as our heart pulsates involuntarily—and, on the other side, active intention, voluntary creation combined with awake consciousness and logical thinking.

The following exercise shows that it is impossible do two different movements at the same time by only using the logical and analytical part of our consciousness. Choose two syllables and create a vocal rhythm in a tempo similar to your heartbeat. For example:

TA KI TA KI TA KI TA KI TA KI TA KI.

Take time to establish this vocal rhythm before you combine it with the following arm movements. Imagine two half circles like bowls in front of you, one on your right, one on your left. Draw these two half circles in the air with your index fingers as you move both arms and combine your movement with the rhythm of your voice. Allow yourself time to enjoy this simple movement. When you are ready, continue to move one arm in the form of the half circle in time with your vocal rhythm, and start drawing a full circle with the other arm at various speeds.

You will most likely experience a loss of control over both arm movements and eventually chaos between your arm movements and your voice. That is because you are trying to do both movements intentionally with your analytical mind. The purpose of this is to demonstrate two very important facts that we will apply to our interaction field:

1. We are not able to perform two or more different movements at the same time, if we are only in the state of logical thinking or analyzing. In our example, one of the two sides will have to proceed on its own accord; we will have to give up voluntary control over it. If the half circle movement is connected with the vocal rhythm in a way that allows it to happen more or less subconsciously, and in trance, we can easily draw our circle intentionally, with

an awake consciousness. Thereby two different realms of our consciousness interact. In fact, we are usually not able to live in two different states of consciousness simultaneously—we are usually in either a trance state or in an awakened-conscious state.

2. If we fall from organized rhythm into chaos, and there is no supportive rhythm from the outside to help us continue, we will sooner or later stop and find ourselves frustrated with the feeling of failure. Chaos is not a safe place if we experience it this way.

But, as we know from nature, chaos is an essential part of creation and evolution. I can still remember what Dr. Koepchen said to me after participating in one of my TA KE TI NA rhythm workshops in Lüdenscheid (Germany): "There seems to be a similarity in human physiology and in the way TA KE TI NA leads its participants into rhythm. In the TA KE TI NA process, as well as in the process of living organizations, *chaos* is an essential part of evolution." Dr. Koepchen then answered the question about how chaos is used to our advantage in TA KE TI NA? "At certain times, every living organism leaves its old order and goes through states of chaos only to stabilize on a new level of order," Dr. Koepchen continued. His words made me reflect more deeply. If chaos is such an important part of evolution, it must play an important role in the rhythmic evolution of each individual. Without knowing the scientific facts, I had created something that mirrors the laws of nature.

How can we make chaos a safe and fruitful place for people entering a musical rhythmic process for the first time? How can we guide them into an experience of chaos and rhythmic order at the same time? Usually we fall out of rhythm because we are distracted from the rhythmic beat pattern we are in. It could be anything from simply looking into someone's eyes to hearing a second rhythmic movement, or even trying to follow that second rhythm. When the inner perception and the audible rhythm lose their connection we inevitably go into chaos. That state is usually accompanied by fear or frustration because our playing or movement becomes blocked—we have lost the basic pulse.

How can we create a field that has the power to lead us into an experience of two or more rhythms at the same time? As we have already seen, we can do two or more rhythms simultaneously only if we use at least two different forms of consciousness at the same time. We could have, for example, a basic step pattern moving in a trancelike manner, following the rhythm on its own while we clap intentionally with our awake consciousness. In order to achieve this, we need a field that allows us to act voluntarily while at the same time allowing us to be in trance, carried by the rhythm.

The Three Dynamics of the TA KE TI NA: Interaction Field

Here are three dynamics that exist in the TA KE TI NA interaction field. They lead us into the simultaneity of several rhythms, and into different realms of our consciousness:

1. BASIC RHYTHM: The connection of a certain body movement (e.g., a specific footstep pattern) with an ongoing basic rhythm that is so simple as to invite easy recognition and effortless memory. The body movement is congruent with the drum signals. You are in rhythm and you are acquiescing to a certain rhythmic form—so you know if you are in or out. That is something that you need to feel and to consciously know at the same time. In TA KE TI NA, the drumbeat is a pulsation from a bass drum (surdo) that plays a repeating sequence of open and closed sounds. For each rhythm there is a special step pattern (derived from tribal and ritual dance) that is directly connected with the drum rhythm. The tempo for all these steps is approximately the tempo of the heartbeat because it seems that we are

able to learn most easily and naturally in this tempo. At the same time, it allows even a quite elderly person to follow the rhythm process for an extended period of time.

2. SUPPORTIVE COMMUNITY: A community that forms a circle and that joins you in synchrony with the same footstep pattern stabilizes your basic rhythm. The circle continues to play, dance, and chant the basic rhythm, even though you may lose your step and fall out of rhythm. But never does everyone fall out at the same moment; there are always some who continue together with the bass drum in the center. You experience the continued basic rhythm, even if you fall out, and, after the first shock and some self blame, you lose the feeling of panic and failure. Most people learn to take it in stride, smile, and return to the ongoing beat.

3. CHALLENGE: The basic beat would soon become boring without the introduction of a second or third rhythmic layer to which participants are invited to join, either by using their voice or by clapping. Such claps occur at precise points in the rhythm, so you must consciously know where to clap. Whenever you operate intentionally from your conscious mind in trying to do two different movements simultaneously, you will fall out. If you allow your stepping to go into a trancelike movement, and stay awake and focused with your second movement, you will begin to open the channel among the conscious, subconscious, and unconscious layers of your mind. Chaos functions as a catalyst in order to reach this state of mind. You allow yourself to go into chaos and listen at the same time to the others as they continue the rhythm. As you open this channel, you will soon access your primal rhythmic imprint, anchored in the silence of your unconscious—a place within you that has no words to speak, but knows everything about being in perfect health.

The Effects of TA KE TI NA

Personal observations and feedback from participants over the past 25 years:

1. The comment has been made that the experience makes one feel as though the pulse rhythm is a best friend. Others said they could easily feel their pulse in all appropriate locations and eventually feel it without touching the pulse itself. I learned that being a "friend" of the heart pulse greatly reduces fear in acute attack situations involving psychosomatic disorders such as asthma or arrhythmia.

Note: After 3–5 TA KE TI NA sets, the quality of the pulse is described by the majority of participants as vital, strong, and slow—around 60 beats/minute. The flexibility of the pulse also seems to increase over the time.

2. Many participants with problems of arrhythmia said their symptoms faded—their pulse became regular. I have seen these effects experienced shortly after a 3-hour TA KE TI NA set. However, lasting change can only be achieved if someone undergoes the TA KE TI NA process over a long period of time.

3. Many participants in my workshops report greater stability of their general health. Research must be done to determine if TA KE TI NA can possibly strengthen the immune system.

4. A long lasting, deep relaxation created by the simultaneity of trance and awake consciousness helps the body unfold its natural healing power.

5.TA KE TI NA also has a psychotherapeutic effects. It has worked very well for patients in psychotic and traumatized states.

As we access our primal rhythmic imprint, we develop musicality, creativity, social awareness, spiritual growth and—as many cases show—greater stability of health.

SOUNDS FOR TRANSCENDENCE: YOGIC TECHNIQUES FOR OPENING THE TENTH GATE

David Shannahoff-Khalsa

Introduction

The term transcendence implies rising above or going beyond the limits of ordinary experience, or exceeding the usual limits. Here the term describes the experience of a non-ordinary state of consciousness, a state where the consciousness of the observer goes beyond the dimensions of the observed finite physical world, the world of time and space. This implies that the mind has access to both multiple dimensions and intelligence.

Limits and boundaries are the construct of the mind of the intellect, the mind that judges, the mind confined to finite reality. It is reasonable to assume that this mind is our root or primary mind. However, it is not unreasonable to assume that it has its limitations. For example, this mind can argue or reason against the existence of a transcendental reality; however, it cannot disprove the existence of a nonmaterial world, or a world beyond our five senses. Undoubtedly this mind has evolved as a tool to cope with the temporal world. Presumably its nature is to disassemble the parts of the whole as distinctive elements of reality and to understand their working interactions.

The prevailing western scientific view is to accept as reality only that which can be defined by words, symbols, or equations, the world amenable to description. An intuitive mind works by different principles, principles yet to be described. This mind struggles to protect its own domain, the world of the undefined, the world without borders and straight lines, the world not easily amenable to the languages of the mind of the intellect. This conflict between the mind of the intellect and the mind of intuition is what creates the schisms of life.

The eternal questions of the soul, death, and our mortal or immortal nature will forever remain a mystery as long as the mind of the intellect alone dominates the experience of human consciousness. It grasps at that which becomes the basis for conventional reality, the world that is familiar, the world that we can discuss. It charts the world of science, the world that can be tested by the "tools of science". But the mandate of science not only requires a better explanation of the "known world" but the pursuit of that which is beyond the realm of ordinary reality. For some reason, western science has excelled at exploring the world of the infinitesimally small particle but has floundered in exploring the nature of the mind and consciousness. This point is made with an example provided by the eminent molecular biologist Francis Crick (1994) in his book *The astonishing hypothesis: The scientific search for the soul.* He concludes that there is no extravehicular soul, only the immensely complex and currently little understood interactive activity of neurons. Thus, man is a machine, and therefore, the mind must be an epiphenomenon of neural activity. Crick's hypothesis is at least as old as its antithesis.

Probably every medical culture, other than that of the western tradition, holds to the antithesis of Crick's hypothesis. Whether it is the world of the medicine man, the ancient or modern Shamanic cults indigenous to most cultures (Harner, 1992), the nonsectarian yogic systems, or the eastern religions that profess a chronobiology of the soul, the concept of soul is elementary.

This paper is not an intellectual argument about the existence of the soul, or transcendental realities, but it is an effort to share the yogic techniques that lead to the experience of transcendental worlds. It is unlikely that science in the 20th century will contribute anything new to the questions of transcendental realities. However, this should not preclude the opportunity for individuals to explore the workings of their own nervous system and consciousness while testing the sacred and ancient yogic techniques that have reliably afforded access to these worlds of consciousness. Perhaps this intricate knowledge will help advance modern medicine.

Sounds captivate and carry the mind. Specific sounds and music are fundamental to yogic medicine. These sounds have been used to transcend ordinary states of consciousness for thousands of years. A theoretical basis for the healing effects of chanted sounds and their effects on consciousness have been discussed (Shannahoff-Khalsa & Bhajan, 1988; Shannahoff-Khalsa & Bhajan, 1992). Shannahoff-Khalsa and Bhajan discuss the mechanistic basis for this system. In the yogic system, a pattern of 84 meridian points on the upper palate (see Figure 1) is known to act as a keyboard for the tongue, where different sounds impart state-specific effects. What is required for the development of the transcendental mind is the correct code.

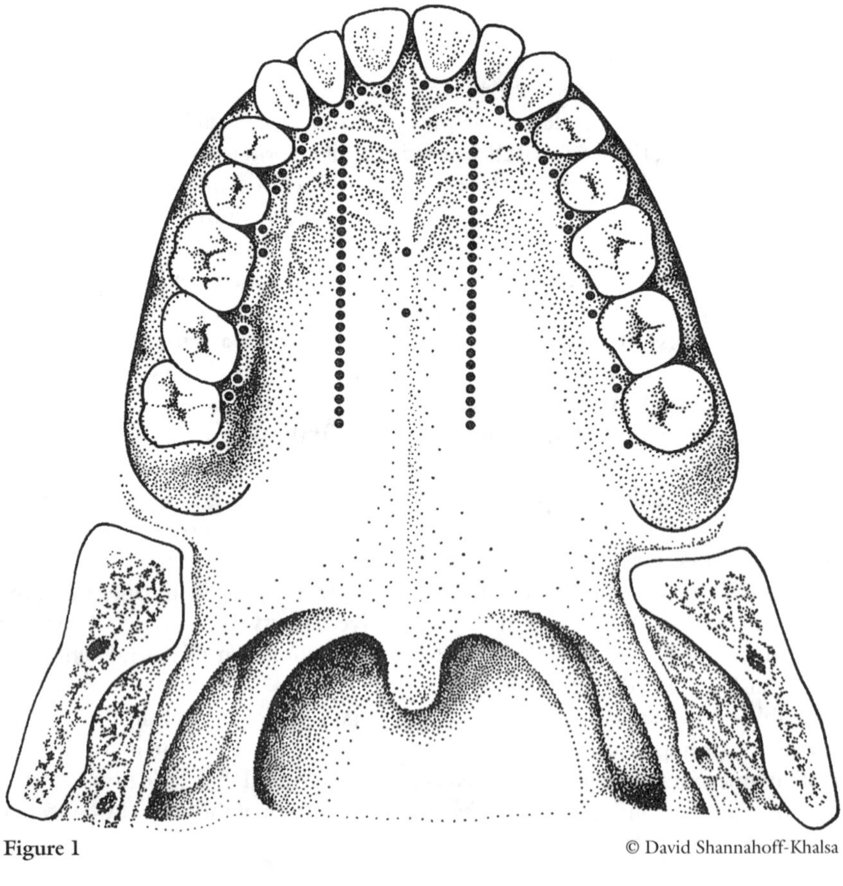

Figure 1

© David Shannahoff-Khalsa

The upper palate is affected by the whole tongue, not just the tip. The 84 meridian points are related to the hypothalamus, and the effect of the tongue on these points is to indirectly stimulate specific regions of the hypothalamus. Signals are thus sent to various areas of the brain where they affect neural activity, brain chemistry, and help induce different states of consciousness. These principles and the related sounds were originally discovered in the systems now called Nad Yoga and Mantra Yoga.

The techniques described here are ancient time-tested techniques that are the result of thousands of years of empirical discipline. They were part of the yogic system before it became taught as today's fragmented specialties, much like today's medicine. This fragmentation eventually led to a breakdown in the original system. The protocol formulated here is advanced but can be employed by the novice. Generally, the time limits are imposed by an individual's capacity and the set maximums. The practice of any techniques should begin with the technique for "getting started". After using the mantra for getting started, either the entire sequence can be practiced or selected techniques; all lead to transcendence. However, this sequence is well balanced. It can be enhanced by starting with three techniques described as:

1. "spine flexing for vitality",
2. "shoulder shrug for increasing metabolism",
3. a sound current technique "stimulating and balancing the 8 centers of consciousness" using the mantra Ek Ong Kar Sat Nam Siri Whahay Guru (Shannahoff-Khalsa & Bhajan, 1992).

Another very useful precursor is called Nabhi Kriya (Bhajan, 1978, pp. 18–19).

Getting Started
Ong Namo Guru Dev Namo

Description of the Technique

This mantra has two parts:

1. "Ong Namo" is chanted with equal emphasis, effort, and time on "Ong" and "Namo" (Ong = Namo). Begin by taking a deep breath through the nose and exhale while chanting "Ong Namo"; the sound of Ong begins with a long "O" with pursed lips, not "ung";

2. "Guru Dev Namo" is chanted after taking a half breath through the mouth and "Dev" and "Namo" are carried a little longer than "Guru". Perform this technique a minimum of 3–5 times before meditating or doing any Kundalini Yoga techniques taught in this series. It can also be used for longer times to help induce a meditative state, in which case it should be chanted until the desired effect is achieved.

When the goal is to "tune it", sit with a straight spine and put the hands in prayer pose applying 10–15 pounds of pressure, hand against hand. The lower part of the thumbs (the bone between the wrist and first thumb joint) touch the sternum without applying pressure to the chest—touching alone is sufficient. The entire thumb also touches along the sternum. This places the hands at the heart center. Keep the fingers pointing up and out at 60 degrees from the ground. Keep the eyes closed and focused at the third eye point—the central point where you can imagine a sun rising on the horizon. Visualize this sun. Let the sounds carry you within your consciousness and experience the vibratory effects of the sounds on your upper palate and throughout your cranium.

The meaning of the mantra is as follows; "Ong" is the universal creative energy, and "Namo" means to bow. So the first part means that you humble yourself to the universal creative energy, the "force" that gives life. "Guru" means that technique or being that takes you from inner darkness into the light of your higher consciousness. "Dev" means divine. So "Guru Dev Namo" means that you bow to the divine wisdom that is awakened from within. This sets a state for healing within and protection from the negative aspects of the mind.

The Ultimate Pranayam
Su Darshan Chakra Kriya

The first written (partial) discussion and description of this technique comes from the writings of Jai Dev in the scriptures of the *Siri Guru Granth Sahib* (Singh, 1964). He says:

> There is One God. By the Grace of the True Guru: The breath is drawn in through the left nostril, it is held in the Sushumna (central meridian of the spine), and exhaled through the right nostril, repeating in the mind the mantra of the Lord's Name 16 times (p. 3645).

The developmental stages of realization and awareness experienced through the practice of this technique are in part described:

> I am powerless, my power has been broken, my unstable mind has been stabilized, and my unadorned soul has been adorned. I drink in the Ambrosial Nectar. Within my mind, I utter the Name of the Primal Lord, the source of all virtue. My vision, that You and I are separate, has melted away. I worship the One who is worthy of being worshipped. I trust the One who is worthy of being trusted. Like water into water, I merge into the Lord. I meditate and contemplate the Luminous, Triumphant Lord. I am lovingly absorbed in the Nirvana of God (p. 3645).

Yogi Bhajan openly taught this technique, initially in Formello, Italy, on December 12, 1990. He comments:

> If you can do this meditation for 62 minutes to start with, and develop it to the point that you can do it 2½ hours per day, it will give you "Nao niddhi, athara siddhi" or the nine precious virtues and 18 occult powers. And in those 27 total virtues of the world lies the entire universe. When practiced 2½ hours every day, it makes a perfect superman out of you. It purifies, it takes care of the human life and brings together all 27 facets of life and makes a human perfect, saintly, successful, and qualified. This meditation also gives one the Pranic power. This kriya never fails. It can give one all the inner happiness, and bring one to a state of ecstasy in life. It will keep all the chakras open so you will not fall into any ditch. It is better to live a life of courage than to live many many years like a coward. Courage is in inner vitality, and if all your chakras are open, you will not be handicapped in vitality. You will get a grip on your life. No matter how bad circumstances are, your intuition will guide your way to happiness, and your vitality shall support you (p. 1990).

This pranayama technique, as a single technique, is the ultimate in meditation techniques. Its multiple facets make it a completely balanced technique. When practiced alone there are no other requirements for other techniques to achieve the full development of the human. For example, the rate of respiration is eventually reduced to less than one breath per minute during practice. This rate produces profound changes in the way the brain functions. This technique changes one's perception of the self and the world. The practitioner develops a consciousness that becomes the living experience of the timelessness of life, transcending time and space. The negative effects and patterns of the subconscious mind are eliminated. This technique helps to overcome the stumbling blocks of the inner world. It helps to cut through inner darkness, and it eliminates both neurotic and psychotic patterns of the mind. According to Yogi Bhajan "You are cleaning your subconscious. You can clean it as fast or as slow as you want. You have to decide how much time you want to devote to getting rid of the fear, anger, insecurity, etc.... the negative thoughts in your subconscious that block your success and prosperity" (p. 1990).

Description of the Technique

Sit with a straight spine on the floor in a cross-legged position, or on a firm chair with both feet flat on the ground. The lower spine (lumbar region) is pressed forward slightly. This spinal posture signals the nervous system to remain alert, it sets a "ready mode".

The eyes are open and focused at the tip of the nose—the end that you cannot see. With eyes focused at the tip, the sides of the nose appear to blur. Some individuals are less able to achieve this eye focus, and practice over time can help to overcome this deficit. This eye position is called "Ajna Band", which means mind lock. Focusing the eyes in this way pressurizes the optic nerve and helps to stabilize thought processes. It is a common element with meditation techniques that are used to tranquilize the mind. Initially the eye muscles may become sore due to a lack of use.

The breathing pattern has three stages:

1. Use the right thumb tip to block off the right nostril (close the nostril by covering the end, not by pushing in the side), keep the four fingers of the right hand pointed up straight, inhale slowly and completely fill the lungs.

2. While holding the breath begin pumping the navel point in and out for a total of 48 pumps while mentally vibrating the sound Whahay Guru 16 times per 48 pumps, with one pump per Wha, one pump per Hay, and one pump per Guru, or 16 x 3 sounds = 48 pumps.

3. Then slowly exhale by closing the left nostril with the end of the index finger. This three stage cycle is repeated. (Note that the reverse pattern of inhaling through the right nostril, holding, and exhaling through the left nostril is *not* performed.) Yogi Bhajan has recommended a counting scheme to maintain the exact numbers of pumps and "Whahay Gurus".

> For counting 1–16 (Whahay Guru's), one (with three pumps), two (with three pumps), three (with three pumps) is counted with the little finger moving slightly three times, four (with three pumps), five (with three pumps), and six (with three pumps) moves the ring finger three times, seven (with three pumps), eight (with three pumps), nine (with three pumps) moves the middle finger three times, ten (with three pumps), eleven (with three pumps), and twelve (with three pumps) moves the index finger three times, thirteen (with three pumps), fourteen (with three pumps), fifteen (with three pumps) moves the thumb slightly for three beats, and sixteen (with three pumps) brings the index finger over to close the left nostril just before exhaling through the right nostril (p. 1990).

When ending this meditation, after the last exhale, inhale and hold the breath for 5–10 seconds and mentally circulate the energy produced, then exhale. Then stretch and shake the entire body for 1 minute to complete the exercise.

The bija mantra Whahay Guru induces a state of great wonder, bliss, and ecstasy, an experience of the totality of the universe, the universal nature of consciousness, and the oneness and unity of creation.

A modified and simpler version of this technique is accomplished by applying only one pump per Whahay Guru, thus yielding 16 pumps corresponding to 16 Whahay Gurus. This version is also less potent, but it is a good place to start if the advanced version is too difficult. An adequate lung capacity can be slowly achieved with the beginner's version. Ultimately, this breath cycle can be reduced to one cycle per minute or less. When respiratory rates of less than one breath/minute are achieved profound changes are more quickly induced.

The difficulty with this technique, beyond lung capacity, is primarily with developing the counting skill and coordination between pumping and sounds, all of which can eventually become a near "automated or second nature" level of processing. While the practitioner is still consciously involved with the pump-sound-counting coordination the technique can be painfully difficult. The time required to become a "learned response" varies amongst individuals and their training and capacities. It can easily take 2–4 weeks to achieve a comfortable level of practice. Eleven minutes is the first plateau of accomplishment, followed by 31 minutes, 62 minutes, and 151 minutes (2 hours & 31 minutes).

Opening the Third Eye
Jo Kirpah Gobind Bhaee

The technique described below is considered one of the most powerful techniques to stimulate and open the third eye. The third eye is related to the activity of the pituitary gland and is also equated with the sixth chakra, or ajna center, the center of the individual mind. Opening of the third eye induces visions of nontemporal events. The mind is not limited to time and space, and the third eye is usually regarded to be the most illustrious psychic energy center. It gives visions of the "unseen", while the 5th chakra gives experiences of the "unheard". One's sense of self and perceived identity is related to the activity of the third eye. A third eye that is closed typically yields a fearful mind, a mind that is out of touch, or without a perceived connection with the universal mind. In this perspective, the experience of life and the essence of spirituality is based on the conscious relationship of individual and universal mind, or the individual psycho-electromagnetic field and the universal psycho-electromagnetic field. The experience of life as that of mystery or mastery reduces to this relationship, and the third eye is pivotal to this experience. Opening of the third eye is a delightful and divine experience. It is central to experiencing the wonder of life and to seeing beyond the temporal nature of human tragedy. Opening the third eye plays a fundamental role in the opening of the tenth gate. This technique helps facilitate both and can build a strong foundation for living in that timeless zone of consciousness.

Description of the Technique

Stand with both feet spread 3 feet apart. Interlace the hands behind the back in "Venus lock" with the left little finger outside of the right little finger and with the right thumb on top of the left thumb for males. Reverse the order for females; left thumb on top of right and the right little finger is outside of the left. This interlock stabilizes the activity of the brain and central nervous system. The eyes remain closed throughout. A tape entitled *Jo Kirpah Gobind Bhaee,* by Master Darshan Singh (available from Golden Temple Enterprises, Espanola, New Mexico) is played. During the vocal segments of the tape only (not during the instrumental portions), the practitioner bends forward with the head coming down towards the knees, simultaneously the arms are raised up over the back to approach being perpendicular to the ground. The legs remain straight and do not bend at the knees. After bringing the head close to the knees, immediately stand up straight with the arms coming back down behind the back. The abdominal/lower back region becomes pivotal to the movement. The head and chest are kept in a straight line. The full motion can become fairly rapid approximating 2 seconds. Therefore, during the vocal portion of the tape, the practitioner can bow about 10 times interspersed with motions of 3, all with a defined sequence guided by the tape. Bowing only during the vocal portions provides the exact and necessary arrhythmic motion to keep this a balanced and paced exercise. For this reason the practice of this exercise is contraindicated without the use of the tape.

The length of practice should be held to 3–5 minutes in the beginning. The practitioner should stretch the back legs carefully before the practice. Caution is given that this exercise can cause extreme soreness to the back of the legs in the beginning if it is not practiced with this caveat in mind. Eventually, the time can be increased to 31 minutes or even 62 minutes maximum once the physical stamina is achieved. Problems with the lower back require additional caution.

Opening the Tenth Gate
Wha Guru

Opening the tenth gate gives access to realms of consciousness beyond time and space. There are realms of the lower world and the upper world, worlds of reality no less real than the one perceived of as time and space. The experience of these worlds, while quite different in terms of natural laws, are no less real to the traveler. It is from within the experience of this world that one gains the experience of their immortality due to the experience of consciousness within the subtle body alone. The technique taught here is specifically employed for the purpose of opening the tube or channel of our being that allows access to these altered states of consciousness and zones of reality. It prepares us for distant out-of-body travel. Additionally, it balances the 10 major zones of the brain to prepare for the flow of energy through the tenth gate. This technique increases absorption of energy through the earth's magnetic field and increases the magnetic field around the crown chakra to provide continuity of flow with the universal psycho-electromagnetic field.

Description of the Technique

Sit on the heels with the knees together in front. The top of the feet are on the ground under the buttocks with the inner sides of the feet parallel. Both arms are over the head with the right hand holding onto the left elbow and the left hand holding on to the right elbow. The fingers of each hand grasp the opposite elbow. A key to the practice is to keep a pressure of the fingers on the elbow regions. This pressure is not light nor too tight to maintain. Each finger and thumb represents an area of the contralateral hemisphere. In the beginning, the most difficult aspect of the technique can be to maintain this pressure. The palms at the eminence of the thumb usually become most sore during practice. However, after several weeks of fairly regular practice this will disappear. Be careful to not allow the arms to just rest on the top of the head. This can cause undue pressure on the cervical vertebrae. The eyes are closed and focused at the third eye. On the inhalation mentally hear the sound of "Wha" as if boulders are rumbling in the earth below. On the exhalation mentally hear "Guru" in a voice like the heavens singing. The Wha and Guru become extended sounds as the breath becomes slow. The breath is through the nose only and becomes slow and deep and can easily be reduced to two per minute or less. The time for practice should first be stabilized at 11 minutes and then slowly progress to a maximum of 62 minutes. An important threshold for experience is around 45 minutes. Even in the beginning of practice around the 62 minute period the practitioner can find him- or herself completely in another world even while maintaining the posture. However, a lay out immediately after the practice can quickly lead to leaving the body and an exploration of the worlds of non-ordinary consciousness. Transitions from time into timelessness and back are facilitated by the practice of this technique.

Harness the Ethers, Master the Elements
Pritvee Heh Akash Heh Guru Ram Das Heh

When the mind can cross the veil of illusion, the barrier of time and space, the ability to master the elements is afforded. The elements, or tattvas (earth, water, fire, air and ether), are imaginary or nebulous qualities until the mind can perceive their interactions and associations in the world where mind and matter are no longer dissociated. Every object of time and space is composed of these five elements. This description is not inconsistent with the world of physics but complementary. A mind that has mastered the elements can master healing.

Description of the Technique

Sit with a straight spine. The eyes are closed and focused at the third eye. The left hand is relaxed in the center of the lap next to the body with the palm up at the level of the second chakra. The right hand is held palm down approximately 3–5 inches over the top of the head like an umbrella. The entire mantra is chanted in one breath. The key is to mentally envision the vibratory effects of the sounds Pritvee Heh at the left hand level and then to experience the sounds of Akash Heh at the right hand level over the crown, and then the sound Guru at the third eye, Ram at the throat chakra, and Das Heh at the heart center. The sounds are chanted with devotion. There is no time limit to this technique.

The Science of the Gong

The perspectives discussed here on the gong are derived from a talk by Yogi Bhajan. His training and insights in turn have come from other yogis using the gong in therapy. Like drumming, the gong has been used to help facilitate transcendence.

The gong is the first and last instrument for the human mind. The structure of the gong is like the sun. There are two types of gongs: one with a raised center, and the second type, which is the flat gong, without a raised center, and the type described here. The flat gong has a flat center that is surrounded by other lines called rhythms along with the outer border. The center, the rhythms, and the border all have different qualities and intensities. The center is the most intense like the sun itself with the rhythms equal to its flare energy and the border equal to its end energy. These intensities are also similar to the light of a candle with its three areas, the center being the hottest.

Before ever playing the gong, the practitioner can tune in to three sacred mantras for guidance and healing to become that protected channel. These three mantras are the

Mangala Charan mantra (Ad Gureh Nameh, Jugad Gureh Nameh, Sat Gureh Nameh, Siri Guru De Veh Nameh), the **Adi Mantra** (Ong Namo Guru Dev Namo), and the bija mantra of the last four lines of the **Mul Mantra** from Jap Ji Sahib, the prayer of Guru Nanak (Ad Sach Jugad Sach Habee Sach Nanak Hosee Bee Sach). The Mangala Charan mantra brings healing, protection, and guidance. The Adi Mantra is a Saraswati mantra "goddess of music" and it is stated that she will never be blissful with the practitioner unless the Adi Mantra is invoked when the gong is played. The third mantra rewrites the destiny for good luck.

The gong is never hit directly on the center or the sides, but with strikes up or down or with a minimal angle and only on the return (when the gong is swinging towards the striker), not when it is moving away. "Hitting" the gong with direct strikes scatters the person. It is like blasting the windshield of a car. When hit on the return, the sound is much more powerful; otherwise the strike reduces the sound. When hit directly, this smashing sound is very dangerous and can damage the heart. If the gong is played correctly the listener cannot have downgrading thoughts. The gong can be used to increase intuition and to affect the pineal-pituitary relationship, the master relationship in the glandular system. Its healing sounds also have a powerful effect on the patterns of neural activity of the brain. The sound of the gong is the master sound or "Adi Nad", the sound of the creator. When used correctly, the gong can be helpful in disengaging the mind of the intellect from the world of ordinary consciousness, thus allowing the individual to merge his/her consciousness with the ethers or out-of-body states of consciousness.

The gong is like a clock where 3, 6, 9, and 12 o'clock all have different effects. When hit below the center, the quality of the sound is an earth sound (equivalent to chakras 1–3). The center is the 4th or heart chakra. Above the center are the rhythms of the 5th, 6th, 7th, and 8th chakras. The balance of prakash and prakirti are maintained by the rays and the border, respectively. Many patterns are possible and this is the choice of the player. The pattern of 2 o'clock and 8 o'clock, or 4 o'clock and 10 o'clock can be intermixed. The player decides which way to take the energy. The player should be able to feel the response going through the people. After you tune in, the response guides you, your body is being used. Twelve o'clock is for loftiness, 6 o'clock is for projecting out to the people for when they are mentally down and tired, 3 o'clock is for raising energy, and 9 o'clock is elevating. The energy of the gong goes by 1.5, 2.5, and 3.5 cycles, or rates of vibration, slow, faster and fastest, respectively.

When starting to play, start around the center. To stop for an emergency, do not touch the gong with the hand, just put the striker into the center to muffle it.

The effects of the gong are unique. There is no defense against the gong. The mind, thoughts, molecules, and the electromagnetic psyche have absolutely no power over this sound. It must be obeyed, the ego, thoughts, psychic formation have no power over it. An individual mind can only resist its effects for 3–90 seconds. After 90 seconds it overtakes every mind. The gong is the only tool with power before the human mind, it supersedes the human mind. The gong produces the basic creative sound, and, from this sound energy, the mind was created. The gong sound is both male and female together.

Acknowledgments

These techniques come from Kundalini Yoga as taught by Raj Yog Guru Ram Das and Yogi Bhajan.

References

Bhajan, Y. (1978). *Kundalini meditation manual for intermediate students.* Pomona, CA.: KRI Publications.

Bhajan, Y. (1990). Videotape, Meditation class presented by Yogi Bhajan, MO65-2, Formello, Italy, 12 December 1990, Golden Temple Enterprises, Espanola, New Mexico.

Crick, F. (1994). *The astonishing hypothesis: The scientific search for the soul.* New York: Scribner's.

Harner, M. (1992). *The way of the shaman.* San Francisco: Harper.

Shannahoff-Khalsa, D. S., Bhajan, Y. (1988). Sound current therapy and self-healing: The ancient science of nad and mantra yoga. *International Journal of Music Dance Art Therapy, 1,* 183–192.

Shannahoff-Khalsa, D. S., Bhajan, Y. (1992). The healing power of sound: Techniques from yogic medicine. In R. Spintge & R. Droh (Eds.), *MusicMedicine* (pp. 179–193). St. Louis, Missouri: MMB Music.

Singh, M. (Translator) (1964). *Siri Guru Granth Sahib.* Amritsar, India: Jaspal Printing Press.